Community Practice in the Network Society

The notion of a network society, structured and organized around information and communication technology (ICT), is seen by many as a significant contributor to 'revolutionary' social changes taking place in an age of globalization. So ingrained is this view in theoretical and policy-making circles that its veracity is seldom challenged. Increasingly, the network society is presented as a space in which people are treated as consumers and sales opportunities. This is a world in which little concern is shown for their rights as citizens or their needs as human beings. Driven primarily by the vested interests of commercial networks eager to stimulate markets, communities and citizens are expected to adapt to the rapid pace of social change or face exclusion.

Using a multi- and inter-disciplinary approach, this book draws on and synthesizes evidence from policy analysts, community ICT practitioners, and researchers from around the world to present a more community-centered vision of the global network society. The book presents a critique of current policy, provides examples of the richness and diversity found in alternative network society practice, and identifies priorities in the emerging community informatics research agenda. It provides evidence supporting the case for the development of more inclusive and participatory pathways to the network society.

Community Practice in the Network Society will be invaluable reading to academics, researchers, and practitioners from a broad range of disciplines interested in community ICT practice, and for community practitioners and researchers wishing to work in this area, whom it is hoped will be motivated and oriented by this book.

Peter Day is a senior lecturer at the School of Computing, Mathematical and Information Sciences at the University of Brighton, UK, a senior research fellow in the Faculty of Informatics and Communication at Central Queensland University, Australia and a director of the Sussex Community Internet Project (SCIP). **Douglas Schuler** is a member of the faculty of the Evergreen State College, USA and has been involved in studying the social implications of technology for over 20 years. He is co-founder of the Seattle Community Network.

Community Practice in the Network Society

Local action/global interaction

Edited by
Peter Day and Douglas Schuler

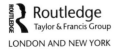
Routledge
Taylor & Francis Group

LONDON AND NEW YORK

First published 2004
by Routledge
11 New Fetter Lane, London EC4P 4EE

Simultaneously published in the USA and Canada
by Routledge
29 West 35th Street, New York, NY 10001

Routledge is an imprint of the Taylor & Francis Group

Typeset in Bembo by
Keystroke, Jacaranda Lodge, Wolverhampton
Printed and bound in Great Britain by
TJ International Ltd, Padstow, Cornwall

British Library Cataloguing in Publication Data
A catalogue record for this book is available from the British Library

Library of Congress Cataloging in Publication Data
A catalog record for this book has been requested

ISBN 0–415–30194–7 (hbk)
ISBN 0–415–30195–5 (pbk)

Contents

Figures and tables

Figures

Tables

Contributors

Abdul Alkalimat is Professor of Sociology and Director of Africana Studies at the University of Toledo (Ohio), where he engineered the only known Internet-based course taught from Africa to students in the USA. He moderates the largest African-American Studies discussion list H-Afro-Am and created and maintains two research websites, one on Malcolm X and one on eBlack Studies. He recently moved his *Introduction to Afro-American Studies: A Peoples College Primer*, for thirty years the most widely used Black Studies curriculum, onto this website.

Ellen Balka's career has been dedicated to the study of technology and society, with an emphasis on women. She is a professor in Simon Fraser University's School of Communication, and is also the director of the Assessment of Technology in Context Design Lab (the ATIC-DL). The ATIC Lab conducts observationally based studies of technology use in field settings.

Oliver Boyd-Barrett is Professor at California State Polytechnic University, Pomona. He has taught and published extensively in the fields of international and educational communications. He has been consultant to various governmental and intergovernmental agencies, including the British Royal Commission on the Press, SHAPE (NATO), and UNESCO. His publications include *The Globalization of News* (Sage), *Contra-Flow in Global News* (Libbey), *The International News Agencies* (Sage), and *Educational Reform in Democratic Spain* (Routledge).

Christina Courtright is currently a PhD student at the School of Library and Information Science of Indiana University, USA. Prior to enrolling, she worked for 12 years in El Salvador as an amateur librarian and information activist. During that time, she worked closely with librarians, policy-makers and development institutions to improve information management and policy throughout El Salvador.

Peter Day is a member of Computer Professionals for Social Responsibility and a senior lecturer at the School of Computing, Mathematical and Information Sciences at the University of Brighton. He has a PhD in community informatics and is co-author of the IBM/CDF sponsored

"COMMIT Report" which critically evaluated UK cross-sectoral community ICT initiatives. He is a Director of the Sussex Community Internet Project (SCIP) and is currently Project Manager of the "Community Network Analysis and ICT: Bridging and building community ties," an Economic and Social Research Council funded project of the "People at the Centre of Communication and Information Technology" program.

Eszter Hargittai is Assistant Professor in the Department of Communication Studies and (by courtesy) in the Department of Sociology, and a Faculty Associate of the Institute for Policy Research at Northwestern University. She is also a Visiting Research Collaborator at the Center for Arts and Cultural Policy Studies at Princeton Univesity. Her research focuses on the social and policy implications of information technologies with particular emphasis on questions of inequality. She holds a PhD in Sociology from Princeton University where she was a Woodrow Wilson Fellow.

Audrey Marshall qualified as a professional librarian in 1978 and has worked in a range of library and information sectors. In the 1990s she worked for the Kings Fund and the Health Education Authority on projects which looked at the uses of new technology for health information. She completed an MA in Information Management at Brighton University in 2000 and is now teaching and researching at the University of Brighton. Audrey also works as a freelance information consultant.

Stewart Marshall is the founding Dean, and a Professor of the Faculty of Informatics and Communication at the Central Queensland University in Australia. Stewart has a wealth of international academic experience, having worked in higher education in England, Papua New Guinea, Australia, and Southern Africa since 1973. His specific research interests focus on the role of ICT in distance education, especially in developing nations. Professor Marshall's publications record includes several books and more than 70 book chapters, conference papers, and refereed articles.

William J. McIver Jr. is Assistant Professor in the School of Information Science and Policy at the University of Albany, State University of New York, USA. He is a specialist in database systems and social informatics. His research has covered the areas of universal service, information needs and uses, human rights, digital government and telemedicine. Bill has a PhD degree in Computer Science from the University of Colorado at Boulder. He is a member of the ACM Special Interest Group on Computers and Society, IEEE Society on Social Implications of Technology, and Computer Professionals for Social Responsibility.

Wayne Miner is completing a graduate degree in information management at the School of Information Science, Syracuse University. He was associate director of CITI and headed up CITI's Center for Excellence in Broadband Applications, spearheading CEBA's cutting-edge broadband applications prototyping projects.

Julia Nosovitch was CITI administrator and budget officer, and holds a master's degree in information management from the School of Information Studies, Syracuse University.

Brian Peterson is currently a product manager at a Canadian technology company. He conducted the field study reported on here during his tenure as a full time employee of the ATIC Design Lab. He studied communications at Simon Fraser University while working at the ATIC DL.

Randal Pinkett is the President and CEO of BCT Partners, a management, technology and policy consulting firm. He has a background in Electrical Engineering and Computer Science, with work experience at Bell Labs and Lucent Technologies. He is actively involved in community technology both as the former principal investigator and co-manager of the Camfield Estates-MIT Creating Community Connection Project. He holds a BS in Electrical Engineering from Rutgers University, an MS in Computer Science from the University of Oxford, England, as a Rhodes Scholar, and an MS in Electrical Engineering, MBA and PhD degrees from MIT.

Scott Robinson has been involved with networking and the introduction of IT into Mexican rural producer organizations since 1994 when the Red de Informacion Rural went online (www.laneta.apc.org/rir). Scott has been involved with Mexico telecenter creation since 1997, and has had numerous articles published online on that topic. He is currently coordinating an IDRC Canada funded telecenter project in Morelos state, Mexico. Scott teaches social anthropology at the undergraduate and graduate levels in the University Metropolitana, Mexico, DF.

Christian Sandvig is an Assistant Professor of Speech Communication at the University of Illinois at Urbana-Champaign. Currently he is also an Information Policy Fellow at the Programme in Comparative Media Law and Policy, Oxford University. His research focuses on the relationships between communication technology, social life, and public policy. He holds a PhD in Communication from Stanford University and is a member of the Computer Professionals for Social Responsibility.

Douglas Schuler is a former chair of Computer Professionals for Social Responsibility and a member of the faculty of the Evergreen State College. He has been involved in the social implications of technology for nearly 20 years. He has published numerous articles and book chapters and has co-edited three books. His *New Community Networks* book published in 1996 was hailed as innovative and indispensable in the field of community technology. He has given presentations in Asia, Europe, North America, and South Africa. Douglas has been a principal organizer at all seven "Directions and Implications of Advanced Computing" symposia.

Richard Sclove is the founder, past Executive Director, and currently an advisory board member of the Loka Institute, a nonprofit organization dedicated to making research, science and technology responsive to democratically decided priorities. He is author of the award-winning book *Democracy and Technology* and has published in many venues, including *Science* magazine; *Technology Review*; *The Chronicle of Higher Education*; *The Washington Post*; *The Christian Science Monitor*, and *Science, Technology and Human Values*. Dr Sclove holds a BA in environmental studies from Hampshire College and, from the Massachusetts Institute of Technology, graduate degrees in nuclear engineering and political science.

Wal Taylor is a Senior Research Fellow at the COIN Internet Academy, Rockhampton, Queensland. A collaboration between the Faculty of Informatics and Communication at Central Queensland University and Rockhampton City Council, COIN operates as a participative action research centre examining the adoption of community ICT in Central Queensland. Dr Taylor has a long history of public agency and community involvement in regional and rural parts of northern and central Queensland. He was awarded Citizen of the Year in 2000, in recognition of his contribution to regional development. With a community informatics PhD, Wal has over 80 publications to his name.

Nicol Turner-Lee is the founder of the Neighborhood Technology Resource Center, a community technology center dedicated to providing individuals and community-based organization with high-speed Internet access and technology education. She is also the Regional Director of the Midwest for One Economy Corporation, a national nonprofit organization committed to providing comprehensive technology solutions to individuals, housing developers and human service providers. She was a former fellow with Northwestern University's Asset Based Community Development Institute, and has published several articles on ways to identify, document and mobilize community assets. She has served as faculty at Northwestern University, North Park College and East-West University. Dr Turner-Lee holds a BA in Sociology from Colgate University, and a graduate degree in sociology from Northwestern University. She also holds a Certificate in Nonprofit Management from the University of Illinois-Chicago.

Murali Venkatesh is an associate professor and Founder-Director of the Community & Information Technology Institute (CITI) at the School of Information Studies, Syracuse University, Syracuse, New York. Dr Venkatesh holds a PhD in telecommunications and information systems from Indiana University, where he was a recipient of the IBM Doctoral Fellowship among others. Dr Venkatesh is currently (AY 02–04) a Senior Research Fellow at the Center for Reflective Community Practice at the Massachusetts Institute of Technology (MIT). He recently guest edited a special issue of *The Information Society* devoted to the development of community technology.

Preface

Information and communication technologies (ICTs) have become critical components of global economic, political, and cultural systems. Such is the significance of this range of technologies that they have become the symbol of the social transformations taking place in what many theorists and policy-makers call the "Network Society". Conceptually ICT are often seen as a significant enabler to the "revolutionary" changes taking place in an age of globalization. As the pace of these socio-economic changes accelerates, fears have emerged that much of the world's population are being excluded from, or forced to adapt to, a rapidly changing social environment not of their own making.

The driving forces behind this new technological landscape are competition and increased profit margins in an increasingly globalized market place. With an apparent willingness to represent the vested interests of commercial capital, policy-makers have shown little concern for the needs of citizens, community and civil society in the information age. In a world of commercial transactions and commodified data flows, people are viewed as consumers of goods and services rather than citizens with the democratic right to shape and influence changes taking place in the world. The future of the network society is being shaped by private and public sector partnerships with little consultation with civil society and community.

Paradoxically, juxtaposed to these exclusionary and elitist processes of techno-economic globalization has been the emergence of a more socially oriented process of globalization. Around the world, citizens in local communities are using ICT to underpin the creation of a participatory and democratic vision of the network society. In contrast to the determinism of the dominant network society culture, in which technical networks are shaping and conditioning human activity, a new public sphere is emerging, in which ICT are being shaped as tools that underpin and support social networks. Embedded in the richness and diversity of community practice globally, a vision of a "Civil Network Society" is emerging, a society where ICT improves the quality of life and reflects the diversity of social networks; where people are viewed as citizens not just as consumers and where heterogeneity is perceived as a strength rather than a weakness.

In much of the "developed" world, especially the US and Europe, academic inquiry related to ICT, unless devoted to "e-commerce," such as "Management Information Systems", or rationalizing public services such as "e-government" is rarely undertaken. Of course, interest among academics and other researchers in the host of issues surrounding the use of computers in society has increased enormously in recent decades. Unfortunately much of this work is tied to the interests of the commercial world and military and is divorced from "real world" threats and opportunities facing people in their local communities. Researchers who are interested in research related to real-world issues are sometimes tolerated but rarely extolled. Few resources are made available for challenging research that seeks to find a more inclusive and socially diverse use of ICT in the global network society. The absence of knowledge and understanding about the relevance of ICT to communities provides little opportunity to support and enhance their local cultural context. A consequence of this is that the richness and diversity of global cultures are under threat from globalized homogenization.

Information and communication technologies have been, and are increasingly being, marketed in the service of efficiency, speed, progress, and, of course, profitability – all in the name of the commercial vision of the network society. The more commonplace side of life – neighborhoods, community, emotions, resistance, human weakness, etc. – play little part in the anodyne network society environment created by the gurus of computerized systems. The message here appears to be: computers are for those who control society, not those who are controlled. Or to put it another way, ICT are intended to maintain the status quo, not to change it.

Using a multi- and interdisciplinary approach to knowledge – one embedded in the social shaping tradition – this book identifies both barriers and pathways to the development of an equitable and effective civil network society. It presents, as an alternative to homogeneity and sanitization, a vision of a civil society based on the richness of human experience, and cultural diversity found in communities around the world. In this way, the book identifies opportunities and challenges facing global community ICT practice and research and discusses the interrelationships and importance of this emergent community-focused discourse.

The themes are reflected in the structure of the book: the broad context for ICT and the network society is discussed in the first section. A variety of case studies from around the world provide a rich and textured background of local community technology projects in the second section. The final section provides theoretical insights, empirical findings, and other intellectual support for the development of the emerging community informatics research agenda.

This situation raises a number of important questions in urgent need of consideration. Why is research that is socially shaped so important in the network society? What can/should academics do? Why do they need to work with people and communities? How could this be a win-win situation? This book illustrates how collaborative community research is flexible and pragmatic, and even though it is generally underfunded it can and is being successfully undertaken around the world. Partnerships based on mutuality, reciprocity, and trust are being forged between some parts of academia and a diverse range of action/advocacy networks and local communities. From these alliances new research paradigms and orientations have emerged.

The authors in this book assume that ICT represents important social opportunities as well as significant threats that cannot be ignored. Ideally we would like to visualize and develop community technology systems that help humanity build and sustain healthy communities, promote social and economic justice, and contribute to a shared knowledge base of community life, but how can such a social vision be achieved? The collective message from the chapter authors in this text provides us with some hope for the future of a network society. By working together in a collaborative and co-operative manner, by sharing experiences and knowledge through discussions that legitimize actions, through communicative action that enables citizens to engage in shaping local community initiatives and enterprises, and finally by demonstrating courage and dedication, sometimes in the face of enormous odds, hugely significant social advances can be made locally that make an impact at the global level.

This volume is a result of the 7th "Directions and Implications of Advanced Computing" (DIAC) Symposium, which was held in Seattle in 2000. DIAC, which is sponsored by Computer Professionals for Social Responsibility (CPSR), was first held in 1987. Its purpose was to help raise awareness of the social implications of computing and was built on the premise that academics do not necessarily have to be "just" academic; as members of society with useful skills and knowledge, they can – and should – play a significant role in society, especially the sectors of society that have fewer resources to draw from. With this in mind DIAC was – and is – intended to provide a forum for the embryonic and relatively unorganized group of academics concerned about the uncritical adoption of computers in society.

Since the symposium we have been working to help bring out the message that computer professionals have a critical role to play in the ongoing deployment of computer technology. It is our contention that knowledge can be served by academics assuming a more active role to the social environment in which knowledge is created. And ICT professionals need not confine themselves to the technical esoterica that has traditionally defined the computer science and information systems enterprise. The story from this book – and elsewhere – demonstrates that important research can be conducted in partnerships with civic and community activists in ways that vastly expand the scope – and relevance – of their practice.

We believe that all people who are interested in the social implications of computing should read this book. This includes community and civil society practitioners, teachers and students, journalists, artists, policy-makers, and – most importantly – citizens. The book tells at least part of the new story about how

ICT might be used more effectively by people in communities, by activists in social movements, by citizens interested in a better future.

We have been fortunate while working on this volume to collaborate with an extremely creative, dedicated, and engaged team of global authors. While we feel that this group is exceptional we are happily aware that they are not alone in their concerns. If the ideas expressed in this book (and the related ideas emanating from around the world) are to become influential in a broad sense it will be because of the efforts and sacrifice of the people working – generally unheralded and with limited resources – with and in communities around the world. We wish you – and all of them – good luck. We hope to be able to work with you in the future in the ongoing struggle to *shape the network society*.

Douglas Schuler, Seattle, Washington, USA
Peter Day, Eastbourne, England, UK

Acknowledgments

We would like to thank a few people. Our families – wives Denise and Terry; children – Nadine and Katie, Reed and Zoe; and grandchildren – Kelsey and Corey – for the love, encouragement, and patience that enabled us to finish. We also acknowledge the support of the UK Economic and Social Research Council (ESRC), through the People at the Centre of Communication and Information Technology (PACCIT) programme, project number RES-328-25-0012, the US National Science Foundation, through the Social Dimensions of Engineering, Science and Technology (SDEST) division through grant 0002547, and the Rockefeller Foundation for its generous grant to DIAC-00, the conference which gave rise to this book. We would also like to thank those from Routledge – Edwina Wellham, Michelle Bacca, Karen Bowler and Claire Gauler – for supporting this project and working with us to see it through. Finally, of course, this work would not even be possible without the great authors and those who assisted them – and the people from around the world who are working for a better community information and communication infrastructure in a "Civil Network Society".

Introduction

Chapter 1

Community practice

An alternative vision of the network society

Peter Day and Douglas Schuler

Introduction

> At a deeper level, the material foundations of society, space and time are being transformed, organized around the space of flows and timeless time. Beyond the metaphorical value of these expressions . . . a major hypothesis is put forward: dominant functions are organized in networks pertaining to a space of flows that links them up around the world, while fragmenting subordinate functions, and people, in the multiple space of places, made of locales increasingly segregated and disconnected from each other.
>
> (Castells, 1996: 476)

The idea that society is going through a process, or processes, of social transformation, in which the hierarchical and class-based power structures of industrial society are giving way to an age of networked social structures, provides us with a thought-provoking point of departure for our considerations of community uses of ICTs for a number of reasons. First, it highlights the major thrust of network society theory. Second, it provides a structural frame within which the practices of communities in contemporary society can be understood. Third, it provides socio-economic context to the changing and challenging environment in which communities often struggle to exist – and in which our journey into *community practice in the network society* occurs.

Before we commence this journey into community practice, however, let us attempt to tease out what Castells' hypothesis (see above) means and why it is of interest to us. We do not intend to spend time here deconstructing notions of "timeless time" and "space of flows." Rather we feel that Castells' comprehensive treatise of social structure and organisation in "the information age" provides the opportunity to consider the possibility of alternative visions. As MacKay illustrates, the concept of "[t]he network of flows is crucial to domination and change in society: interconnected, global, capitalist networks organize economic activity using technology and information, and are the main source of power in society" (MacKay, 2001: 35). However, information supports social processes across a wide range of cultures, in many ways, at many social levels, and whilst networks provide the organizational structure for these processes, it is important to recognize that information communication technologies (ICTs) have been pivotal in assisting the speed of these developments. They provide the basis for understanding the very nature of what is commonly perceived as the network society.

"[W]ithout its technological tools," Castells argues, "society cannot be understood or represented" (1996: 5). Indeed, one of the prime elements of the space of flows – linking and organizing the dominant functions around the world, e.g. "flows of capital, flows of information, flows of technology, flows of organizational interaction, flows of images, sounds, and symbols" (Castells, 1996: 412) – is ICTs. The other two elements, according to Castells, are: interconnected nodes and hubs – where strategically important network functions and activities are performed by organizations in a geographic location and the interactions and transactions of the various network elements are co-ordinated, respectively, and the spatial organization of dominant, managerial elites that manage and direct network functions and activities. Through the combination of these three elements can be found what Castells describes as the "material form of support of dominant processes and functions" of the network society (1996: 412).

Castells' comprehensive analysis of the "space of flows" (1996, 1997 and 1998) illustrates that the dominant social processes and functions in the network society are embedded in a techno-economic agenda. Although often accompanied by the logic of economic rationalism – an approach driven by human agency – this agenda often appears to be rooted in technological determinism. This is not to say that Castells' analysis is deterministic, although some authors question this (MacKay, 2001: 35), rather that the dominant functions and activities, as he portrays them are clearly driven by a techno-economic agenda, and can be viewed as being disconnected and segregated from society. Interestingly, as can be seen from the quote at the start of this chapter, Castells posits this situation the other way around, i.e. that the techno-economic agenda – or "space of flows" – is society and that individual locales are increasingly disconnected and segregated from one another. Such an analysis is not uncommon among network theorists, e.g. a similar perspective can be found in social network theory, where the rise of "networked individualism" – "sparsely-knit, linking individuals with little regards to space" – is heralded at what appears to be the expense of local, geographic communities (Wellman, 2002: 10).

We do not challenge the perspectives put forward by colleagues such as Castells and Wellman, indeed we believe they have much to offer in describing the unfolding of events in communities across the globe. In so doing, they make a significant contribution to the development of the global community knowledge landscape. However, rather than focusing on the dominant societal processes and functions and the technological development that supports them, we take another path to understanding human activity in the network society and invoke Rosenbrock's Lushai Hills metaphor (1990) to assist us. Rosenbrock, who once lived and worked in India, uses the metaphor in his seminal defence of alternative technological systems in manufacturing industry. Criticizing the "one best way" approach of Taylorism and espousing a human-centred approach to technological design and development, Rosenbrock recalls an expedition he once made through the Lushai Hills.

> Climbing upwards in this way, one would reach a fork where two streams joined, and a choice had to be made. No reliable information could be obtained from the map, and no general overview was possible to guide the choice, which was based only on what could be seen within a few yards, or on any general predisposition to go towards the right or the left. . . . Having climbed high up the side of the valley, one would pause and camp for the night. . . . Then it was possible to feel a sense of achievement: to have climbed so high and to be able to look back over the lower country out of which one had come. And it was easy to believe that all the choices, which had been made along the way were justified by the outcome, and were the only right choices to be made. This self-congratulation might have of course been quite unwarranted. Some other route might have led to still higher ground, and done so more easily. But if so, the knowledge was hidden, and the complacency uncontradicted.
>
> (Rosenbrock, 1990: 123–124)

Although it is now well over a decade later, the central theme of the Rosenbrock metaphor is as germane to the development of information and communication systems and applications in the network society as it was to systems design back then. No matter how far the current path of technological knowledge has taken society in terms of its overall development, there remains the potential that other paths exist – following other directions of scientific and technological development – that might lead to richer, friendlier, and more fertile levels of social development. There are always other truths as yet unknown to us, other technological paths as yet untravelled, other social landscapes as yet unseen, and other voices as yet unheard.

Today, in the network society, the dominant perspective, the dominant voice and the dominant agenda, is what Castells calls the "space of flows" – the techno-economic agenda – and what many academics, industrialists, and policy-makers insist citizens of the world have no alternative but to accommodate, accept, and change for. In rejecting, but learning from, this approach, we chose a path from, to, and between communities as our starting point on this alternative journey of understanding the network society. We do not accept that Castells' view of the "multiple space of places" consisting of disconnected locales in which people and functions are fragmented and subordinate to the "space of flows" is an acceptable vision of human existence.

There is evidence enough to illustrate a growing social reaction against such a world view. An indication of the potential power of this reaction can be witnessed in the anti-war movement, which mobilized people in communities from all over the world to engage in an activity that for many, probably the majority, was totally new and even alien to them, i.e. collective protest, on this occasion, protest against what they perceived to be the injustice of the US/UK invasion of Iraq. Similarly, the developing anti-globalization and environmental movements are embedded in networks of social and cultural diversity. In all these networks, ICTs have played a central role in the production and sharing of information that sustains communicative network planning, development, and activities. This social phenomenon points to the re-emergence of social movements, civil society, and community networking in the information age and illustrates a developing counter-culture to the hegemony of Castells' "space of flows."

This then is the starting point of our journey. If, as van Dijk argues, a network society is a society "in which social and media networks are shaping its prime mode of organization and most important structures" (van Dijk, 1999: 248), the following questions become central to our deliberations. What do community practices tells us about the nature of the network society? What does the network society tells us about the nature of community practice? We believe that the critical evaluation undertaken through the stories of community networkers – both academic and practicing – in this book merits critical consideration at all levels and across all sectors of society. Our purpose then in editing this book is to engage practitioners, policy-makers, and academics in an ongoing and fruitful dialogue about *community practice in the network society*.

In this chapter we seek to provide context for such an exchange of ideas, as well as introducing the chapters that follow. However, in order to consider alternative paths in the network society, e.g. those currently explored by the emerging Indymedia[1] movement globally (Morris, 2004), it is necessary to understand how and why we arrived at our present location. Accordingly, before considering *community practice in the network society*, we turn our attention to the historical developments that led to the emergence of the network society. Interestingly, changes in dominant social structures, the centrality of ICTs, and the primacy of information as a socio-economic resource to these processes provide much of the foundations for the information society discourse and it is here that our brief historical journey begins.

Birth of the information society

Theoretical perspectives

In an assessment of the information society literature, Duff *et al.* identify 1960s Japan as the birthplace of contemporary information society philosophy. Apparently, the term was adopted to describe the growing influence of information and ICTs in Japanese organizations (1996). However, it was through the works of Daniel Bell that the concept of an information society developed a resonance in academic circles. Although Bell is best known for his venture in forecasting the post-industrial society (1973), his seminal treatise focused on three inter-related social phenomena that find import in contemporary society: (1) the power of computers, (2) the centrality of theoretical knowledge as the axis around which new technology, economic growth, and the stratification of society was being organized, and (3) the emergence of a new socio-economic order.

By the end of the decade Bell's post-industrialism had emphatically embraced the emerging information society discourse. He argued that control of information technologies had political, as well as technical, implications (1979); that the development of a new social framework would be based on tele-communications (1980); and that these events heralded the emergence of a new socio-economic order. The information society, according to Bell, was represented by a shift from manufacturing to services; the domination of science- and technology-based industries; and the advent of new social stratification through the rise of a new technical elite (1987). In Bell's theories on post-industrialism and his subsequent information society theory, the early roots of what has now become network society theory can be identified.

Policy perspectives

Underlining the importance of theoretical knowledge in modern society, Garnham explains that as Bell was developing and polishing his *venture in social forecasting* during the 1970s/80s, the basic tenet of the information society discourse had started to permeate the thinking of Western policy-makers (1994). However, it was not theoretical knowledge that led to a growth in popular awareness of the information society. Illustrating the existence of a mutuality between theoretical and policy knowledge, this accolade is often attributed to former Vice-President Al Gore, who used the metaphor of an information superhighway in exemplifying the wide ranging socio-economic communi-cations potential – to the USA – of a national information infrastructure (NII) in a speech to the Press Club of America (1993). Interestingly, the NII vision itself predates the Gore speech and can be traced to what Dutton calls an optimistic vision of domestic and business electronic services piggybacking on the development of online interactive computer systems and cable television projects in late 1960s America (1997). Problems with the uptake of interactive cable television and commercial videotext services, in the early 1980s, led to a waning of the vision until resurrected in the early 1990s (Gore, 1991).

In Europe, one of the most significant early pan-European developments was the 1983 agreement to fund the First Framework Programme. €3.75 billion were made available between 1984 and 1987 to stimulate research and develop-ment (R&D) and provide a coherent strategy for the development of EC science and technology. Flagship of the First Framework was the European Strategic Programme for Research and Development in Information Technology (Esprit), the most striking achievement of which was – an early indicator of the significance that would soon be placed on networking – the construction of a culture of co-operative transnational networks, which placed Europe's IT industrialists and researchers ahead of governments in terms of European integration (Federal Trust, 1995).

The techno-economic nature of these early policy interventions were maintained as NII (US) and Information Society (Europe) strategic policies were developed and assumed greater social significance. In developing its NII strategy, the Clinton/Gore administration advocated the social and economic importance of new telecommunication infrastructures. They believed ICTs would impact significantly on the way people worked, learnt, and interacted with one another. To this end they created a policy agenda to turn the vision into reality. A high-level Information Infrastructure Task Force (IITF) was established to co-ordinate the Federal Government's activities. IITF was assisted by an "Advisory Council," which aimed to involve the private sector in the process of policy development (Kubicek and Dutton, 1997). In September 1993 the vision plan, *Agenda for Action* was published (IITF, 1993). This was followed a year later by a progress report and two related publications covering a wide range of applications (IITF, 1994 a, b and c). Broadly speaking, the rationale of the NII strategy was that ICTs would increase the competitiveness of the US economy, reduce administrative costs, and make government more efficient and responsive (Kalil, 1997).

Europe adopted a similar approach. *Growth, Competitiveness, Employment: The Challenges and Ways forward into the 21st Century* (Commission of the EC, 1993), also known as the *Delors White Paper* – after the European Commissioner that presented it – promoted the development of a high-quality Trans-European Network as central to Europe's survival in the twenty-first century. Technical interoperability, further deregulation, and increased competition were also identified as essential elements of the transition to an information society. Surprised by the public enthusiasm for Gore's NII initiative (Kubicek and Dutton, 1997), the European Commission established a High-Level Group – drawn principally from key industrialists and financiers – chaired by Commissioner Martin Bangemann, to consider the specific measures needed to develop a European *infostructure*. The group's report, which became known as the *Bangemann Report*, emphasized market mechanisms as the motivating power to take Europe into the *Information Age* (Commission of the EC, 1994a). Just three weeks after the June presentation of the *Bangemann Report*, an Action Plan was presented to the European Parliament, outlining the European approach to the information society (Commission of the EC, 1994b).

The development and establishment of the formal information society policy mechanisms in both the US and Europe show a number of interesting commonalities and differences.[2] However, the fact that both policy mechanisms comprised high-level "experts" from public and private sectors illustrates the high level of inherent techno-economic determinism that existed during this period of information society policy making. As Moore notes, "There can be few other examples of technological change stimulating formal policy creation in order to bring about social change" (Moore, 2000: 2). The success of policy in seeking to stimulate such social change in response to techno-economic developments can be gauged in the pervasiveness of a commonly held public perception that current ICT trends represent the "way of the future" to which everyone has to adapt – even though they are often unable to explain why they hold this view. The lack of any citizen involvement in the development of a public role for ICTs has enabled technology experts to influence social policy development, unchallenged by public scrutiny, in a way that would be unacceptable in other aspects of the public arena (Sclove, 1995).

Networking the information society

There is little doubt that ICTs are currently employed and utilized in ways that significantly influence society's structure and organization but in whose interest are these changes taking place? In order to address this question it is necessary to understand the motivation behind recent technological developments. Our brief exploration of early policy developments illustrated how what became known as the information society was triggered by the combined efforts of private enterprise and governments seeking to create markets for a vast range of ICT-related goods and services and in so doing revitalize economies and competitive advantage. The unquestioning belief of this increasingly common form of partnership in market forces as the driving power behind all social development was – and still is – often accompanied by an uncritical acceptance of the inevitability of the ICT revolution.

> The information society is on its way. A "digital revolution" is triggering structural change comparable to last century's industrial revolution with the corresponding high economic stakes. The process cannot be stopped and will lead eventually to a knowledge-based economy.
>
> (Commission of the EC, 1994b)

Techno-economic determinism of the network society

This public/private sector shaping of network society developments without engagement with, or participation of, civil society has led to an unquestioning public acceptance of present techno-economic policies. As Castells observes,

> Our exploration of emergent social structures across domains of human activity and experience leads to an overarching conclusion: as a historical trend, dominant functions and processes in the information age are increasingly organized around networks. Networks constitute the new social morphology of our societies, and the diffusion of networking logic substantially modifies the operation and outcomes in processes of production, experience, power, and culture. While the networking form of social

organization has existed in other times and spaces, the new information technology paradigm provides the material basis for its pervasive expansion throughout the entire social structure.

(1996: 469)

In these few sentences Castells exemplifies the now commonly held view that society has entered an information age in which networks, usually facilitated by an ICT infrastructure, form the dominant social structures in the world in which we live. Certainly the notion that most levels of human activity are interlinked as networks in some way or another is accepted without as much as a second thought in most commercial, policy, and academic circles. Indeed, this perspective has formed the basis of the development of the inter-linked information and network society discourses for more than a quarter of a decade.

However, the notion – usually proffered by "experts" – that there is no alternative to the current techno-economic direction of network society developments and that people, their cultures, and society in general just have to adapt is both deterministic and undemocratic. In fact, this apparent social transformation poses a fundamental question that demands an unequivocal answer. Is it not reasonable to expect, in a democracy, that citizens of the "digital revolution" have the right to be involved in determining and shaping its development?

Freeman (1994) contextualizes the kind of technological determinism and "expertise" found in much modern socio-technological policy planning and implementation by pointing to the maximization of profit as the prime goal behind the selection and adoption of new technologies in capitalist economies. It requires no enormous conceptual leap to understand how "experts," can shape the design and development of ICTs through publicly and privately funded research and development programs, whether it be to suit the purposes and commercial interests of transnational corporations, the policy agenda of malleable governments or the vested interests of a science-technology community financed and indebted to private/public capital. These factors, together with the absence of any citizen participation in the policy process, dispel the common myth of the neutrality of technology. In the dominant network society paradigm, most technological development is, in fact, undertaken on behalf of a range of vested interests. None of these involve individual citizens, their representative organizations of civil society, or the communities in which they live.

Searching for the network society's Lushai Hills

Where the public and/or private sectors have sought to engage with citizens at community level, this normally takes the form of initiatives funded through short-term grant competition and that are top-down in nature. With some honourable exceptions, it is becoming increasingly clear that the lessons of previous research in this area have yet to be fully understood. The organizational cultures and practices of sponsoring organizations and funding agencies can have a detrimental effect on and stifle active community involvement (Day and Harris, 1997) and the "bureaucratization of authority, professional power and expertise" frequently prevents active participation (Sanderson, 1999).

The philosophy of funders and sponsors of community ICT initiatives is also an area worthy of consideration. Usually, development programs provide support for the purpose of facilitating access to ICTs. However, Clement and Shade are highly critical of many of these programs. "Thus, it is ironic that most notions of access have typically relied on models that are solely technology driven, and not socially constructed" (1996). There is often little consideration in such programs – beyond access for access's sake – of how ICTs might be useful in supporting, developing, and sustaining community life. It is for this reason that we now turn our attention to what we mean by community. In addition, because community is a social construct, we also consider what we mean by *community practice in the network society*.

Understanding community

Developing a clear picture of what is meant by the term community is not an easy undertaking. The UK-based Community Development Foundation (CDF), when grappling with just this issue, highlighted tensions between "wide and narrow definitions of community" (Chanan *et al.*, 2000: 4). Showing how governments have a tendency to use large geographical boundaries, e.g. city/town or electoral ward perimeters, CDF argued that smaller areas and more scattered groupings provide more natural points of reference for people when they think about what *they* mean by community. Identity – a sense of belonging – with a locality or with areas of interest/practice are therefore acknowledged as crucial elements in determining community.

Communities are not like organizational structures, the boundaries of which can be identified, measured, and quantified: they are hard to pin down. Because they often comprise such a diverse range of organizations, agencies, groups, networks, individuals, activities, and cultures, community is frequently a contested space. They are abstract constructs that depend on the subjective and emotional loyalties of community members. This might explain why – as Jewkes and Murcott suggest – many researchers studying community give up in frustration (1996). Creating an unambiguous definition of community with which everyone can agree is a complex sociological task that has exercised academics and policy makers, somewhat unsuccessfully, for decades. Rather than duplicating these attempts for a hard and fast definition, we draw on the work of Butcher (1993) to provide a starting point for our discussion. Relating community to public policy issues Butcher uses three distinct but interrelated *senses of community*, each of which is broad and flexible enough to accommodate the subjectivity of most interpretations, and each of which is relevant to the network society context – *descriptive community, community as value* and *active community*.

Descriptive community, which draws on the word's etymological origins of having "something in common," provides our first sense of community. This "something in common" might be location: such as neighborhood, village, town, etc., but might also be interest or practice: such as activity, ethnicity, religion, sexual orientation, etc. At this point we highlight our belief that the distinction between these two community commonalities need not be and usually are not mutually exclusive. Indeed geographic communities often comprise different cultures and it is not uncommon for groups and individuals to share knowledge and draw from each other's experiences, creating new forms of common interests as a consequence (Warburton, 1998). The Seattle Community Network (SCN) is an excellent example of how diversity of culture, value, and belief systems can, through the synthesis of collective activities and communal communications, learn from and contribute to each other in a manner the product of which is greater than the sum of its parts (Schuler, 1996). Of course, the opposite can be and often is true. The contested nature of community means that conflict can and does arise. However, healthy, sustainable communities learn to manage and learn from such conflict through the development of *community values*.

The idea that healthy communities require certain shared values – solidarity, participation, and coherence – provides the second sense of community. Although these community values are open to interpretation, the principles upon which they are established provide the value base of community initiatives and policies. Solidarity encourages friendliness, builds allegiances, and inspires loyalty through mutual support and collaboration in relationships. Participation enables citizens to contribute to and engage in the aspirations and activities of the collective community life. Coherence connects individuals to the community, encouraging comprehension of themselves and their social environments, whilst developing a communal knowledge base. In an exposition of SCN (1996), Schuler represents core community values as a network, highlighting how each value influences and is related to the others. A weakness in one is a weakness in the whole. Healthy communities require strong core values, which should be embedded in the planning and development of all community activities and services.

However, it is important to understand that communal should not subsume individual. To build and sustain healthy communities through shared *community values*, a balance is required between adequate amounts of privacy, autonomy, and localism. Shared public spaces, community associations, and activities providing the opportunity to engage with one another need to be tempered with spaces offering both privacy and respect for the diversity of cultural principles. The potentially contested nature of such diverse social environment, cultures, and belief systems in a network society require community members to respect and celebrate the social richness of community life if they are to co-exist in the same geographical space and share social experiences.

Community values then are the social product of individual citizens living in and identifying with a specific "something," often but not always a geographical space. The collective community comprises individual community members that have developed an inherent interest in each other. In addition to sharing the same geographical space and social experiences, in healthy communities members learn to respect and celebrate the richness and diversity of human interests. Diversity then, distinguishes the individual from the collective but at the same time contributes to that collective.

It is through this sense of belonging to – of identifying with – a local community that people engage in community activities. The *active community* – the third sense of community – refers to collective action by community members embracing one or more communal values. Such activities are normally undertaken purposively through the vehicle of groups, networks, and organizations that constitute a community's social capital, social structures that are significant to any discussion of community. Community and voluntary sector groups and organizations form the bedrock of community life through the planning, organization, provision, and support of community activities and services. Although usually under-resourced and over-stretched the community and voluntary sector play a significant role in building and sustaining community.

The significance of community policy

Although community and voluntary sector groups are the cornerstone of community life, the daily pressures for survival on such groups often means that enabling *active community* is a major task, and a shared value base between citizens, local civil society, and community policy-makers is desirable. However, distrust of bureaucrats and politicians often means that achieving this shared value base is problematic, especially between citizens/community groups and the mechanisms of local governance. Nonetheless, in the same way that community policy can create environments that block the development of healthy communities, so too can it create the circumstances to assist their development. By understanding what "community" means to local people at local level, it should be possible to develop policies that are meaningful and germane to people in those communities.

Although many different forms of *active community* exist, especially in more affluent areas – where local resources, knowledge, and expertise often exist in abundance – it should be remembered that not all communities possess the wherewithal required to facilitate, support, or sustain community engagement. Marginalized or socially excluded peoples often require more direct involvement from community policy mechanisms than where healthy community already exists. Despite the need for support, however, community policy mechanisms should be predicated on the notion that community practices, i.e. services, activities, functions, and processes, need to be embedded in the aspirations, needs, and culture of the people involved. Ownership and identity, then, are crucial elements in building healthy community. To achieve such a state of embeddedness for community policy, we propose the following policy framework.

Community policy should: (1) understand and meet community needs; (2) work in partnership with active community groups and organizations; (3) be based on one or more community value, i.e. solidarity, participation, and coherence; (4) prioritize the needs of the community's socially excluded, marginalized, disadvantaged, and oppressed; (5) valorize and celebrate cultural diversity; and (6) reflect a commitment to the objectives of community autonomy and responsibility for community initiatives.

Of course, all this is based on the normative assumptions that community is a desirable social goal, and that a function of policy is to facilitate community building, renewal, and sustainability. Where healthy communities exist, the role of policy should be to support and sustain their existence and when appropriate, facilitate community renewal. Where community is being eroded or does not exist, policy should encourage community building. By this we mean policy should facilitate: capacity building, community activity, and community involvement. Building capacity means stimulating the processes through which communities acquire and hone the skills to manage and develop an environment of community. Capacity building can relate not only to skills, knowledge, and expertise among individual community members but can also apply to developing, supporting, and sustaining organizational skills, knowledge, and expertise in community groups, networks, and institutions. Community organizations such as these – often referred to as a community's social capital – are the main driving forces in planning, organizing, providing, and supporting community activities and services, and in developing and nurturing community values. Community involvement is the achievement of broader participation in the activities and processes of community life and is a prerequisite to achieving healthy communities.

Community practice

We have argued that the development of community policies is dependent on building, sustaining, and renewing healthy active communities. We contend that the implementation of community policies requires changes in the mind-sets of those involved in community governance – both policy-makers and bureaucrats. This is a theme to which we will return in the final chapter. Achieving such changes requires new and distinctive methods and techniques (Glen, 1993). Glen describes such processes as *community practice*, which is distinct from but related to community practices. The latter, as some of the chapters in this volume illustrate, relate to specific community activities and services. This book is a collection of examples of praxis, as opposed to theory. Community practice on the other hand is the theory behind such community praxis. It is a method for promoting policies that encourage the planning, building, and sustainability of healthy communities and usually involves some or all of the following components:

(1) The sustained involvement of paid community workers; (2) A broad range of professionals who are increasingly using community work methods in their work; (3) The efforts of self-managed community groups themselves, and (4) Managerial attempts at reviving, restructuring and relocating services to encourage community access and involvement in the planning and delivery of services.

(Glen, 1993: 22)

Describing the symbiotic relationship between community practice and community policies, where each is related to and promotes the other, Glen identifies three community practice approaches: (1) community services approach, (2) community development, and (3) community action.

The last two operate at grassroots level. Community development concerns itself with the empowerment of communities to define and meet their own needs. It focuses on the promotion of community self-help. Community action comprises planning, and mobilization and involves campaigning for community interests and community policies to achieve community goals. This sometimes involves the employment of conflict tactics in the community interest. The community service approach focuses on the development of community-oriented organizations and services. It involves both philanthropic and compulsory forms of assistance to people in need.[3]

It is important to note that due to the wide range of agencies, organizations, groups, and partnerships involved in community practice, approaches can be "top-down" – i.e. promoted and/or provided by local authorities, charities, and voluntary bodies – in a "doing to" manner. Or they may emanate from within local communities, i.e. "bottom-up" in a "being done by" manner. Usually, top-down facilities and initiatives tend to be associated with the community services approach. As community practices move toward a more action-oriented approach, so they tend to adopt a more bottom-up attitude.

No matter what the composition of local partnerships or the complexion of the approach being employed, community practice should be viewed as a framework of three interrelated elements that assist in identifying, understanding, and fulfilling community need. Within a network society context, community practice requires the subordination of ICT systems, artefacts, and services to meeting those needs as a crucial contribution to building healthy, empowered, and active community.

Structure of the book

When we started to plan this book, which is presented in three parts, we were eager that it should result in something more than a presentation of international case studies, as absorbing as that would be. It is for this purpose that we have framed community ICT practice within a critical evaluation of the techno-economic nature of dominant network society policy, practice and theory.

The network society – issues and exigencies

Our evaluation is picked up and expanded on in Part I, which critiques the dominant network society paradigm and provides an analytical background for understanding the challenges faced by communities utilizing the Internet as a tool for civic networking and community building. Providing insights into the US dominance of global cyberspace Oliver Boyd-Barrett warns, in Chapter 2, against overstating the positive social change potential of the Internet. The Internet, he concludes, is as likely to be harnessed by the forces of oppression as it is to be utilized by non-elites worldwide in support of communicative action. Developing a critique of the global economy Boyd-Barrett identifies the limitations of, and threats to, using the Internet as a public sphere. He then provides some balance to his argument by introducing a range of alternative, civil society-based news organizations that contribute to public sphere activity.

In Chapter 3 Richard Sclove outlines a number of ways in which the commercially driven Internet is detrimental to civil society and democratic self-governance. Discussing the erosion of local economies, face-to-face community vibrancy, and capacities for local self-governance, he introduces what he calls the "Cybernetic Wal-Mart Effect." Both local civil society and individual citizens are being weakened, relative to global market forces and multinational corporations, as a consequence of the growing commercialization of the Internet. Sclove concludes by proposing several actions that communities can adopt to reduce Internet-induced harm, while redesigning the Internet in a more civically responsible form.

Continuing the theme of commercialization of the Internet in Chapter 4, Christian Sandvig compares the creation of property rights in and on the Internet Domain Name System with a similar situation that faced broadcasting in the United States in the 1920s and early 1930s. To Sandvig, both instances demonstrate the consequences that result when policy choices are constrained to the unquestioned, unguided assumptions of the marketplace as normalized default. Current DNS policy, he argues, robs local communities of an important symbolic resource: their names. Chapter 5 by Eszter Hargittai concludes this part of the book by reasoning that search engine results, the layout of portal sites, and the way people are directed from one site to another influences the type of content found and viewed online. Since big portal sites are driven by a need to make a profit, their decisions on what content to feature are not necessarily based on the quality and relevance of the websites they present to users. Considering the implications of this situation for not-for-profits, who have fewer resources to spend promoting their online presence, Hargittai concludes by suggesting ways in which they might also gain exposure to relevant audiences without large expenditures.

Snapshots of community practice

Part II provides snapshots of community practice in the network society, identifying issues and problems encountered by community ICT initiatives operating in the current milieu. Insights into initiatives, programs, and projects contributing to the emergence of a new form of public sphere within and between local communities across the globe are provided. The first chapter by Audrey Marshall explores the idea of social inclusion in relation to information and health in the network society. Drawing parallels between the so-called "digital divide" and the problem of health inequalities, often called the "health divide," Marshall contends that ICTs can contribute positively to health communication. However, in order to play a positive part in tackling social inequalities a more democratic approach is required. Observing that the success of community health ICT initiatives is dependent on addressing local community need, Marshall concludes that the participation of local people should be central to their design and development.

Scott Robinson points to the dramatic rollout of cybercafés in many parts of Latin America as evidence of the digital divide in Chapter 7. Critical of the vested interests driving information society programs and development in Latin America, Robinson argues that while cybercafés may offer practical, micro-entrepreneurial solutions to government inaction, users of these commercial services employ the digital tools in a frivolous fashion, chatting, surfing porn sites, and using email. Countering this by describing the social conscience, local heart, and commitment to generating local content online plus training programs for users in Telecenters, Robinson discusses how such initiatives are often hampered by the lack of online incentives that are geared to meeting local community needs and culturally appropriate contents.

Christina Courtright provides another critical assessment of information society strategy in Latin America in Chapter 8. She describes a participatory action research program in El Salvador during 1998 and 1999. Using case studies, consultations, and focus groups, the program identified both problems and strengths relating to the digital revolution and proposed a series of sector-based projects aimed at leveraging existing resources and producing sustainable change. Describing and critically evaluating the process and outcomes of this program, Courtright propounds a number of significant research questions related to international and local development challenges in a digital world.

The experience of the African American community in the information age forms the heart of the arguments presented by Abdul Alkalimat in Chapter 9. Alkalimat asserts that most African Americans are being excluded from the social transformation currently underway, and that missing out on the redefinition of standards for social life – they are literacy, job readiness, upward social mobility, and social power – may be permanent. The chapter reports on an action-research project designed to explore ways in which the everyday life of African American communities can become the content of their virtual community identity, and by so doing can create a bridge over the digital divide. Based in Toledo, Ohio (USA) the project is a joint effort by the Africana Studies Program at the University of Toledo and the Murchison Community Center.

An emerging community technology research agenda

Part III considers issues relating to the emerging significance of the community technology research agenda in the network society discourse. Authors examine the implications, consequences, and contribution of research to *community practice in the network society* and vice versa, and in so doing, illustrate the importance of the community technology practice, policy, and research nexus (Day, 2001).

Chapter 10 reports on the qualitative results of a mixed method field study of Internet use at a public library branch Internet site in Vancouver, British Columbia (Canada). Observations of patron use of public access Internet terminals, conducted by Ellen Balka and Brian Peterson, are discussed in relation to Canadian public policy goals of citizenship and social cohesion. Results to date suggest that the goal of supporting citizenship via public access to the Internet is not being achieved. Despite this, it is suggested that some degree of social cohesion is being achieved, although the mechanisms through which this is being realized vary markedly from the vision promoted by the Canadian government. Highlighting a need to move beyond an infrastructure "field of dreams" mentality, Balka and Peterson conclude that the Canadian government needs to direct attention towards the development of social facilitation and social programs.

Chapter 11 by Bill McIver provides a conceptual and historical overview of the development of applicable human rights concepts and presents frameworks that might be used to implement and enforce the human right to communicate. McIver claims that issues of access to the Internet can be analyzed within formal and well-established human rights frameworks deriving from the United Nations 1948 Universal Declaration of Human Rights. He concludes by asserting that by adopting a human rights perspective, policy-makers will have an appropriate framework for addressing human needs in the network society, e.g. addressing the digital divide and universal service.

Highlighting the significance of meaningful partnerships between community practice and research, Nicol Turner-Lee and Randal Pinkett examine the integration of community technology and community building in Chapter 12. The chapter compares, contrasts, and shares the lessons from asset-based community development activities at Northwest Tower, in Chicago, Illinois, and Roxbury, Massachusetts. At both locations tenants collaborated with academic researchers on a range of community building through community technology initiatives. The purpose of both projects was to identify the critical success factors for integrating a community technology and community-building initiative in a low-income housing development, and its surrounding environs.

Murali Venkatesh, Julia Nosovitch and Wayne Miner examine participation by potential users of a community network, based on advanced information and communications technology, in the context of five individual projects in Chapter 13. The community network is being developed for use by public institutions, community-based organizations and small business entities in economically depressed geographical communities. Impediments to user participation, which affect some organizations more than others, are identified, as is the significance of the broader social context in which the developmental effort occurs. The chapter concludes with an examination of the role of power and vested interests in the network's development.

In the final chapter of Part III (Chapter 14), Wal Taylor and Stuart Marshall propose a framework for the development of a Community Informatics Systems (CIS). Community informatics, they propose, is an ideal meeting place for inter-disciplinary research and cross-sectoral practice: a location where, through the fusion of appropriate expertise, knowledge can be turned into action. Arguing that new forms of partnership and community engagement are at the heart of higher education in the network society the chapter concludes by introducing a framework designed to stimulate discussion around the development of community/university partnerships from which innovative and socially meaningful CIS research and practice can emerge.

Conclusion

It is clear from the evidence presented in the pages of this book that a widespread interest in community ICT practice is emerging, but are these efforts destined to blaze temporarily and burn out or do they signal the beginning of new significant social forces? The protean nature of the medium and its potential for inexpensive and ubiquitous access to information and communication suggests rich potential for civic uses. In the book's concluding chapter (Chapter 15) Peter Day and Douglas Schuler develop a vision for community-centric pathways to network society development.

As a number of authors suggest here, the obstacles will be great. Many forms of community technologies are emerging as communities seek to achieve a diverse range of social goals. Social movements across the world are utilizing ICTs to support and sustain their communication, organization, mobilization, and activation processes. Just how solid, durable, effective, equitable, and socially meaningful the local action and global interaction of community practice and social movements in the network society will be in shaping our social environments is as yet unclear. The journey has begun, the implications of the decisions we make now, at each fork along the path to the network society Lushai Hills, will begin to unfold in the months and years ahead.

Notes

1   Although an area of related interest to our considerations, space precludes a detailed examination of Indymedia here.

2   For a more detailed consideration of the commonalities and differences in US and European information society policy development, see Day (2001).

3   Often refers to both statutory and voluntary services.

Part I

The network society

Issues and exigencies

Chapter 2

Globalization, cyberspace and the public sphere

Oliver Boyd-Barrett

Introduction

This volume's title and tone promises analysis of positive application of network technologies to social development. In another contribution to a recent volume (Schuler and Day, 2003), my goal had been to set limits on such optimism. In effect, I argued, if one's goal is social, political, and economic improvement, then network technologies do not really present a compelling starting point. That argument was made prior to the attacks on the World Trade Center in New York and on the Pentagon in Washington DC, on September 11, 2001, which represented the beginning, symbolic and actual, of a new chapter – an extraordinarily tragic chapter – in global order. 9/11 and the events that it set in train endorse my cautions against over-emphasizing network technologies as a compelling starting point for significant change. These technologies buttress the agencies of centralized power in its bid for global domination, at the cost of significant retrenchment of civil liberties (in the name of "freedom"). And yet, network technologies *also* constitute a uniquely important forum for open and independent discussion, analysis, and protest, but for how long?

What better time, then, to revisit the concept of the "public sphere" than when the machinery of US democracy appears co-opted and subverted by a governing alliance of financial institutions, major corporations, military, politicians, and bureaucratic mandarins in partnership, as necessary, with their international subalterns? Of course, this is not new in US history: President Rutherford B. Hayes complained after the 1876 election: "This is a government of the people, by the people, and for the people no longer. It is a government of corporations, by corporations, and for corporations" (quoted in Korten, 2001: 65). What has changed is the scale of the problem under mature corporate capitalism and US superpower status.

One cannot assume that the governing alliance will achieve any inclusive, long-term vision of global good in its response to the "terrorist threat." The perils faced by peoples of developed and developing worlds alike would be clearer to all had mainstream, privately owned and advertiser-supported media the capability of sustained, independent focus. Capable, that is, of selecting and framing issues independent of official spin fed them without interruption, free of cost or other inhibition, by political and other elite actors for the purpose of maintaining wealth, status, and power. The concept of "public sphere" in this context becomes much more than a useful conceptual tool for the reformulation of media structures in post-communist Russia and Eastern Europe, or for critical examination of the shortcomings of both state-controlled and private media worldwide. It stands at the heart of any and all strategies for the restoration and reformulation of meaningful democracy in the United States, itself a critical first step towards the resuscitation or establishment of democracy in any other part of the globe.

US global cyberspace

The starting point for my companion chapter was a world deeply divided, half of whose population, according to United Nations Development Program statistics (see UNDP reports for 1999–2002) subsist on less than $2 a day (an *extremely* pusillanimous definition of poverty). A significant feature of wealth distribution is a substantial, widening gap between "haves" and "have-nots" between and within nations. The UNDP 2001 report (p. 17) referenced a study of 77 countries with 82 percent of the world's people, showing that between the 1950s and the 1990s, in-country inequality rose in 45 of the countries and fell in 16. In 2002, 1 percent of the world's people received as much income as the poorest 57 percent. Some 55 countries experienced *negative* annual income growth per capita during "boom-time" 1990s. The 2001–3 recession increased that number. Several not-inconsiderable improvements in global justice are less impressive than they at first appear. What value has the increasing number of countries that hold multi-party elections (140 out of nearly 200 in 2000) if only a third of voters say their country is governed by the will of the people (UNDP, 2002: 1)? The introduction of democracy at local (national) level too often signifies accession to a highly inequitable, undemocratic global economic system.

Huge disparities persist in access to media, with approximately half of village households in India, for example, lacking access to computer, telephone, television, or radio. Of the world's 500 million Internet users 72 percent live in high-income OECD countries with 14 percent of the world's population. A starting point for remedy of such injustice is UNDP's 1999 recommendation for a framework of global governance based on ethics, equity, inclusion, human security, sustainability, and development, all in the pursuit of freedom *from* discrimination, want, fear, injustice, violation of the rule of law, exploitation of labor; and freedom *of* thought and speech; realization of human potential, participation in decision-making. Media's potential contribution to achievement of these UNDP goals is to offer to all peoples of this world the benefits of greater inter-connectivity, community, capacity, meaningful content, creativity, collaboration, and better access to cash resources.

Globalization references the extension of politics, economics, culture, and trade beyond legal territorial boundaries. While nothing new, it is the transformations in the forms of globalization over time that are interesting. The current "neo-liberal" manifestation dating from the 1980s has three outstanding features: transnational corporations, inclusive reach, and dependence on communications and information technologies. World business activity in 2000 was dominated by a handful of major economies, notably the United States, Japan and Great Britain, accounting for over half of global economic activity (see Boyd-Barrett, 2003b). North America and Western Europe accounted for 80 percent of the world's top 1,000 corporations. Eighty-five percent of the world's 60,000 transnational corporations and their 500,000 foreign affiliates were registered in developed (OECD) countries. Knowledge-based industries represented 11 percent of top companies and accounted for up to half of US business output by the mid-1990s. American companies Microsoft, Hewlett Packard, Sun Microsystems, Oracle, Intel, IBM, Compaq, Dell, AOL/Time Warner, Cisco, and Lucent dominated the global markets for operator systems, computer chips, computer and PC hardware manufacture, Internet access, computer server systems, and telecommunications equipment. Outsourcing by US computer companies contributed significantly to other economies like India and Ireland. Additionally, the USA was lead exporter of high-tech products, selling $206 billion worth to other countries – as much as the next two leading exporters combined, Japan and Germany (UNDP, 2001: 42). According to a year 2000 *Wireless* magazine survey quoted by UNDP, 2001 (p. 45), the USA had 13 "technology hubs" – locations that matter most in new digital geography – more than three and four times as many as the next national technology leaders (UK and Germany).

The communications and information industries include traditional or "old" media such as voice telephone, newspapers, cinema, and television, and "new" electronic and digital media – including satellite, mobile and wireless broadband telephony, the Internet, and the Internet "backbone." Increasingly the two sectors have come together in response to major trends. These include digitization, convergence, fusion (the merger of "common carrier" and "gatekeeper" models of content delivery), deregulation, privatization, concentration, "competitivization" (a cycle of competition, triggered by technology innovation or regulatory reform, followed by market concentration and oligopoly), commercialization, internationalization of market share, Americanization of content and business strategy, and neo-liberal style democratization (usually leading to privatization and deregulation). There has been intense accumulation and concentration of capital investment in communications within and across national borders: this is evident to varying degrees in content, content formats, patents, hardware, business models, and management practices. Through computing the USA provides the digital infrastructure upon which global industry, in general, and communications, in particular, have come to depend.

US leadership in communications and information technologies contributed significantly to US strategic reaction to a period of severe vulnerability for the country's global power during the 1970s. In essence, the strategy involved (1) control of developing nations, undermining their previous, unsuccessful policies of nationalization and import substitution by debt management and the imposition of "structural adjustment" conditions in return for lending (in collaboration with the World Bank, International Monetary Fund and World Trade Organization), (2) enhanced trade liberalization and expansion of transnational corporations, (3) destruction of the Soviet Union through a process that has been described by President Carter's national security advisor Z. Brzezinski (1998) as entrapment in Afghanistan, and (4) aggressive ideological campaigning on behalf of corporate capitalism through ideological hegemony, media globalization, Hollywood product, and advertising. Communications technologies proved vital, underpinning global communications networks for global business and regulatory institutional control, also for post-Vietnam military dominance in battlefield awareness, precision-guided weaponry, and "missile shield" technology. Communications represented an export industry dominated by US corporations, and the exploitation of increased demand for US news and entertainment products in the wake of media privatization, deregulation, and proliferation throughout the world. Computer and information technologies prove vital to the next waves of US technology dominance in such fields as biotechnology and nanotechnology.

Critiquing the public sphere

The work of Habermas (see Calhoun, 1998) has been particularly influential in identifying the properties of a "rational" public sphere, that is to say, a forum, physical or otherwise, in which people can come together to exchange ideas and views pertaining to matters that have as their focus the good of society as a whole, as opposed to the good of mere private interest. Habermas drew inspiration from the eighteenth-century salons of Paris and the coffee houses of London. These institutions, he argued, reflected the emergence of a new bourgeoisie or middle class, and established an awareness of the world not reflective solely of the interests of nobility, aristocracy, or church. This public sphere was far from perfect. Working classes, peasantry, women, were not well represented. Yet the discourses of salon and coffee house – integrated with opinions and information disseminated through pamphlets, periodicals, and broadsheets about arts and, when authorities allowed, politics – focused on matters of public concern, and were independent of government, church, private interest, and the interests of capital, while contributing to more enlightened governance. Recognition of quality or force of argument lay not in *who* was arguing a point of view, their status, property, or role, but on the compelling *rationality* of their argument.

Whatever approximation to the ideal public sphere that the eighteenth-century coffee houses represented was progressively corrupted by the success of power-holders in controlling or managing public opinion. Newspapers became institutionalized, accommodated the interests of the authorities and, driven by profit motive, aspired to reach ever higher circulations (new technology allowed larger print runs), and increase revenue from advertising. Newspapers no longer addressed to particular groups, were no longer embedded in specific social contexts; their communications became increasingly one-way rather than dialogic, given to spectacle as much as to substance, to political positioning rather than reasoned debate.

Habermas' concept of a rational public sphere and his narrative of a consistent decline is open to question. Calhoun (1997), quoting Schudson (1995), argues that the active participation of citizens in public discourse and politics has ebbed and flowed without linear trend over time. One may also critique the concept of "reason" in the Habermas model: who determines the criteria for "rational"? Calhoun notes that the concept of public sphere also presupposes fixity of participant identities prior to debate, rather than allowing that identity, solidarity, and culture are shaped *through* debate.

That the press (in print and electronic forms) contributes to public sphere or civil society is intrinsic to classic theories of democracy that overlap with notions of public sphere. Curran (1992) assessed the performance of both privately owned, and state or publicly owned media against criteria of classic democracy. The proclaimed "watchdog" role of the press, that it should represent the interests of the public by critically monitoring the doings of government, is conventionally applied to the *state* whereas, Curran argued, abuse of the public interest is as likely to result from the operations of private *capital*. It is difficult to set up publicly owned watchdogs that are truly free of state intervention. Possibly the best-known institution of this kind is the British Broadcasting Corporation. Despite "arm's-length distancing" of corporation and state, various sources of state interference over the BBC persist, not least state power to set the license fee and appoint the chairman of the board of governors. Nor are private press watchdogs free of external influence: increasingly they are owned by large conglomerates which pursue selfish economic interests that are often politically partisan. Because they are motivated by profit, information and opinion may not be as important to them as entertainment or diversion. This in turn affects the culture of audience expectation, and forces publicly owned media to compete for audiences using the same strategies and deceptions as commercial media.

Curran also considers the "fourth estate" role of a free press namely, that it should exist as an autonomous civic power within society, a check and balance against other powers. The main weakness of media performance against this criterion is that media are increasingly unable to represent civil society. Processes of privatization and deregulation enhance oligopolization of media. These leave media to the mercy of market forces; competition leads to concentration, and this reduces diversity of content and ideology, audience choice, and public control. Oligopolization increases costs of market entry, reduces diversity of expression, positions audiences merely as different categories of consumer. Also serving to reduce diversity is the organization of journalism as a profession, including routine news "beats" and a tradition of reporting that focuses on *events* rather than processes and on the activities of *elite* nations and people.

A third press role assessed by Curran is the importance of media as the purveyors of information, arguably a basic necessity for a flourishing public sphere. Here too, there are problems. The selective influence of advertising on the markets that media choose to target, and the means by which audience attention is hailed, reduces the diversity of ideas. Information does not come from neutral sources; much of it derives from institutions, both state and private, whose purpose is to manipulate public opinion. The media and their sources set agendas that highlight certain issues while hiding others from public attention, and they "frame" the issues that they do cover within elite-defined frameworks of value and ideology. Information, therefore, is not independent of its function of representation (of people, institutions, and ideas).

A fourth criterion has to do with the independence of journalists, and their ability through professionally responsible practices to represent and nourish a public sphere. Reference has already been made to routinization of news, agenda-setting, and framing. In addition, journalists work within constrained cultures that are hierarchically organized, within which they aspire to career advancement; they are told what to report, they do not determine how stories eventually appear. There are significant problems about the extent of dependence of news consumers on these professional "mediators" and the lack of opportunity available to most people to achieve un-mediated expression through traditional media.

Internet towards a public sphere

Does the Internet constitute a public sphere, or contribute to one? Indisputably, the Internet has provided a powerful new means of expression to individuals and institutions. Some 10 percent of the world's total population (at the time of writing early in 2003) are Internet users, and the proportion is rising. The Internet gives users access to millions of different websites, including those of established media, sites originating from any part of the world, accessible from any part of the world, and including sites of alternative or Internet-only publishers. It permits users to access information (data, script, audio, and moving image) in ways that were barely conceivable in pre-Internet days. Users can quickly compare how a given news story is covered across a range of international newspapers, at a tiny fraction of the cost, time, and hassle that it would once have taken. They can access sites that specialize in specific themes, issues, or points of view that bring together a vast range of relevant sources and hyperlinks to other sites. They can easily access archival material. Users can construct their own portfolios of news and information, and many sites make it possible for them to do precisely that. They can access both primary and secondary sources in any of the major media forms including text, audio, and video.

The Internet is less easy to censor than traditional print and broadcast media. Users can set up their own sites; some such sites attract visitor numbers that exceed the total circulation of many a local daily newspaper in the United States. Users can engage in direct one-to-one or small group conversation at will with other users, regardless of time or place; they can often pass comment on what they have read and post their comments for others to read; they can elect to receive regular, automatically disseminated updates or newsletters that save them the trouble of having to remember to log on to particular sites. Existing small-circulation publications oftentimes greatly expand their audience by establishing institutional websites, and articles posted on these often turn up in searches conducted by people who had previously no knowledge of the existence of these publications. The efficiency of search engines, therefore, greatly magnifies the potential reach of minority as of other writings.

There is a downside. Most people have little time to spare over and above family and/or work commitments. Most Internet users who access news and information sites depend on established sources, whether these be the welcome pages of their internet service providers, or the sites of well-known mainstream news "brands." These have many if not all the limitations of existing commercial news media. Most are owned by giant conglomerations. Their sites typically benefit from relatively abundant resources, needed to attract and hold the attention of mass audiences. Most depend on advertising revenue to cover their costs, although few have achieved a profitable business model. Portals and search machines also depend on advertising revenue, and advertising considerations influence the structure in which information is provided or search results reported. The costs of getting online for many people around the world are still considerable, including computer acquisition (hardware and software), access to a telephone line, or simply the fees to access machines at "Internet cafes." The structure of the web still reflects its origin, with half of the user population and the websites they use based in the USA. Content is most likely to be in English. In the USA and elsewhere most consumers will likely end up accessing the web via Internet service providers selected or even owned by the phone company or cable operator that provides service in their area, providers that constitute oligopolistic corporations at national level, while enjoying local market monopolies. These distribution networks will set limitations on the structure of access to the web (Lessig, 2002).

Through the web there are very many alternatives to mainstream media provision of news and information. These contribute significantly to diversity. But the mainstream media, by power of their audience size, brand name, and privileged access to authority, still have the power to "validate" information items and perspectives and thus to marginalize others. The profusion of alternatives, their relative newness, and lack of audience familiarity may contribute to a climate in which such sources are regarded as less credible or trustworthy. In addition, many states, such as China, have found ways of restricting or limiting access to the Internet or of sanctioning forms of provision or use of which they disapprove, and in almost all states there are moves to increase the powers of security and police forces to monitor Internet traffic.

Case study of the Internet as public sphere

Whatever the limitations of the Internet, events at the turn of the twenty-first century have demonstrated its profound contribution to the public sphere, one that helps compensate for staggering failures on the part of mainstream media. Here, I will make reference to one example: the Internet as source of a new range of voices in international news provision.

International news and social justice

For over 150 years, major networks of collection and supply of international news for the benefit of the "retail" national and provincial news media were the major international news agencies, based in the world's leading centers of political and economic power, notably New York, London, Paris (see Boyd-Barrett, 1980, 2003a; Boyd-Barrett and Rantanen, 2003). At the time of writing the major international news agencies are Agence France Press (AFP) (French), Associated Press (American), and Reuters (based in London); each organization has been around for over 150 years (if one accepts Havas as direct predecessor to AFP). Reuters is also the world's major economic and financial news agency (followed by Bloomberg of New York, also covering general news). Associated Press and Reuters operate the world's leading private suppliers of television news film (APTV and Reuters Television International). For many decades these agencies or their predecessors nurtured and entered into exclusive contracts with a network of national news agencies. The typical national news agency was a consortium of local news media, perhaps with some government involvement, exercising a monopoly on the gathering and supply of nationally relevant news for national and provincial "retail" news media. The global network of international news agencies, working in unequal partnership with the national news agencies to whom the international agencies supplied their international news in exchange for national news, often on an exclusive or near-exclusive basis, showed remarkable persistence and robustness. In recent decades its influence has been undermined by international broadcasters such as CNN that maintain significant international reporting strength and easily accessible news.

The global news agency network provided global news to news media around the world, at a price that was affordable. It helped compensate for the fact that few of the world's media could afford their own international correspondents, and even those that could usually maintained only a handful of correspondents scattered across a few countries. The major agencies on the other hand had news bureaus in almost every country of the world. The shortcomings of this system were various. It was unequal. Why should the media of a country like Bolivia in South America, for example, depend for its supply of world news on the judgments of editors based in New York, Paris, or London or on organizations headquartered in those cities? Inevitably, the news was selective: certain countries or regions, topics, or issues were favored over others. Judgments as to what was newsworthy reflected the news criteria and rituals of Anglo-Saxon journalism traditions, in the service, first and foremost, of the world's major print and broadcast news media and other clients – sources of revenue that were concentrated mainly in the developed world countries. Earlier attempts to develop alternatives, sponsored by UNESCO or similar humanitarian sources, such as the Caribbean News Agency, Pan African News Agency, or InterPress Service, etc., experienced considerable difficulty; many failed or are failing.

The Internet encouraged the development of a new generation of alternatives, representing a broader range of perspectives and practices, in many cases approximating a news philosophy more reflective of goals of social justice than earlier alternatives, or operating more like the "watchdog" or "fourth estate" models of the press than wealthy mainstream media in the developed world. What follows is a list of some of these. The list shows that state and capital do not always have to be the major or dominating sources of inspiration, finance, or operation for news agencies, whether national or international, although all sites are challenged to find a business model that permits them to survive. In some instances, especially where the news services are intended for "retail" news media, significant subscriptions are required to access full services.

All-Africa.com

This is an advertising-supported Internet service, registered in Mauritius with offices in Washington DC and Johannesburg, and involves the collation of news reports from over 100 African news providers, including mainstream national newspapers and news agencies (extending to archives of the Pan-African News Agency, PANA, and the South Africa Press Association, SAPA). The service distributes 700 stories daily, has 400,000 archived articles, although 90 percent of its clientele reside outside the African continent. It has a four-tiered revenue stream: advertisements, transactions, information sales, technology services. It claims a readership of 4.5 million.

EcoNews Africa

A not-for-profit international non-governmental organization registered in the Republic of Kenya. Founded in 1992, EcoNews provides analysis of global environment and development issues from an African perspective and reports on local, national, and regional activities that contribute to global solutions.

Globalvision News Network (GVNews.Net)

GVNews.Net is a global syndicate of more than 240 independent news organizations that provides local news affiliates with a global outlet for their reporting and converts local news content to standardized digital formats for syndication into new global media markets. Revenue is shared back with participating news organizations. It claims to offset the dominant, largely Anglo-American organizations delivering most of the news that is now found on the Internet and elsewhere. Its "Daily Edition" shadows and supplements world news reporting of mainstream news outlets. Its "News Alerts" and "Intelligence Reports" are emailed, and Internet-distributed newsletters are provided to paying subscribers. In 2002, GVNews.Net launched "Global News Feed" providing access to over 3,000 news items each day from 150 cities worldwide (Karr, 2002).

Independent Media Center or Indymedia (www.indymedia.org)

Indymedia is a progressive network of more than 80 separate independent media collectives in 30 countries. The first center was established in Seattle in 1999, to provide alternative coverage of the World Trade Organization (WTO) protests. Each center operates independently of the global network. According to Peterson (2002) any person can go to an Indymedia website and publish an article, photos, video, or audio clips, anonymously if they wish. Each center, she says, is a collective, "with open membership and all decisions are made by the consensus process. Each collective is comprised of several working groups, which coordinate different aspects of the website or work together on common projects." Unlike establishment media, in which content is determined by a small group of people (editorial, executives, and advertisers), the information of independent media centers is controlled by the people who produce the information.

Indo-Asian News Service (eians.com)

Formerly India Abroad News Service, this was conceived by Gopal Raju, founder of the *India Abroad* weekly newspaper, in 1986. The original purpose was to enhance the flow of news and information between India and North America, a goal that has extended to enhancement of information flows between India and the Middle East and the Indian diasporas worldwide. It now claims to be India's "first multinational and multilingual wire service," claiming among its clients every major newspaper group in India and subscribers in many other countries.

IRINnews.org

This is a product of the United Nations Integrated Regional Information Networks (IRIN), which is part of the UN Office for the Co-ordination of

Humanitarian Affairs (OCHA), and funded by financial contributions from donor governments and/or institutions. It has English and French language services that are specialized according to region (in Africa, the Great Lakes, East Africa, Horn of Africa, Southern Africa, West Africa; and Central Asia) and themes (children, governance, economy, environment, food security, gender, health, human rights, peace and security, refugees). It seeks to strengthen "universal access to timely, strategic and non-partisan information so as to enhance the capacity of the humanitarian community to understand, respond to and avert emergencies." In addition to its own multimedia, information officers, and freelance journalists, reports come from governments, aid workers, civil societies, disaster specialists, and members of the public, and cover the "full range of humanitarian issues from the abuse of human rights to the environments."

OneWorld (oneworld.net)

One World is a non-profit network whose mission is to harness the democratic potential of the Internet to promote sustainable development, human rights, and an end to world poverty. It claims the world's leading web portal (founded in 1995) on global social justice, bringing together a partnership of over 1,250 NGOs worldwide, ranging from United Nations agencies, Amnesty International, and Greenpeace to grassroots groups. The content of OneWorld.net is edited by ten One World centers in both the South and the North. According to its publicity manager, Glen Tarman (2002), One World editors add value and enhance user experience by repackaging content from partner websites into sections such as world news, special reports, campaigns, and database content by theme and topic. One World grew out of a small UK-based charity, One World Broadcasting Trust (OWBT), which seeks to encourage the media, especially broadcasting, to promote awareness of human rights and global development issues. It came into being as NGOs were beginning to initiate a web presence and advised many small NGOs on the development of their sites. From November 2001, One World has also distributed through Yahoo!, the first non-profit world news syndication to a corporate web portal, for which it provides original stories by One World editors on the basis of sources among NGO partners.

The Panos Institute (panos.org.uk)

Panos was founded in 1986 as an independent non-profit organization, with offices in London, Paris, Washington, Kathmandu, Kampala, Addis, Haiti, and Dakar. It now owns Gemini News Service, a long-established alternative news agency. Its London website describes itself as a source of news, opinions, and perspectives from developing countries. It works to "stimulate debate on global environment and development issues" and seeks to "amplify the voices of the poor and marginalized." It provides features, topic and issue briefings, written by correspondents from the countries covered, then edited and distributed from London. It supports communities to undertake their own journalistic reports on developmental issues.

Stratfor.com

A private provider of intelligence, analysis and forecasting, founded in 1995, Stratfor.com is associated with the Center for Geopolitical Studies, established by George Friedman. Its aim is to help decision-makers worldwide "convert facts into understanding and information into actionable knowledge." Its employees are described as business and intelligence professionals with backgrounds in the military, academia, and think tanks, as well as journalists and editors. It claims more than 35,000 subscribers worldwide. Services include confidential consulting on "existing or potential competitive and security threats that global companies and/or nation states may face in specific markets or regions."

WorldNetDaily.com

Representing a commercial "alternative" Internet news source, it was in fact founded in 1997 as an Internet project of the non-profit Western Journalism Center. Based in southern Oregon, it claims to attract nearly two million unique visitors a month and more than 40 million pageviews. Its website proclaims a "watchdog" role on government – "to expose corruption, fraud, waste and abuse wherever and whenever it is found."

Conclusion

The examples that I have quoted hardly constitute an exhaustive list – far from it. But they illustrate important features of the new online world of news gathering and dissemination. First of all, they represent a broader range of business models than the time-honored division of commercial versus state sources of funding that have characterized "old media." In doing so, they collectively resemble the Habermas "public sphere." Many encourage reader dialogue with site editors and auditors; the capacity of broadband does not require the highly selective choices that are characteristic of mainstream media "letters to the editor." Second, they suggest the possibility of a radically different and broader range of voices and concerns than those provided by mainstream media. Consider, if you will, the many national news agencies that UNESCO has helped to establish in the developing world over several decades. Many were committed to fostering news portfolios that were to be radically different from those of existing, first world media. Nonetheless they slipped quickly into established, conventional Anglo-Saxon journalistic traditions; many have failed or are failing. When we look at what is available on the Internet, on the other hand, we quickly find, as above, many organizations that operate extensive international news operations and clearly present their audiences with news portfolios that cannot be found in existing mainstream media, dealing with issues that are barely covered in the mainstream, from perspectives that are barely represented in the mainstream. My list has not focused on special-issue sites, or on sites that provide critical perspectives from within established national boundaries. But had it done so, I would have provided many examples of sites that have played a major role in helping to contest, for example, the strategies of "total spectrum dominance" that are currently pursued by the USA, sites that have helped mobilize millions of people to street expression of their opposition to US warmongering, and sites that have radically redefined Establishment accounts of the meaning and origins of 9/11 (see Boyd-Barrett, 2003c). These sites help expose, I believe, the uncomfortably close alliances that exist between mainstream media and national and international corporate, plutocratic, and military elites. And they have demonstrated this to a far larger number of people than it has been possible to reach in the past. Rather than working in the splendid competitive isolation of mainstream media, they work much more collaboratively, sharing information, and providing links to other sites. Not least, they have contributed to the finding of solutions to the problems with which they deal.

The Internet is probably the best representative yet known of "network technologies" in the digital age. It is true that these technologies are first and foremost of benefit to the existing structures of power in the world. In particular, they are part responsible for securing US superpower status and part responsible for maintaining US military and political advantage in a period of energy crisis and the "war on terrorism." At the same time, the Internet has provided a forum, historically unequalled, for the expression of new and marginalized voices, and this chapter has looked at some of the ways in which the Internet, for at least a period of time, has come to represent the most significant vehicle for critiques of hegemonic discourses, even though the benefits are accessible to only a modest proportion of the world's population. Thus, the Internet recalls earlier debates about the "public sphere" and controversial narratives of a "decline" in the public sphere and of traditional media's contribution to such a decline. At this precise moment that I write, the Internet is both magnificent in its unequalled extension of communicative power to non-elites of the world, while simultaneously vulnerable to the ominous gathering of the forces of hegemonic oppression.

Chapter 3

Cybersobriety

How a commercially driven Internet
threatens the foundations of democratic
self-governance and what to do about it[1]

Richard E. Sclove

Competing technological myths

With technology supercharging the new century, two myths vie for supremacy
in the United States. The first might be christened "Genesis, Chapter 51":

> And finally it came to pass that God repented of the punishment which
> God had meted out to Eve and Adam. And God gave unto Eve and Adam
> and all of their descendants as a gift unto them forever a new Garden, which
> was full of all manner of wondrous things. And these included all the
> knowledge from the Tree of Life of which people were needful in order
> to make for themselves lives of peace, grace, and abundance. And God
> saw that it was good. And also God gave unto Eve and Adam and all of
> their descendants the ability to share knowledge among themselves, to
> communicate easily among themselves no matter where or how far apart
> they might variously journey, to form themselves into groups howsoever
> they might wish, and to produce as though in an instant all the things
> necessary for their comfort and enjoyment. And the name for this new
> Garden of knowledge-without-limit which the Lord God gave unto all the
> people living upon the face of the Earth was Cyberspace.

The second myth follows a far bleaker script, "Net Wars, Episode 1 – The
Empire Is Assembled":

> Long, long ago, on a planet far, far away (Earth, 1992–1995). Noble
> visionaries struggle to create an Internet grounded in principles of universal
> access, free speech, personal privacy, and support for civic uses. Over-
> whelmed by the financial and political power of businesses jockeying for
> advantage in the emerging global tele-economy, their heroic efforts fail.
> Their symbolic moment of defeat is February 1996, when the US Congress
> enacts the Telecommunications Policy Act ("the best law money could buy,"
> according to embittered survivors of the visionary cause). The Internet is
> swiftly recreated as a medium dominated and driven by commercial
> interests.

Adherents of Genesis 51 herald the Internet and other new communication technologies as forces that will educate and empower individuals, expand wealth, and reinvigorate democracy. The Net-War critics insist that a heavily commercialized Internet will cement social inequality and hierarchy. Their chief complaint: Internet access is skewed toward the socially advantaged, while the poorest among us are shut out. Provided this racial and class bias can be overcome, this critique goes, the Internet's positive democratic potential will unfold.[2]

Who is right, the optimists or skeptics? Most likely both, but also, in significant and disturbing ways, neither. Each ignores potential avenues by which an Internet driven by powerful commercial interests can undermine the foundations of democratic self-governance. Moreover, unless preventive measures are taken, the dangers would be just as great, if not greater, in the event that universal, affordable access to the Internet is actually achieved.

The Internet has, of course, yielded a variety of striking social and political benefits. Certain forms of information about government, commerce, and the world generally are becoming much more widely available. People can communicate with one another and organize in exciting new ways. Rural areas have access to data and services that once were to be had only in metropolitan centers. Dissidents struggling under authoritarian foreign regimes are able to circumvent censorship.

Moreover, the goal of forging a more equitable society, in which the benefits of electronic networking are available to the poor, *is* vitally important. But "universal and affordable access," as currently formulated, is a faulty prescription for realizing that objective. Under current policy regimes – and given the dynamics of social and technological change that I shall shortly describe – the quest for universal access could easily overshoot the mark into an *over-wired world*. Before long we may find ourselves living in a society of *inescapable, compulsory access*. The erosion of conventional, offline modes of social and economic interaction could not only force people to use the Internet involuntarily, but would also produce a host of other personal and civic harms.

Consider the history of another powerfully seductive, personal technology. The United States has more or less achieved universal, affordable access to private automobiles, with some profoundly positive – and profoundly negative – results. Automobiles have supported personal mobility and freedom, as well as the expansion of vast industries. But the proliferation of cars and trucks has also constrained us to endure daily traffic jams, air pollution, the ill effects of suburban sprawl, tens of thousands of annual road fatalities, and dependence on non-renewable and insecure sources of imported oil. In the process, we have created a society in which owning an automobile and driving upwards of 10,000 miles a year has become, for most Americans, not at all a voluntary option. This exemplifies what cultural iconoclast Ivan Illich calls "radical monopoly." Automotive technology and its supporting institutions have rendered alternative modes of existence inaccessible, thereby imposing use of a car as compulsory (Sclove and Scheuer, 1996; Illich, 1973).

If we now have second thoughts about how our society achieved universal access to the automobile, there are sound reasons to suspect that we will feel every bit as ambivalent about the manner in which we are pursuing universal Internet access. On the other hand, a technology's contradictory social consequences need not be accepted whole cloth. Wise policies governing the design and use of a technology can encourage its benign effects and lessen the deleterious ones. Unwise policies can do the opposite.

In the United States no popular clamor for building a new road system pressured Congress to pass the Interstate Highway Act in 1956. Only about half of American families owned a car. Everyone else depended on public transportation. Auto-makers, road-builders, and realtors who saw profits in developing suburban subdivisions, however, all lobbied Congress aggressively. In response, lawmakers created the Highway Trust Fund, earmarking taxes from gasoline sales for highway construction. Public transit systems, unable to compete with subsidized automobiles, rapidly atrophied. Soon more Americans were forced to buy a car to shop or to hold a job. So the tremendous social transformation that followed hinged upon the political muscle of powerful business interests and external compulsion – not simply the free choices of consumers and certainly not any inexorable internal logic of technological development (Flink, 1988: 358–373).

Western European nations, in contrast, opted for different public policies governing transportation systems (ibid.: 373–376). The results include networks of bicycle lanes and public transit systems that are comparatively comfortable, extensive, and easy to use.

Democratic impacts

The Internet's commercial development poses a political issue that may prove at least as defining for our social future as did the politics of automobile use. For instance, in 2001 US President George W. Bush and the Congress extended the Internet Tax Freedom Act of 1998 for two years, continuing to exempt most online commerce from sales tax (Hardesty, 2001b). President Bush (like President Clinton before him), along with some leading US congressmen, wants to permanently exempt e-commerce from existing sales taxes. Critics counter that the loss of revenue to state and local governments would endanger schools, roads, and other essential public functions. The Internet tax policies that Congress is continuing to debate will profoundly influence the democratic structure of our society for decades to come.

Unfortunately, to date that debate has been narrowly preoccupied with economic considerations. Such a single-minded focus is dangerously short-sighted. When fundamental impacts on democracy and civil society are at stake, they too should occupy a central position in policy deliberations. Here I am thinking of "democracy" in the broad sense that the philosopher John Dewey (1954) envisioned it – as a form of social organization in which all people have opportunities to develop their capacities as independent moral agents and to influence the basic, shared circumstances of their lives.

The larger issues of democracy extend far beyond the prevailing economic calculations about how businesses, consumers, and governments can most profitably cash in on the Internet. Do we, as a society, have the civic maturity to acknowledge the emerging virtues of cyberspace, inquire into the offsetting liabilities to democracy, and then implement public policies that will enhance the former while minimizing the latter?[3] Probably not, as I shall explain. Still, there are feasible fall-back actions that can reduce Internet-induced harm, while building an organized social base that will make it possible in the future to redesign the Internet in a form more responsive to democratic values.

To think through the Internet's civic liabilities, let's start with an elementary question that should be applied to any technology-inspired vision: *"Suppose that vision is fully realized, what would be the problems?"* In this case, what would be the problems with universal access to a commercially driven Internet?

The Cybernetic Wal-Mart Effect

> This little piggy went to market,
> Another piggy shopped online from home,
> The second piggy paid no sales tax,
> So why do both feel disempowered and alone?

Consider the case of electronic commerce. Businesses going online can prove a boon for consumers. But as this trend deepens, what does it mean for democracy and civic life? Among the first casualties might be local economies, by which I mean local capacities to produce enough goods and services to meet a fair share of local needs. In our own lifetime, Wal-Mart has become a symbol for the malling of America, which has wiped out many individual mom-and-pop retail stores. I'm concerned that the Internet can extend this trend via a "Cybernetic Wal-Mart Effect."

Imagine what happens when a Wal-Mart store opens on the outskirts of a town. Suppose that half the residents start to do one-third of their shopping at Wal-Mart. That means they still do two-thirds of their shopping downtown, while the remaining half of the population does all its shopping downtown. Thus everyone wants downtown to remain vibrant. However, if half the people do a third of their shopping at Wal-Mart, you've extracted about 16.7 percent of the revenue from the downtown and neighborhood economy. If profit margins aren't high, that's enough to start shutting down the downtown. Here we have a perverse market dynamic – a loss to the entire community that not a single person wanted. And it is a coercive, self-reinforcing dynamic. Once the downtown starts to shut down, people who preferred to shop there by default must now switch to Wal-Mart. Social scientists call this a "collective action problem" – a situation in which private rationality produces a socially irrational outcome (e.g. Hardin, 1982).

The Cybernetic Wal-Mart Effect – as more and more commerce goes online – aggravates the conventional "Wal-Mart" dynamic. Online, you're not just competing with Wal-Mart, you're competing with the full global marketplace. Moreover, Wal-Marts basically threaten mom-and-pop retail shops. Online commerce can spread out into every sector of the economy, including local manufacturers, business suppliers, and even service providers, such as accountants and lawyers (e.g. Tedeschi, 2000a).

Assuredly, some local businesses will thrive and grow by going online themselves. But the advertising economies of scale in attracting customers to a select number of hot websites suggest that before long the global economy will consolidate into a smaller number of prominent, large, very un-local enterprises. As an analyst from a leading Internet consulting firm explained to the *New York Times* in 1999: "It's not a pretty picture for local merchants. . . . National players have the deep pockets to create [Web] sites with the best user experience and market them. And the mom-and-pops don't have that."[4]

Consumers versus citizens

If we are thinking of ourselves solely as consumers, this Cybernetic Wal-Mart Effect is not a problem. But the catch is that we are *not* simply consumers. We are also family members, friends, local community members, and workers. From the standpoint of democratic politics, above all we are citizens.

As consumers, we always want to know, "Is this the best deal for me?" But when we assume the posture of democratic citizens, we pause and remember that we are more than acquisitive egoists. As citizens, we seek to act as moral agents committed to advancing the common good, and we ask a broader question: "Does this proposed change serve the overall well being of everyone in our society, including our first-order interest in preserving and improving the character of our democracy?"

Viewed from this democratic citizen's perspective, the Cybernetic Wal-Mart Effect is problematic. Remember that it propagates through a coercive, self-reinforcing dynamic. My online shopping contributes to shrinking the local economy, *forcing* you to go online because local alternatives are no longer available. That dynamic, which forecloses your option of choosing a locally oriented way of life or of choosing to remain offline, represents an entirely involuntary imposition.

But the anti-democratic implications of the Cybernetic Wal-Mart Effect reach further. Eviscerating a local economy weakens local cultural and community vibrancy. That's bad in its own right. But it's also bad for democracy, because as social bonds weaken, people relinquish mutual understanding and the capacity for collective action. Those are essential foundations of a workable democracy (Bowles and Gintis, 1986).

The destruction of local economies furthermore translates into greater local dependence on national and global market forces and on distant corporate headquarters – powers that communities can't control. The locus of effective political intervention thus shifts toward more distant power centers. Everyday citizens can't be as effective in these distant centers as in smaller political settings, so democracy is further impaired.

Serfing the Net

Businesses, moreover, are using computer networks to consolidate high-level managerial control over their expanding global operations. As a result, corporations are becoming ever more empowered relative to individual workers, trade unions, and even national governments. As a cover story in *Business Week* boasted some years ago, new "stateless" megacorporations are "leaping boundaries" to intimidate labor unions, elude domestic political opposition, threaten meddling government officials with plant closure and capital flight, and "sidestep regulatory hurdles."[5]

In addition, the volume and speed of electronic transfers in the global financial system heightens the threat of capital flight. Manuel Castells vividly describes how global electronic networks both alter and deepen the politically coercive implications inherent in this threat:

> It is only in the late twentieth century that the world economy was able to become truly global on the basis of the new infrastructure provided by information and communication technologies . . . . A global economy is a historically new reality . . . it is an economy with the capacity to work as a unit in real time on a planetary scale . . . . Capital flows become at the same time global and increasingly autonomous *vis-à-vis* the actual performance of economies.
>
> (Castells, 1996: 92–93)

Here is an entirely new twist to the issue, transforming financial instabilities that were formerly localized and episodic into the chronic condition of the entire world economy. With capital soaring aloft in perpetual global motion, national governments that formally feared capital "flight" must now compete for transitory capital "alight." This constrains what elected leaders dare say and do, further compromising the democratic process for determining national policies (Sclove, 1995: 237–238).

The perils and irony of "friction-free capitalism"

Cybervisionaries such as Microsoft chairman Bill Gates have waxed ecstatic in describing the coming wonders of Internet-enabled "friction-free capitalism." In *The Road Ahead* Gates (1995: 181) writes that: "We'll find ourselves in a new world of low-friction, low-overhead capitalism, in which market information will be plentiful and transaction costs low. It will be a shopper's heaven."

In Gates' view capitalism will become low-friction when market information is "plentiful." But early indications are that the kind of information that is becoming available, and its distribution, both reflect biases of social power and wealth. In a general way, information pertinent to buying and selling is becoming more accessible to both producers and consumers. But access to other kinds of information continues to reflect distinct power asymmetries. For instance, businesses are electronically assembling statistical profiles on the performance of individual employees and personal consumer habits as never before. In contrast, worker and citizen abilities to penetrate the veils of corporate managerial secrecy and proprietary information are not remotely keeping pace. Corporations and financial institutions can snoop into your life in ways that you most definitely cannot snoop back (Guernsey, 1999; Garfinkel, 2000; Tedeschi, 2000b).

The implications for open and informed democratic deliberation are not cheering. The proprietary nature of corporate strategic planning decisions puts governments, workers, and citizens several years behind businesses, in terms of access to information about impending, socially consequential innovations. Businesses can use their inside information to devise and deploy technological or social *faits accomplis*, or to lobby government, long before anyone else even knows what's afoot (Sclove, 1995: 210, 276–277 n.42). This looks less like friction-free capitalism and more like information-free politics – ironic in a self-stylized "Information Society."

Moreover, the economic historian Karl Polanyi, in his classic book *The Great Transformation*, argued compellingly that whenever conditions have approximated the ideal of friction-free, self-regulating markets, the consequences have proven calamitous:

> To allow the market mechanism to be sole director of the fate of human beings and their natural environment . . . would result in the demolition of society. . . . Robbed of the protective covering of cultural institutions, human beings would perish from the effects of social exposure. . . . Nature would be reduced to its elements, neighborhoods and landscapes defiled. . . . [N]o society could stand the effects of such a system.
>
> (Polanyi, 1957: 73)

Polanyi showed, in particular, how the subjection of human labor to unregulated market imperatives produced horrendous social and economic hardship during the centuries in which Britain became an industrial powerhouse. His insights are absolutely pertinent today. Contemporary capitalism is only humanly tolerable to the extent that a combination of inefficiencies and social regulations protect people and the natural world from the relentless hyperexploitation that friction-free capitalism would otherwise enact.

Initial glimpses of the inhumane results of electronically enabled capitalism are already well in evidence. As new technologies disengage jobs from factories, offices, and other specific work locations and from traditional daily rhythms, the work lives of millions are accelerating out of control (Robinson and Godbey, 1997: 38–42; Schor, 1997; Harmon, 1998). Social occasions and family meals are increasingly interrupted by cell phone calls and pager signals. Commuter automobiles and airline seats are reconfigured as mobile offices, as we take up lives of multitasking. Bill Gates (1999) unselfconsciously encapsulates the frenzied *zeitgeist* in his latest book title, *Business @ the Speed of Thought.*

Virtual community as coercive compensation

At first glance, it might appear that the benefits of electronic "virtual communities" will offset the destructive civic impacts of electronic commerce run amok. Communities based on electronic communications, such as email or electronic chat rooms, unquestionably have social merit. They can, for example, prove a liberating boon to people with physical disabilities. They also offer us a chance to link up with others who share our obscure passions and hobbies. Virtual communities thus seem unproblematic, indeed commendable – if joining them is a free choice. But will that choice remain free?

Imagine, for example, increasing numbers of workers telecommuting from home at odd hours of the day or night, the electronic erosion of local economies, and ever more people voluntarily spending time participating in electronic communities. You might just find, when you do want to hang out with family or friends or just stroll down to a local gathering spot, that no one else is around. For one reason or another, they're all online. So, whether you like it or not, you too have to log on to a virtual social life.

Like the Cybernetic Wal-Mart Effect, this turn to virtual communities can potentially exhibit a pathological social logic that I call "coercive compensation." Initial adoption of such a technology erodes a prior social practice or way of life, compelling more people to adopt the new technology not by choice but by default, as compensation. But this only aggravates the initial dynamic. Thus without anyone necessarily realizing it, the new technology is latently responsible for *eliminating* the desirable way of life for which it is ostensibly compensatory. And yet we may cling to, identify with, and even vigorously defend the very technology that is the ultimate source of our pain.

Once a society is gripped by this coercive logic, how different will we be from the infamous drunk in Antoine de Saint-Exupéry's *The Little Prince* (1943: 42–43), who guzzled booze because he wanted to forget. Forget what? Why, that he was ashamed of drinking! In the updated version:

> *Little Prince:* "Why do you spend so much time online?"
> *Cybernaut:* "In order to shop! For companionship. To be where the action is!"
> *Little Prince:* "But wouldn't it sometimes be nice to stroll downtown for that?"
> *Cybernaut:* "Oh, no thank you. The Internet has already half-destroyed downtown. Now excuse me while I log back on."

The dynamics of coercive compensation can swiftly generate extreme outcomes in part because they incorporate what systems theorists call positive feedback loops. That is, the output of a process (some people opting to shop, work, or socialize online at times of their choosing) circles back into the original process as input (reduced face-to-face social activity), generating more output (more and more people compelled compensatorily to spend ever more time socializing online). A little generates more, more generates a *lot* more. Systems with positive feedback loops can easily burst limits and grow cancerously.[6]

Virtual apartheid

Internet users tend, in addition, to sort themselves out into like-minded enclaves. In its proper place, that is fine. But if time spent in homogeneous online chat rooms substitutes for mingling in face-to-face public spaces with diverse groups of people, democracy is, once again, in trouble. Democratic self-governance is only possible if people from diverse backgrounds and ways of life know something about one another's lives and develop some cross-cutting social bonds. So sorting ourselves into electronic interest groups may erode our capacity for forging fair and effective social compromises. Toward the extreme, such segregation could degenerate into a world of attack ads, scapegoating, and polarization – the kinds of social trends historically associated more closely with fascism and apartheid than with a robustly democratic civil society (Sunstein, 2001).

Moreover, cyberspace does not alter the reality that no matter how far our words and imaginations fly, our bodies remain anchored in physical locations. Indeed, all of our political jurisdictions are territorially defined – local, county, regional, national, and so forth. If cyberspace disengages our social bonds from geography, how will we find common ground on public school policies, services for the elderly, and public safety if we know nothing about our physical neighbors' lives?

The loss of habitat for citizenship

Only a few years ago, cyberspace was a commerce-free zone. The prevailing ethos was that any commercial come-on whatsoever was intolerable. The occasional transgressor was instantaneously subject to vicious, retaliatory verbal attack. Today, of course, it is all but impossible to browse the World Wide Web without being bombarded by flashing animated advertisements, unsolicited commercial pop-up screens, smarmy requests for personal information, and "sticky" (hard-to-exit) websites. Even many "virtual communities" are sponsored by corporations and managed primarily to shape consumer wants and capture market share (Werry, 1999).

Or consider the *New York Times*, the United States' *de facto* newspaper of record. The front page of a typical printed copy of the *Times* – I happen to have on hand, Friday, October 25, 2002 – includes an imposing 243 square inches of news text, news headlines, and accompanying illustrations. At the very bottom of the page there is one miniscule advertisement (occupying 1/10th of a square inch of space), giving a telephone number for ordering home-delivery of the newspaper. Thus less than 1/10th of 1 percent of the printed *Times'* front page is occupied by advertising. This page is a kind of national civic space, affording readers an opportunity to experience themselves as citizens, not consumers.

Now log on to the same day's *New York Times* homepage on the World Wide Web. Compared with the front-page print version, the average article on the homepage has shriveled from 8.5 paragraphs down to a single-sentence teaser. There are eighteen commercial advertisements, each with an accompanying color graphic or logo. The upper left-hand corner, right next to the famous gothic-font *New York Times* logo, displays a graphical box with a Java-animated ad for an online employment service. (Yes, that's the same boxed corner that in the *Times'* printed version displays the motto "All the News That's Fit to Print." The *Times* has quietly banished that time-honored slogan from its homepage.) Measured in square inches, the *Times* Web homepage is 16 percent advertising – an advertising-to-content ratio comparable to that of US prime-time commercial television. This is substantially commercial space, not civic space.

This commercial onslaught may itself weaken the social foundations of democratic citizenship. The latter does not demand that we each act on the basis of our higher, less-egoistic citizen-self all the time, or even most of the time. But it does demand that *most of us* exhibit our citizen-selves *some of the time*, and especially when important public decisions about the basic character of our society are at stake (Barber, 1984: xiv, 151). That can only happen if neither our consumer-selves nor worker-selves overpower and engulf our citizen-selves. We must be able to function as other-regarding, democratic citizens during those critical moments when it counts (and to recognize when we confront such moments). But to do so, there is a certain minimum amount of space and time that we need in our lives to experience ourselves and others as something more than mere drudging workers, self-promoting careerists, or acquisitive consumers.

So, guess what happens if cyberspace continues to evolve into an ever-more compulsory, commercially dominated medium? From a societal point of view, the shared time and space, both online and off, in which to experience others as citizens appreciably contracts. And with that, our own propensities to exhibit civic virtues likewise shrink.

On being no place at once

Meanwhile, an ever-more compulsory cybernetic lifestyle threatens to accelerate life on the job and off, distract and fragment our moment-to-moment existence, and alienate us bodily and psychologically from our immediate physical environment. Some of us are already spread simultaneously so thin among so many places that we exist constantly in an emotional state of "being no place at once." In effect, attention deficit disorder is being upgraded from psychological impairment to societal norm. According to a leading scholarly study of how Americans use their time, recent stressful trends of this sort mean that "many Americans never experience anything fully, never live in the moment" (Robinson and Godbey, 1997: 39).

That could cripple our capacity for committed personal relationships, as well as our willingness to act personally and politically to protect the environment (cf. Bowers 2000: 48–75). It's also likely to challenge our patience with the necessarily slow pace of democratic deliberation, to reduce our experience of meaning in daily life, and – given all of the above – to impair our moral development and discourage our personal participation in civic affairs.

From an Eastern perspective, being-no-place-at-once is antithetical to the here-and-now, single-pointed attention and subtle awareness that Buddhists, for example, consider essential to clear vision, compassionate knowing, human emancipation, and enlightenment (Goldstein, 1976; Nhat Hanh, 1987). From a Western perspective, it offers a final example of how far removed a society is from the classical democratic ideals of Jean-Jacques Rousseau, Thomas Jefferson, John Stuart Mill, and John Dewey if it is ruled by a hyper-commercialized Internet. Independent moral judgment, civic obligation, democratic deliberation, self-government, and the common good atrophy. In their place, we find compulsion, power asymmetry, friction-free capitalism, and the commodification of just about everything.

Inescapable, compulsory access

Devising public policies to prevent or remedy such negative impacts, while still preserving the Internet's notable social benefits, is not particularly difficult. But the odds are against such remedies actually being adopted anytime soon.

We would be wise, for example, to amend the guiding policy mantra of seeking "universal and affordable Internet access." That slogan is advertised as an essential requirement for social equity. But those who stand to benefit most unequivocally from its promotion are not the poor or disadvantaged minorities. They are the corporations that hope to stake their fortunes on an infinitely expanding cybermarket. For example, Eric Schmidt, a recent CEO of software giant Novell, has praised the idea of federal subsidies to help low-income Americans purchase computers and Internet connections. But he also concedes: "This is all clearly self-serving at some level because all of us in the industry benefit by having more customers" (quoted in Lacey, 2000).

The likely outcome of enshrining universal access as an unqualified social good will be a world of inescapable, compulsory access, in which cherished offline modes of life become more expensive, less available, or in some cases extinct. At that point, lack of Internet access *will* constitute "deprivation."

This poses a particularly poignant dilemma for low-income communities. As Internet access becomes functionally compulsory, tangible penalties will emerge and escalate steadily for the unwired. On the other hand, some working-class and low-income communities have preserved more vibrant face-to-face social networks than their more affluent neighbors. This amounts to an endangered reserve of social capital, an essential foundation for political efficacy and economic revitalization. Going online, especially if it entails coercion into using the Internet excessively, at the wrong times, or in the wrong ways, could destroy those vital community ties.

A preferable public policy for all of us might be "universally affordable, *voluntary* access to online and *offline* life" for the following reasons:

- "Voluntary," because whether and when to go online should be protected as a matter of free and informed personal choice.
- "Offline" – as well as online – life, to underscore that it is as essential to ensure equitable accessibility to an immense variety of offline choices as to the Internet itself.

Unless offline life is protected as a set of viable, attractive options, the phrase "voluntary access" could gradually ring hollow. How would you feel about an interstate highway system that had plenty of roadways and on-ramps but no off-ramps? We need a cyberspace where the on-ramps are universally accessible without becoming compulsory, entailing that place-based settings are nurtured and protected so that they too remain "universally and affordably accessible."

Capturing benefits, limiting harm

As for other policy remedies, the simplest way to hold electronic commerce in balance with local economies – and thus to limit the erosion of civic vitality and democratic self-governance – would be to place a modest tax on electronic commerce and mail-order catalog sales. Some of the revenue could, in turn, be rebated to localities to invest in rejuvenating local economies and civic life. The rationale for such a tax is simple and compelling: unlimited e-commerce poses fundamental social and political harms that are not reflected in market prices. Current public policy irrationally *encourages* a Cybernetic Wal-Mart Effect by exempting most out-of-state purchases from state and local sales tax (Sclove, 2000).

The democratically damaging effects of excessive international monetary flows – which are currently at least several hundred times greater in financial terms than the international flow of goods and services – can in principle be limited by adopting a variant of the so-called Tobin tax. Proposed two decades ago by Nobel Prize-winning economist James Tobin, the tax would levy a small charge on all international foreign exchange transactions. Tobin originally envisioned setting the levy at 0.5 to 1 percent, which he estimated would damp down short-run speculation and threats of capital flight, without adversely affecting long-range productive investments.[7] As in the preceding case of an e-commerce tax, a portion of the resulting tax revenue could be rebated to national governments or international civic institutions for reinvestment in local economies and activities supporting democratic civil society.

Taxing e-commerce and global financial exchanges would, of course, go against the prevailing US anti-tax ethos. But these proposed taxes differ from conventional income, property, or sales taxes in being targeted specifically to activities that will otherwise produce basic social and democratic harm. In that sense they are akin to "sin taxes" or "green taxes" – taxes targeted to reduce socially or environmentally harmful activity.

Like green taxes, these are also taxes that *preserve and expand* treasured and essential social options. Green taxes do so by helping to preserve non-renewable resources, clear air, clean water, parks and other green spaces, wilderness areas, fragile ecosystems, and endangered species. Analogously, the taxes that I espouse would help preserve personal choice and freedom, local economies, community vibrancy, face-to-face conviviality, civil society, and the tradition of democratic self-governance. (Indeed, if the revenue from these taxes were to grow appreciably, it would become practicable to offset them by reducing conventional sales, income or property tax rates.)

Stronger labor laws could protect workers from intrusive work surveillance, and reimburse them for the escalating number of hours now worked without additional pay, a trend exacerbated by email and other new technologies. Local communities could preserve time for face-to-face activities by reviving some version of the old "blue laws"[8] – in effect, augmenting existing holiday and weekend time, during which large numbers of residents would be off work and free to participate in social and civic events. Communities could also time voluntary weekly "TV-free" and "computer-free" periods to coincide with some of the new vacation time.[9]

A prohibition or tax on third-party advertising on the Internet would be a straightforward way to roll back commercialization and preserve habitat for citizenship. It sounds unthinkable – until you remember that less than a decade ago it was the idea of commercial advertising on the Internet that was unthinkable.

In addition, everyone deserves a direct say, or real effective representation, in the crucial processes of *designing, evaluating, and governing the new telecommunications systems*. New technologies are profoundly affecting daily life and the basic character of our political institutions – as much, say, as any amendment to the Constitution. Yet business, government, military, and university research leaders are normally the only players permitted to participate in technology policy-making at the national level. Those who pay for these technical innovations (that's everybody through their tax dollars and consumer purchases) and those who are affected (which is also everybody) have, unless one happens to be in one of the privileged groups above, no effective representation in deciding these policies (Sclove, 1998; McChesney, 1999: 119–185).

Conclusion

It's time to bring due process, fairness, and much broader public participation into decisions regarding powerful new technologies. Businesses could be offered tax breaks for including representatives of affected public groups in their processes for conducting research, product design, and strategic planning. All government advisory boards for science and technology should include strong, diverse representation of public-interest groups, affected workers, and ordinary citizens. Congress and federal agencies could emulate governments around the world that have begun assembling panels of everyday citizens to cross-examine experts, deliberate among themselves, and then announce their own technology policy recommendations at a national press conference. Congress should also shift a small portion of federal research support to help researchers and community groups, working as full partners, to answer communities' own most pressing questions. Empowered by such "community-based research," citizens could much more easily participate in technology policy decisions (Sclove, 1995: 205–230; Sclove, 1996; Sclove et al., 1998; Sclove, 1999).

So yes, it is technically, economically, and socially possible to develop and use information technologies in humane, just, wise, and democratic ways. Of course, during the height of the Internet mania, the idea that such measures would seriously be considered seemed impossible. During those giddy and greedy, wild-eyed days of yore (1999–2000), voices of caution were simply laughed on to the sidelines. The subsequent collapse of the dot.com stock market bubble, followed by protracted economic recession and general stock market meltdown, has inflicted hardship on millions of workers and investors. But it also somewhat improves the odds on taking a more measured societal approach to the Internet's ongoing evolution.

Still, overall the prospects for a more civically oriented development of cyberspace remain limited in the short run. Internet mania may have collapsed, but the nation's infatuation with laissez-faire economics, our limited societal readiness or institutional capacity for examining technologies critically, and a decided pro-Internet bias of the media all endure.[10] (Media outlets of all kinds have a considerable financial stake in the Internet and the success of e-commerce.) Politicians and regulators remain subject to substantial pressure to make sure technology policies back corporate visions – and little pressured indeed to attend to the democratic or social repercussions.

That doesn't provide much ground for immediate optimism. Nevertheless, there are important fall-back steps that can be taken now to reduce, and one day reverse, Internet-induced social and civic harm. Wise communities, for example, will act now to protect their local economies from the Internet's encroachment. The practical beauty of seeking greater local economic self-reliance is that any county, city, or neighborhood can pursue it, and no permission is necessary from state or national governments. Successful examples abound. As of 1996, for example, there were 450 community-supported organic farms in the United

States (up from just two only ten years earlier); more than 2,000 community development corporations; 10,000 worker-owned companies (up from 1,600 in 1974); and 47,000 consumer, housing, and other co-ops (Alperovitz, 1996; see also Shuman, 1998; Sclove, 1995: 127–135, 161–179, 212–216, 237).

The self-designated "slow food movement" (www.slowfood.com) is a modest but heartening example of a bottom-up, international endeavor to combat the relentless fragmentation and speed-up of the pace of life.

Local communities can't, acting by themselves, do much to prevent nation-wide or global over-wiring. But residents can organize at the local level to prevent some of the locally experienced ill effects. For example, one can counter-pose community networking, neighborhood telecommuting-and-civic centers, and responsible voluntary Internet uses versus the export of scarce local dollars to far-flung cybershops and coercively compensatory uses (Schuler, 2001). Or counterpose child-centric versus computer-centric school curricula (Cordes and Miller, 2000; Bowers, 2000: 109–195). Above all, communities must decide which aspects of face-to-face, place-based life they most treasure, and then make vigorous efforts to enhance and protect what they treasure from the predatory ravages of a rampantly over-commercialized Internet and over-wired world.

Meanwhile, some subsidiary battles related to the policies I have suggested may well be winnable, even now. For instance, some state, county, and local governments support taxes on e-commerce to protect local services from a dramatic loss of revenue. They could prove strong allies in lobbying for taxes on online sales (e.g. Associated Press, 2000; Hardesty, 2001a). Deployed judiciously, the Internet itself can be of assistance: many non-profit organizations, grass-roots groups, and trade unions are using the Net to co-ordinate their actions with one another, providing some counterweight to global corporate hyperem-powerment.[11]

Later, when the novelty of our over-wired lives wears thin, advocating for more sensible Internet policies will prove less lonely. The challenge then will be to restore or reinvent opportunities for a vibrant, place-based social and civic life. At that point, a critically aware, organized political base will be essential to insist upon change and to help design and implement it. The time to begin building that base is now, and the obvious means is to fight right now for sensible policies, despite the odds against immediate, sweeping success. Even efforts that fail will raise public awareness of the technological and social choices before us.

In the long term, history provides reason for hope. Consider Copenhagen. Denmark initially overdosed on automobiles in much the same way as the United States. Photographs of downtown Copenhagen in the early 1960s show all the old-time plazas converted into open-air parking lots, all the streets choked with traffic. But the Danes came to their senses and gradually began taking their streets and plazas back from the car. Today Copenhagen – and every city and town in Denmark – has a car-free, downtown pedestrian area (Gehl and Gemzøe, 1996). There's a lesson here. We human beings do sometimes get carried away with our technical virtuosity. But we can be just as socially creative in correcting our errors – when we're ready. In the case of the Internet, the sooner, the better.

Notes

1 This is an abridged version of a longer study. For comments on earlier drafts and related public presentations, the author is grateful to Gary Chapman, Katrina Kay, Larry Kirkman, Howard Rheingold, Douglas Schuler, and Marcie Sclove. Colleen Cordes especially provided detailed substantive criticism as well as extensive editorial help. Preparation of this study was assisted financially by a grant from the Foundation for Deep Ecology and by general support to the Loka Institute from the Albert A. List Foundation, the John D. & Catherine T. MacArthur Foundation, and the Menemsha Fund.

2 Critical perspectives on the US Telecommunications Policy Act of 1996 include, for example, Computer Professionals for Social Responsibility, 2001; and the Benton Foundation, 1997. On public-interest group concern with unequal social access to the Internet see, for example, the Digital Divide Network website at http://www.digitaldividenetwork.org.

3 The importance of a robust civil society is discussed in Wolfe, 1989; Skocpol and Fiorina, 1999; and Putnam, 2000.

4 Lisa Allen of Forrester Research, quoted in Tedeschi, 1999.

5 Holstein *et al.*, 1990. See also Mander and Goldsmith, 1996.

6 This is a point overlooked by measured techno-optimists, such as Mitchell, 1999, e.g. pp. 72–73, 90–91.

7 See Felix, 1995; and the Tobin Tax Initiative website at http://www.ceedweb. org/iirp/.

8 US "blue laws" formerly restricted or prohibited various kinds of commercial activity on Sundays. "All 50 [US] states had such laws . . . as late as 1961; by 1996, only 13 did" (Lagerfeld, 1998: 67). The revived blue laws I envision would carve out new, shared free (including commerce-free) time on a weekly basis, not necessarily on Sundays. E.g. establishing work-free and commerce-free time one or two weekday evenings each week might be civically helpful.

9 The non-profit TV-Turnoff Network http://www.tvfa.org/ has set a precedent in successfully sponsoring annual, voluntary one-week moratoria on TV-watching in communities across the United States, as well as other programs to promote reduced hours of television-watching.

10 Regarding the United States' "limited institutional capacity" for examining technologies critically, it does not help that a Republican-dominated Congress abolished the Congress's own 23-year-old Office of Technology Assessment in 1995 (Bimber and Guston, 1997).

11 For information on trade union use of the Internet see, for example, Turner, 2000.

Chapter 4

Welcome to 1927

The creation of property rights and Internet domain name policy in historical perspective

Christian Sandvig

Consider, if you will, the story of a young communication system. It has fantastic potential to connect us in a vast network across great distances. It allows us to communicate in ways that have never before been possible. As a new technology, it seems wild and untamed, different. Only the younger generation and the technologically inclined seem to be able to fully understand it. The government has asserted that developing it is a national priority. It seems to hold great promise in advancing education – with increased access to it, the average person can obtain a wealth of information in ways that have never before been possible. No one is sure how to make money from it, but many are trying. As a communication system, it has both military and commercial applications, but the bulk of users seem content to just roam around: sending messages to friends, exploring, learning, and entertaining themselves.

This communication medium is radio, the site: the Unites States, the year: 1920 – although this description could also be of the Internet circa 1998. Both early radio and the early Internet share the characteristics above. By understanding the development of radio broadcasting in the USA eighty years ago, we can gain insight into the issues currently pertinent to the Internet today. Others have pointed out that the development of early radio resembles the Internet (e.g. Hargittai, 1998, 2000) and this chapter extends that approach by specifically considering the creation of property in both media, to consider how the creation of property rights functions as a system of control. Both radio and the Internet rely on the commodification of valuable resources, and parts of both systems utilize the marketplace to allocate these resources. In fact, the public policy decisions in each of these two periods are often unnecessarily constrained by the marketplace. For each, the market serves as a false default: the choice to use a marketplace model to allocate these resources seems to be not the product of intentional thought with due consideration for the consequences which result, but merely the unquestioned norm. This is a false default because there is no "natural" market in these contexts – it takes considerable work to commodify intangibles such as radio broadcast licenses and Internet domain names. Through a discussion of these two moments in history, this chapter will show that the incentives of the market in each case lead to outcomes that are inconsistent with the public interest – even inconsistent with the goals advanced by those who chose the market mechanism in the first place. In addition, the choice of a market mechanism for resource allocation places long-term constraints on the future shape of the system, chiefly in the form of property rights. This results in the disenfranchisement of those without the necessary property or capital to participate.

Political pathways to a technical system

The activity of broadcasting in the United States, first systematized in radio and then later inherited by television, can be best understood not as a technological breakthrough, but as a political struggle that defined a scope and a structure for the technological breakthrough. In the study of technology, a wide range of scholarship has embraced the political nature of technological development (see, e.g., Winner, 1980; Hughes, 1983; Bijker *et al.*, 1987). As a series of historical analyses have explained, the early period of radio broadcasting leading to government regulation is one marked by a competition between differing visions of what "radio" was to become (Douglas, 1987; McChesney, 1993; Smulyan, 1994). This chapter will discuss the creation of property in early radio broadcast policy, and then use this framework to analyze the creation of property that occurred on the Internet in the late 1990s.

Systems of communication are considered here first and foremost "as economic entities with both a direct economic role as creators of surplus value through commodity production and exchange and an indirect role . . . in the creation of surplus value within other sectors of commodity production" (Garnham, 1990: 30). As Garnham states, these systems are not isolated in one branch of the traditional trichotomy of relatively autonomous economic, ideological, and political spheres. These systems are economic, but fundamentally constructed through a political process with ideological baggage throughout.

Perhaps contrary to expectations, comparisons of the Internet to radio (or television) broadcasting are only slightly limited by the differences in the technical characteristics of each medium. Although technologies are fundamentally shaped by social processes, in analyzing them it is useful to consider some parts as "technical" or "physical" (after Vincenti, 1995; we leave the argument that everything technical is best understood as social for other authors). Let us assume that both radio and the Internet have some degree of structure that is technically imposed – an example would be the propagation characteristics of radio waves or the (currently) maximum known transmission capacity of a fiber-optic cable. As many have noted, atop this base structure of technology lies a framework of decisions often made in deference to technical necessity, but within which, in reality, there is considerable leeway (cf. Hughes, 1983). An example would be the specific size of spectrum dedicated to one AM radio channel (or the specification for the length of a datagram on the Internet). The degree of leeway can vary, by decision, from small to large. Some decisions may be heavily influenced by current technological limitations, or perceived limitations, while others are more clearly political choices. Political, economic, and ideological considerations play some role, be it small or large, in each of these decisions.

The creation of property in broadcasting, 1920

Let us begin with radio, and reflect back to the 1920s. From the earliest public statements discussing the life of radio as a new technology, clear instances of legislative intent and words of caution about the direction of the system stand out. In perhaps one of the most often-quoted statements made about early radio, "at the Third National Radio Conference [in 1923], Herbert Hoover declaimed that "the quickest way to kill broadcasting would be to use it for direct advertising . . .'" (Smulyan, 1994: 41). Indeed, "[m]any observers of early broadcast radio . . . worried about the influence of commercialism" (ibid.: 125). In the wake of the Elk Hills and Teapot Dome scandals involving public resources such as oil on public lands, conservation-minded activists insisted on adding language to the Radio Act of 1927 that explicitly defined the broadcast license to provide "for the use of . . . channels, but not the ownership thereof" (Barnouw, 1966: 195–196). If the aims of the period were to create a technological system of communication that was (1) free of direct advertising, (2) not dominated by commercialism, and (3) not based on the private ownership of the spectrum, or radio "channels," how did what we presently know as broadcasting emerge? The system that arose from these intentions is (1) dominated by "direct" advertising, (2) almost without exception commercial in nature, and (3) based in action if not in statute on the buying and selling of the broadcast license. It is this system that passed intact from radio to television and is still with us today.

Commodifying the air

Broadcasting is organized in the United States around the commodification of airwaves and audience. This is the structure on which all debates of broadcast policy rest. The government, on the basis of the Radio Acts of 1912 and 1927 and the later Communications Act of 1934, is in the business of creating private property in the form of the broadcast license. Arguments about the value of that property and the rights of property owners are then used in the regulatory system to advance one interest over another. Thomas Streeter's critique of US broadcasting policy provides this rich framework for understanding the creation of property as a key causal agent in defining the resulting structure of the system of communication we know as broadcasting (1996). As Streeter and other historians of early radio have noted (Douglas, 1987; Smulyan, 1994), property may be the most profound form of control over commercial broadcasting.

Missing from usual consideration of broadcasting is the acknowledgement that the commercial constitution of broadcasting as a property issue is notably artificial – which is to say, political. All private property is a form of social agreement, as there is nothing about ownership in nature, yet popular conception holds that governmental control is in opposition to some "natural" state of the uninhibited market. Through a brief consideration of property it can be seen that the "natural" state of the broadcasting market is no such thing. The creation of private property in the spectrum, the audience, and the broadcasting license created the broadcasting industry in the form that we know it. Control need not mean the control of a central body or the subjugation of the medium to a cogent master plan. Structuring broadcasting in terms of property is controlling because it sets the scope of the industry and the framework within which we consider the broadcast media. The discursive structure of broadcast policy does not acknowledge this form of control, but assumes it as a foundation.

In the tumultuous world of early radio, *c.* 1920, the primary participants in the spectrum were amateurs who sought to use the medium for entertainment, military interests who sought to co-ordinate the fleet, and businesses, which initially only saw radio as a means to relay point-to-point messages. Amateur interests had been severely curtailed the decade before by the Radio Act of 1912, and there was rising commercial interest in radio as a mass medium (Douglas, 1987: 236). However, in the 1920s the final framework that radio would take was far from certain. Broadcasting stations were spreading, despite having ". . . little idea of how to finance either their program needs or operating costs" (Smulyan, 1994: 40). Streeter's analysis of the political economy of broadcasting rests upon the idea that to locate and understand the creation of property in broadcasting is to make great strides toward understanding broadcasting as a system. Quite aside from the organization of broadcasting as a monopoly, oligopoly, or competitive system are the needs that must be met for broadcasting to be commercial in any form. Namely, broadcasting must be constituted as something that can be bought, owned, and sold. Streeter refers to this system as "postmodern property," in that the existence of the property in question rests solely on our conception of it. Unlike land there is no physical form for a television channel, and a license is an idea more than a piece of paper. We have socially constructed a system wherein the broadcasting license, spectrum, and audience are entities with borders drawn around them. Streeter defines the urge to view corporate stewardship in co-operation with governmental control as the ideal solution to managing a resource as "corporate liberalism." A full review of this philosophy is beyond the scope of this chapter, but the key is to note that the corporate liberal impulse led to the enactment of property-based policies that, once in place, became normalized, and thus invisible. While contemplating the electromagnetic spectrum as a scarce resource, the government ceded priority to corporate interests because in the face of scarcity they were told that only a well-capitalized private system would lead to full utilization. In this manner the corporate stewards locked out independents and educators.

After the establishment of a fiduciary system of accountability based on a transferable license and a government regulator constrained by property rights, the idea of "owning" a license was normalized. Any backlash against the behavior of business interests was then met by attempts to "regulate the results of the growing commercialism," rather than to "strengthen the alternatives" (Smulyan, 1994: 126). Policy initiatives such as the Radio Acts had set up a system wherein broadcasters were to be corporate interests, and their business was to be the purchase and sale of broadcast licenses and audiences. Structurally, incentives were built into the system for these businesses to be responsive to advertisers who funded their operations, and there is ample evidence of this occurring (Smulyan, 1994: 129; Sterling and Kittross, 1990: ch. 4).

Lessons learned from early broadcasting

What could have changed this situation to bring the results in radio in line with the three goals for the radio stated earlier? That is, a radio system free of direct advertising and *de facto* spectrum ownership, with ample participation by non-commercial broadcasters. Clearly, a greater attention to the creation of property during the policy process would have been a great step forward in allowing the architects of modern broadcasting to understand the system they were constructing. The policy process at the time, however, was confused by the aura of expertise surrounding key decisions. Radio was little understood, and the majority of the experts available represented business interests. In hindsight, it is hard to accept that policy-makers did not see that the creation of transferable license properties would tend to systematically push out non-profit, non-commercial, alternative interests. In fact, they may have realized this, but they felt that commercial interests could somehow "rise above" the system of incentives present in the structure. As there were feelings in Congress that educational broadcasting was important and that "direct" advertising was a mistake, this was thought to be the direction that broadcasters would voluntarily choose, although these goals were never clearly codified in law and broadcasters would not be forced by explicit legislation to follow them (cf. Barnouw, 1966: 200). We see today that these were not reasonable expectations: in the years of broadcasting since the structure was established that would favor only commercial participants and reward them for commodifying mass audiences, the broadcaster that spurns these incentives to promote diverse programming (and as a result, forsakes profits) is rare to non-existent. The early expectation that broadcasters, despite the market structure's reward system, would somehow choose to ignore the profit motive is not sound logic. While keeping this scenario from radio in mind, let us turn now from the past to the present and examine the Internet with property rights in mind.

The creation of property on the Internet, 2000

There is no direct parallel to licensing on the Internet, as you do not require government permission to transmit, and there is no license to obtain. The case of domain name registration examined here is not meant to *exactly* parallel the fiduciary license system of radio. It is, however, illustrative of the foundation of assumptions about how a communication medium should work that can be inherited across history. There is still little awareness of the forces and incentives unleashed by the creation of a property right.

At the time of early radio broadcast regulation during which this system was established, there was little to no awareness of the future audiences radio would reach. Decisions made very early in the process of radio broadcasting had large consequences as the decades passed. In the current excitement surrounding the Internet, we have the opportunity to discover and address the marketplace as an assumption relatively early in the medium's development process. Domain name registration is useful, then, as an example of a system for the allocation of resources that is still young and very much in flux. It allows a case where (like radio broadcast licensing) control was ceded to the marketplace with little reasoned discussion, and it allows us to see how little, in many respects, our approach to new media has changed over the last seventy years.

The early domain name system

Briefly, the story of the domain name as property begins twenty years ago, when the Internet consisted of about 20 interconnected research networks, of which ARPANET was the oldest (Leiner *et al.*, 1998). As the fledgling network continued to expand and add nodes, it became clear that for each computer to have a unique name was impractical as the words left available for new nodes became scarce. In 1981, a system of "name domains" was proposed (Mills, 1981). In 1983, the engineers under government contract to develop the network proposed the establishment of six top-level domains (TLDs).[1] "The motivation," explained a memorandum, "is to provide an organization[al] name that is free of undesirable semantics" (Postel and Reynolds, 1984: 1). All addresses on the network would be divided into six domains: government (gov), education (edu), commercial (com), military (mil), organization (org), and older DARPA hosts (formerly "arpa"). If an organization had over 50 computers, and could demonstrate that it possessed the technical ability to manage its own network address table, it could register with the publicly funded Network Information Center at no charge (ibid.: 5). The organization would choose one of the six TLDs, and pick a unique word within that domain to identify itself (e.g. "stanford" within the TLD "edu").

Provision was also made at this time for the use of two-letter TLDs based on the International Standards Organization Codes for the Representation of Names and Countries: United States = us, France = fr, Japan = jp, etc. These domains, later called "country code" domain names, represented an additional hierarchy within which organizations could list themselves, but this second system tied to physical places would prove slow to develop and comparatively unpopular in the US. It may be that as the Internet promised to make geographic distances irrelevant, referents to geography went against the grain, from the early pioneers to the users of today. Restricting the Internet to geographic addressing boundaries may make it seem less potent; as historian Carolyn Marvin stated of past communication media, "The more any medium triumphed over distance, time, and embodied presence, the more exciting it was" (Marvin, 1988: 194).

On the other hand, that the country code domains exist at all indicates the importance of geography – as Klein (2002) notes, any category system might have been used. US preference against the use of country code domains may be a way to remind the world that the Internet was a US creation. Indeed, initial US control of the administration of every country's Internet namespace gave the US government a unique symbolic authority that the rest of the world might rightly resent. It is this control that led the People's Republic of China (.cn) to propose in 1995 that the Taiwan, Republic of China domain name be revoked (.tw), and later that the Hong Kong domain name (.hk) become a subsidiary domain to .cn. Control of country code domains effectively created a Palestinian state on the Internet in 2000 (with the addition of .ps) and reassigned the control of Afghanistani Internet space (.af) to the Karzai government in 2003. To try and sidestep the many political problems inherent in defining the identities of nation-states, domain name administrators have lately claimed the country code domains are not political at all: administrators now strive to simply reproduce a UN standard list of geographic territories.

It is important to stress that as the entire domain name system developed, it also seemed to be a clear-cut technical matter of addressing. As the network grew during the 1990s, particularly after the advent of the World Wide Web in 1992, it began to creep into the public's awareness. Two additional gTLDs (global TLDs) were added: "net" for computers of network service providers, and "int" for organizations "established by international treaty" (Postel, 1994: 2). The DNS architects perceived that everything had been resolved, permanently. In 1994, an engineering document proclaimed boldly, "It is extremely unlikely that any other TLDs will be created" (ibid.: 1).

Privatization and commercialization

During this period, military sites spun off the publicly accessible network (to become "milnet"), DARPA ceded control to the National Science Foundation (NSF), and the NSF began to implement policies for commercialization (Hart et al., 1992). NSF prohibited commercial traffic on the "backbone," or long-distance portion of the network, but actively encouraged it on the local and regional hubs. By blocking business from the NSF backbone, this strategy successfully stimulated private investment by companies such as PSI, UUNET, and ANS CO+RE in long-distance network capacity to get around the backbone restrictions, as hoped by the NSF. Later, the NSF ceased to underwrite the backbone network entirely and turned its attentions to issues of inter-connection, among others. These privatizations were fraught with problems (see Kesan and Shah, 2001).

In January of 1993, NSF privatized the domain name system by granting little-known Network Solutions, Inc. a five-year contract to provide registration and other DNS-related services (Network Solutions, 1993). Network Solutions was to administer domains under the "generic" (or non-geographic) TLDs "gov," "edu," "com," "net," and "org." Although Network Solutions was initially paid directly by the NSF for these services, a cost-plus-fixed-fee price for the registration of a second-level domain name was eventually introduced to defray costs (Network Solutions, 1995). Effective September, 1995 all would-be registrants must pay $50 per year, with two years payable upon initial registration. Procedures to transfer the domain names between parties had been in place for some time, cementing the nature of the names as commodities – if something can be exchanged, it can be bought and sold. At the time, no one predicted that this somewhat arcane technical addressing system, government contract, and its related fee would soon become so important.

A new real estate born

The popularity of the Internet rose dramatically in the mid-1990s. Commercial enterprises began to pour onto the network, and every business wanted a name for itself. US firms, unwilling to be associated with the geographic hierarchy, sought second-level domains like "cbs" under the only generic TLD of the possible seven provided explicitly for commerce, "com." By 1997, one million unique words were registered as second-level domains by Network Solutions. Three years later, ten million domains had been registered (Network Solutions, 2000). In the first rush to register, even unpunctuated combinations of common words were snapped up. For instance, the domain "americascheeseexperts.com" was registered by Kraft Foods in these early days, but has now lapsed (CNET, 1996). While the fairly arbitrary $50 fee per year of registration had seemed reasonable in 1993, with the large increase in demand, Network Solutions' projected revenue under the NSF contract went from $6.5 million in 1995 to $44 million for 1996 to a projected $70 million in 1998 (Clausing, 1998b).

Industry began to realize the value of these domain name "properties," in a marketplace that was termed "cyberspace real estate" (Aguilar, 1996). Corporate interests with deep pockets began to buy not only a domain name for every product line they carried, but also any word they might conceivably have need of in the future. In one example, consumer-product giant Procter & Gamble "launched a flurry of domain name registration[s] . . . that included not only many of its prized brand names, including clearasil.com and charmin.com, but also a host of generic names, like babydiapers.com and cough.com" (Dunn, 1996). The company collected over 100 names in all (including "diarrhea" and "pimples") in a manner that the press termed a "land grab" (Aguilar, 1996).

Smaller entrepreneurs were not to be left out. Any far-sighted individual with $100 could profit if he could think of a name anyone might need in the future. Entrepreneurs set up domain-name "brokerage houses" where pooled capital

Table 4.1 Sample domain name sale prices

Year	Domain	Price
1996	slate.com	$10,000
1996	television.com	$50,000*
1997	business.com	$150,000
1997	porno.com	$42,000
1998	altavista.com	$3,300,000
1999	business.com	$7,500,000
1999	wine.com	$3,000,000
1999	wallstreet.com	$1,030,000
2000	loans.com	$3,000,000

Sources: Hakala and Rickard, 1996; ".com," 1996; Wingfield, 1996; Lee, 1999; Pollack, 1999; Associated Press, 2000.

* Price offered, not taken.

allowed the purchase of thousands of names, with the profits split among investors. Early entrants in this area were *bestdomains.com* and *domainwise.com*. One such domain broker has named itself "I [for Internet] GoldRush" and has the motto "mining the net" (http://www.igoldrush.com/). Domain name speculation has even spilled over into the geographical hierarchy, with brokers purchasing the names of cities. When non-Internet-savvy municipalities woke up to the value of using the network and attempted to establish an Internet presence, they found their city's name already taken, and held by a party looking to sell to the highest bidder (Silberman, 1997).

Scarcity has drastically inflated prices above the $50 fee initially charged by Network Solutions, if inflation is even a reasonable construct to use in this situation – as the concrete value of a second-level domain name is arguable. Brokers often set "minimum bids" of $500, while at the upper end of the spectrum, several agreements have been reached for amounts over $1 million. Table 4.1 lists a sample of domain name sales reported by the press that were considered noteworthy at the time reported.

Normalizing the DNS, with property comes power

During the explosion of "cyberspace real estate," it was clear to some that there was little reason for the present scarcity of the ethereal domain names. A monopoly by Network Solutions on the basis of a US government contract seemed increasingly absurd in the context of a global Internet. A consortium of companies and user groups secured a partnership with the World Intellectual Property Organization and the International Telecommunications Union and formed an international body that planned to introduce several additional top-level domains, known as the Global Top-Level Domain Memorandum of Understanding, or gTLD-MoU (Internet Assigned Numbers Authority, 1997).

Confusing the issue slightly was the fact that the international body had no authority to do so, but a counter-argument might be that Network Solutions has none either (Harmon, 1998). No one was sure what body could grant authority over this international infrastructure. Still, the technical function of translating domain names to the IP addresses that allow data to be routed to the appropriate computers would need to be performed.

By the end of the 1990s controversy ensued. The Network Solutions monopoly on domain name registration ended and the protection of the rights of property owners took center stage. Although this was surprising to many, it is entirely consistent with the history of radio policy.

Playing for the "control of cyberspace"

While ending scarcity by increasing the number of available TLDs seemed to many to be of paramount importance (Froomkin, 1999), in February 1998 the Clinton administration issued a proposal to introduce only one new domain name, and forced the international consortium to back down by refusing to acknowledge its authority to participate in the naming system (US Dept. of Commerce, 1998). It is illustrative that the debate surrounding this issue was phrased as a battle for "the control of cyberspace," although control over the handful of generic top-level domain names does not imply actual control over the network-only over the ability for data to reach hosts registered under those domains (Harmon, 1998).

The discursive framework surrounding property rights is so prevalent in our culture that this issue seems to be one of crucial control, even if it is of less technical or practical significance. In examining the case of the Internet's DNS, we see another example of the largely unintended creation of property on a grand scale, and then surprise being expressed by many parties at the actions of actors in the system who are merely following incentives set up by the system. Reliance on property as a model is so naturalized to us that it permeates our lives and we immediately consider speculation in Internet address codes to be "real estate." These domain name registrations are agreements to direct data to specific computers upon receipt of a series of words and punctuation characters. They have no physical form, and are transferred among owners by asking the registering body that they be transferred. Yet the price of the registration fee (which, even when at the 2002 price of about $30, has been described as arbitrarily high considering the actual work involved by the registrar) is multiplied many times because of the evocative, symbolic, or connotative meanings corporations hope these names will bring them. By instituting a structure for these names based on a property system of commodification, just as occurred in radio, non-profit, non-commercial users are relegated to second-class Internet addresses because first, they are priced out of the system of value and second, those who secure a domain name first can reap the monetary rewards as value accrues to the name due to scarcity – all reminiscent of the radio broadcast license.

At the beginning of the century, corporate liberalism led legislators to assume that full utilization of a scarce resource could only be realized by sufficiently capitalized and expert private entities. At the end of 1998, US officials had reached the same conclusion about a new medium: the private sector would administer name registration, as envisioned by a Department of Commerce (1998) proposal (also see Clausing, 1997a, 1997c, 1998c; US House of Representatives, 1998: 203–300). In 1998, the director of the American Intellectual Property Law Association testified approvingly before congress that:

> any effort to design the Internet of the future should involve . . . a recognition that the private sector is best equipped to administer and maintain the domain name system . . . we are pleased that the [Department of Commerce] Green Paper is largely consonant with [this] principle . . .
>
> (US House of Representatives, 1999a: 236)

The creation of an impartial international body (the Internet Corporation for Assigned Names and Numbers, or ICANN) was advanced to organize the system that would evolve, but the primary goals of the system would be to protect two property interests: the property rights of current domain name holders, and the property rights of those who hold another type of property, the trademark.

Trademark law and corporate control

Trademark concerns grew in the late 1990s to consume more and more domain name policy attention. After the heady speculation of the early days, courts of many nations have begun to apply trademark rights to the DNS, ICANN implemented a dispute resolution policy to address claims by trademark owners, and in the US a 1999 amendment to the Lanham Act provided statutory relief for "bad-faith" registration of trademarked names. Further, concerns of trademark holders were often cited to quash proposals to introduce additional TLDs to alleviate scarcity (US House of Representatives, 1999a: 216, 258; 1999b: 213).

In this manner, a major goal of domain name policy has been the protection of trademark property rights; yet this goal as it has been addressed is irrational when considered in a broader context. First, direct conflation of trademarks and domain names makes little sense: domain names have fallen into the role of a directory system, and this combined with scarcity drives much of the inflation in value noted earlier. In even a small local area, company and service names are not expected to be unique (Mitchell et al., 1997: 264), this is why trademarks are justifiably limited to geographic areas and (ideally) particular product types. Generic TLDs, on the contrary, are not limited by product domain or by geographic area. More important, however, the Internet has more than one function. While it may be an emerging electronic marketplace, it is also a medium for a broad range of other forms of communication, and these different forms of communication imply different policy goals (Heiskanen, 1999: 34). Even if we acknowledge that the protection of intellectual property rights such as trademark is a legitimate goal of government regulation of the marketplace, the Internet can be more than a marketplace. Any given word or string that might be registered as a domain name might be conceptualized in a commercial context, but it might also be used in another way. In the US, when policy-makers assign trademark rights priority in discussions of domain names, this conflicts with the freedom of speech right of those who do not own trademarks and non-commercial communicators.

We can see, then, that the trademark property right in this instance only accelerates the force of the marketplace to consolidate control among those with capital – the capital and legal resources to register trademarks in many countries and enforce them through lawsuits. Although early radio had nothing comparable to trademark, trademark as applied to date on the Internet reinforces the notion that this is a medium for commerce and a place for commodification of the audience.

While we imagine that the Internet is not like the one-way media of the past, the dominant frame of policy debate to date places the user of the Internet as a consumer of commercial messages, exactly like television and radio. Even very well-reasoned proposals to reconcile the DNS with trademark interests tend to assume the Internet is a marketplace, and only a marketplace – because these are the goals foregrounded by approaching the topic from trademark law (e.g. Burk, 1995; Gigante, 1997; Nathenson, 1997; Shaw, 1997). As the President of the International Trademark Association testified before the US Congress:

> The fundamental question . . . is how to protect consumers' interests in locating the brand or vendor of their choice on the Internet without being misled or confused, and how to protect companies from having their brand equity eroded or commandeered in an electronic environment.
> (US House of Representatives, 1999a: 243)

Alarmingly, even those on the opposite side of the debate from corporate interests use the language of consumerism (e.g. Ralph Nader's objections to ICANN; see US House of Representatives, 1999b: 134). Broadly, many objections to a corporate agenda are more often phrased in terms of consumerism than as appeals to the interests of "citizens" or "the public."

Community practice in the network society

These maneuverings in obscure, international technical bodies may at first seem divorced from the everyday practice of community media. However, the organization of communication systems must allow and support community participation as a first precondition for community media to exist. As the story of early radio in the US teaches, the historical development of communication technology has often been a story of community, educational, and not-for-profit voices being pushed aside. Examples abound in the US alone: educational broadcasters were explicitly marginalized in the early regulation of radio. In television, only about 170 current US licensees are non-commercial (out of approximately 1,700 total), even among these non-commercial licensees public television in the US now closely resembles commercial television. New prospects for low-powered community and educational "microradio" were eviscerated by Congress in 2000. Does the Internet need to be another in this series of defeats?

As discussed in this chapter, the development of the Internet's domain name system to date sets the stage for another community media loss. The continuing artificial scarcity in the Internet namespace and the privileged position given to trademark holders means that any given word in an Internet address will most likely belong to whoever can pay the highest price. Community organizations can work to change this state of affairs by directly participating in domain name policy, and by supporting a domain name structure that is consistent with the communication needs of not-for-profit organizations, community media groups, and other non-commercial organizations. For more information on participating directly in domain name policy, see the Computer Professionals for Social Responsibility (CPSR) Working Group on Domain Names (http://www.cpsr. org/dns), the watchdog group ICANN Watch (http://www.icannwatch.org/), and the Internet Democracy Project (http://www.internetdemocracyproject. org/), a joint effort of American Civil Liberties Union, the Electronic Frontier Foundation, and CPSR. To support alternative domain name structures, consider participating in the Open Root Server Confederation (http://www.open-rsc. org/) and encouraging non-commercial organizations to register domain names under TLDs that explicitly demarcate a space for non-commercial participation. These include .org, but also two new domains that began operation at the end of 2001: the cooperative domain .coop (http://www.nic.coop/) and the museum domain .museum (http://www.nic.museum/).

Conclusion

In the 1920s, property rights were constructed in the ether, and any discussion of radio is now constrained to what these rights allow or forbid. Today, property rights have been constructed in the domain name system of the Internet, with preference being given to those that own another form of property – trademark. The grand hopes many have held out for the Internet's future do not seem compatible with a network where participation devolves quickly into a question of what properties you own, what symbols you can afford.

Surely the NSF did not intend to exclude those with fewer financial resources from prime addresses on the Internet, just as it seems the US government did not particularly intend to produce the system of broadcasting we have today when constructing it in the 1920s. The power of grand assumptions about the marketplace and property is great, particularly in the United States – it is an imperative that we now learn to step outside these assumptions. Our goals should direct the development of legal structures of control, and not vice versa. As Streeter states, "the principal question for media policy in the United States should be, How do we, as a matter of democratic choice, want to organize our popular communications, our means of producing and distributing culture and information?" (1996: 318).

If we allow the lessons of early radio and the present day Internet to inform policy decisions in the future, it is still possible to construct a communication system that excels where past media have fallen short, and meets our goals, whatever they may be. Unlike the long-established broadcast media, it may not be too late to implement policy goals for the Internet independent of the market structure now in place with only a minimum of effort rather than a radical restructuring. A communication system organized around the ownership of various forms of constructed property and dominated by the interests of the owners is not the best result, the inevitable result, or even a more rational result, it is instead the false default that will persist if we continue to think that creating property is not a policy intervention. One can only hope that it is not too late to set our goals for the Internet independent of the structure now in place.

Acknowledgment

A portion of this research was kindly supported by a Markle Foundation Information Policy Fellowship at the Programme in Comparative Media Law and Policy, Oxford University, and by a visiting research fellowship at the Oxford Internet Institute. An earlier version of this paper was presented to the Union for Democratic Communications on June 13, 1998. I would like to thank Ted Glasser, François Bar, Elissa Lee, Hernan Galperin, Karin Wahl-Jorgensen, and Larry Bensky for their helpful comments.

Notes

1   For a broader overview of the domain name system's background, see Mills (1981), Su and Postel (1982), Mockapetris (1983, 1987), Postel (1983, 1994), and Postel and Reynolds (1984). For a discussion of Internet histories, see Guice (1998).

Chapter 5

The changing online landscape

From free-for-all to commercial gatekeeping

Eszter Hargittai

Introduction

Each day, millions of people across the world turn to the Web to find information about countless topics. Given the vast amount of material available online, users rely on intermediaries to channel them toward content. Whether through the use of search engines, directory listings, or links supplied by favorite destinations, people often rely on content aggregators and third-party sites to help them find information of interest. The majority of these intermediary sites are for-profit ventures. Does the commercial nature of these sites influence what types of content are most easily accessible to users? Is all content on the Web created equal? Or are there ways in which some materials online get more exposure than other content regardless of relevance and quality? And do such differences limit the level of content diversity that is realistically within the reach of most users? When considering the Web's implications for a global civil network society, it is important to recognize the institutional factors that may influence how users benefit from this global medium.

The mass diffusion of the Internet across the world has led many to speculate about the potential effects of the new medium on society at large. Enthusiasts have heralded the potential gains resulting from use of the technology suggesting that it will reduce inequality by lowering the barriers to information, allowing people of all backgrounds to improve their human capital, expand their social networks, be more direct participants in the political process, search for and find jobs, have better access to health information, and otherwise improve their opportunities and enhance their life chances (e.g. Anderson *et al.*, 1995). Some have gone as far as to say that the Internet will lead to "universal liberty," a new overarching tolerance and the "restoration of ethics" (Barlow, 1997). In contrast, skeptics have warned against the potential costs of such a technology due to its ability to overwhelm us with often useless information (Rochlin, 1998; Shenk, 1997) and isolate us from our social networks leading to loneliness and possibly even depression (Nie, 2001; Nie and Erbring, 2000).

Historical studies (Carey, 1988; Marvin, 1988; Pool, 1983) suggest that understanding how technologies are adopted involves two levels of analysis. First, we need to look at users and what characteristics at the individual level shape how different segments of the population adopt a medium. Second, we must recognize that the institutional structure of a communication medium is not preordained, rather, it is situated in a particular economic and legal environment. Consequently, it is wrong to make blanket claims about the Internet's potential implications for society without considering the myriad of factors that influence how technologies are adopted in society. In this vein, it is also incorrect to assume that simply having access to the Internet will improve people's life chances. There are numerous institutional factors that influence how a communication medium diffuses across the population and to what uses it is put. From hardware manufacturers to content creators, from federal regulators to local government policy-makers, from university administrators to corporate managers, lots of institutional players are contributing to the emerging shape of the new medium. In this chapter, I focus on one institutional level variable, namely, the evolution of business interests online and how this influences people's use of the medium.

Studies have looked at how people use the Internet (for a review, see DiMaggio et al., 2001) and in particular what types of content users view online (e.g. Howard et al., 2001). There is a separate body of literature that looks at how people use information retrieval systems and, in particular, how people search for information on the Web (for a review of this literature, see Jansen and Pooch, 2001). However, these two areas of inquiry exist in isolation from each other. There has been little discussion of how people's online actions may be influenced not only by their interests but also by their abilities to find various types of content online (Hargittai, 2002). Does the way in which content is organized, presented, and distributed online influence people's ability to find their way to material on the Web? In this chapter, I look at the evolution of point-of-entry sites and the most popular search engines online to show how various business strategies have shaped the ways in which content is presented to users and how these business decisions influence users' everyday online actions.

Much of the promise of the Internet for global communities is based more on the person-to-person communication possibilities afforded by the medium rather than the information retrieval aspect of the network. However, in order to participate in civil society and find networks of interest, users need to have the ability to find the relevant types of groups and communities with which they want to be involved. In this respect, the nuances of information retrieval become an important component of who may be able to find and join communities and how far reaching these interactions can be. In this chapter I look at what processes mediate what online information reaches users.

The changing online landscape

The promise of the Web

Billions of Web pages are available on the Web for public use (Bergmann, 2002; Lake, 2000). Any individual or organization with the know-how to create a site can contribute content to the public Web. The technicalities of making such content as available to users as the most popular Web sites are more or less the same. The Internet has the potential to create arenas for more voices than any other previous communication medium by dramatically reducing the cost of the replication and distribution of information. Writers, musicians, visual artists no longer have to rely on large production agencies and distributors to get their work out to the public. Politicians and activists have the potential to reach citizens without having to go through media giants or the difficulty of pamphleteering step by step impeded by geographical limits.

The facility associated with the use of the network – both with respect to posting and retrieving information – has led to much enthusiasm about its potential to connect members of marginalized groups, to give voices to those without many resources, and to provide information to those in remote locations lacking access to more mainstream media outlets. By allowing a vast reduction in the replication and distribution costs of a product – whether text-based, audio, video, or multi-media – the Web puts product dissemination within the reach of the individual. This reduces the salience of the gate that functions between the creator of information and its materialization. Not only can a person create a product easily, it is also possible to make numerous copies of it available at very low cost. Moreover, because it is no longer necessary to transport these items physically, it is also nearly effortless to allow access to the product from various geographic locations.

The challenge of reaching audiences

Information abundance sometimes exacerbates the problem of attention scarcity. Ironically, even people who have recognized the importance of attention scarcity have suggested that any individual will be able to sidestep organizations and corporate packaging in an attempt to receive attention (Goldhaber, 1997). In contrast, I emphasize that attention scarcity leads individual creators of content to rely on online gatekeepers to channel their material toward users and leads users to rely on such services to find their way to content on the Web. Web services that categorize online information – search engines, point-of-entry sites – can be considered gatekeepers on the World Wide Web.

The term "gatekeeper" refers to points that function as gates blocking the flow of some material while allowing other information to pass through (White, 1950). Studies on industries that make cultural products (Hirsch, 1972; Lopes, 1992; Peterson and Berger, 1975; Powell, 1985) have explored the role of gatekeepers in influencing the type of products that are produced and distributed on the market. With previous media, the costs of production were so high that a vitally important gatekeeping step concerned the decision about what products should be produced. Individual creators of cultural products had to go through both producers *and* distributors of their products to get attention on the market. The final link in the distribution chain – supermarket rack jobbers, disk jockeys, movie critics, book review editors – can be a key figure in allocating people's attention to material. Although there may be less emphasis on these inter-mediaries in the online world when it comes to producing and making available content, the final step of reaching audiences remains a crucial part of garnering attention for one's material.

Although there may be numerous high-quality sites on the Web, there is no guarantee that anyone will find their way to them. The central concern is no longer what is produced, but what consumers hear and know about. Accordingly, gatekeeping activity still occurs online, but now takes place at the level of information exposure. Its location has shifted from the decision about what should be produced to control of what materials get to consumers and of what material they become aware. In this vein, it is important to distinguish between content that is merely present on the Web in contrast to content to which users are easily exposed. "Available" content is material that is present online but which should be distinguished from "accessible" content which is realistically within the reach of users.

The rise of search engines and portal sites

Due to the ease with which users could add content to the Web, thanks to the rise in the number of users, and as a result of an increasing number of organiza-tions embracing the Web as a communication tool, the amount of content available online has risen exponentially. In 1995, there were approximately ten thousand Web sites (Prettejohn, 1996); by 2003 this number had grown to more than thirty-five million (Netcraft, 2003). Not surprisingly, services that help users find their way to content of interest are crucial to the Web's ability to be a useful tool for people.

As the amount of Web content skyrocketed, search engines became increasingly important in sifting through online material. The first search engines appeared in the mid-1990s and several of them came out of research universities (see Table 5.1 for dates and information about origins). In many cases, academic research settings sponsored their creation and their one goal was to help people better navigate Web content.

Initially, these sites functioned in one of two ways. Some provided the option of openly searching the Web's content (e.g. WebCrawler and Lycos) while others organized information into Web directories and people could access content by clicking on categorized links (e.g. Yahoo). The former relied on computer programs whereas the latter were manually compiled. At this point the one goal seemed to be to feature interesting and high-quality content. In time, the ventures left academic settings and became profit-seeking commercial enterprises.

Another source of popular portal sites were the default home pages that came up during the use of the most popular browsing software applications, Netscape Navigator and Internet Explorer. At first, those sites offered little more than software upgrades, but soon they grew into much more than a place to download

Table 5.1 The launch date of some major search engines and their original institutional affiliations

Search engine	Launch year	Original affiliation
Lycos	1994	Carnegie Mellon University
WebCrawler	1994	University of Washington
Yahoo!	1994	Stanford University
Altavista	1995	Digital Equipment Corporation
Excite	1995	Excite, Inc.
Infoseek	1995	Private
HotBot	1996	Wired Ventures
Google	1998	Stanford University (Google, Inc. by the time of launch)

an application. In 1998, the Microsoft Corporation made a conscious effort to consolidate all of its online ventures into one site at MSN.com, creating a massive one-stop point-of-entry site (Broersma, 1998).

Strategies for profitability

Government support for media content is rare in the United States. (Although the Web is an international medium, all of the most popular search engines and portal sites originated in the United States, thus the focus on that one country.) This left the burden of financing these online ventures to other potential sources. The model in the 1990s was to turn to corporate sponsorship. Alternatives could have included individual subscription fees or funding by private foundations. Most online services were funded through advertisements, by venture capitalists, or through corporate cross-subsidization where the profitable division of a company covered the costs of the online undertaking. In order to legitimate funding, Web sites had to attract and keep visitors and encourage them to stay and revisit frequently.

To achieve this, search engines and portal sites expanded their repertoire of services beyond simply pointing people to content elsewhere on the Web. Instead, they changed their business models to the goal of keeping users on their sites as long as possible. By contracting with large content providers they offered sports information, entertainment news, current events, and many other services (e.g. free email accounts and space for personal home pages) all under one roof. As Lycos openly proclaimed: "The Company seeks to draw a large number of viewers to its Websites by providing a one-stop destination for identifying, selecting and accessing resources, services, content and information on the Web" (Lycos, 1998).

The online landscape had clearly changed. For example, contrast the launch of Lycos by academics and the launch of Yahoo by students in 1994 with the launch of Go.com in 1999 as a joint profit-seeking venture between the Disney Corporation and the Infoseek Corporation. In just five years the commercial nature of search engines and big portal sites became unmistakable. The focus was no longer to simply offer guidance to the rest of the Web and point users to other sites. Instead, the goals of the newer sites became to keep users on their own territory as long as possible maximizing revenue from advertisements presented to users while on the host site.

However, no one such site could ever offer access to all of online content. In fact, any one search engine is only able to index a small percentage of the Web and even combined they can only account for a portion of online material (Lawrence and Giles, 1999). This means that only a fragment of what is publicly available online is realistically within the reach of users. If a site is not indexed or does not get pointers in a Web directory it can easily fall into oblivion, never to be seen by any users.

According to one survey, 85 percent of users have ever used a search engine (Pew, 2002) suggesting that the majority of Web users turn to content aggregators at least part of the time to locate material online. By 1999, search engines and portal sites dominated the list of most popular Web sites, garnering traffic from millions of unique visitors each month. Often users are locked into whatever portal is the default setting when they buy their computers. Research by Netscape in 1998 showed that 50–60 percent of users did not change their default browser homepage (Guglielmo, 1998) leaving them with a prepackaged site from a provider. America Online constitutes a special case in that AOL users are not only presented with a very specific AOL-sponsored content box when they first log on, there are other proprietary AOL services that users have to sidestep to find Web sites not related to the service provider.

All in all, what service provider one uses and, accordingly, what content first shows up on one's browser has a potential significant effect on users' online actions. This phenomenon can be summed up by the term: *default homepage advantage*. Most users do not choose their default homepages – the computer manufacturer, their service provider, or their employer or library does. Many users do not change the settings, leaving the default homepage advantage in the hands of corporate entities. The goal of these actors is to benefit from driving users' eyeballs to particular content whose prominence they can influence via their default homepage advantage.

The implications of commercial interests online

To understand whether different types of content are given equal opportunity to reach audiences, we must consider how sites achieve good rankings on search engine result lists and prominent positions on portals and directories. For the most part such decisions are proprietary information and companies do not disclose the details of their search engine algorithms or how they make decisions about directory listings. Nonetheless, it is possible to collect some information about site practices and get some idea of the role of commercial interests in how content is categorized and presented online.

The strategies described here do not pertain to explicit graphical advertisements displayed on Web pages. Rather, they all involve the role of financial incentives in search engines and directory placements. There are several ways in which sites can achieve good positioning by paying a fee (this is often referred to as pay-for-placement). Most search engines now have various sponsored programs where site owners can purchase a particular position after certain specified search terms. For example, one can contract to be placed in the list of "Sponsored Links" (e.g. on Google in 2003) or "Sponsor Match" (e.g. on Yahoo in 2003) after users run a search on a particular term. However, these "sponsored link" designations are sometimes quite ambiguous on search engines and even when they are clearly noted users do not necessarily notice them or know that they are the result of behind-the-scenes financial arrangements. Sites vary considerably in how prominent they make the fact that a particular result came up because of sponsorship and not necessarily because of overall relevance to the search query.

Undoubtedly, the entry of the private sector into the Internet world encouraged its wide spread and the growth in online content. Search engines and portal sites assist millions of users every day in finding information online. So why is it a problem that commercial interests sometimes guide the content selection on popular sites? The concern is that search engines that are guided by profit motives may point people away from the most relevant and best-quality sites in favor of those that have paid the highest bids for placement on the results page regardless of their quality and specific relevance to the search query.

Analyses of large-scale search engine usage data suggest that users mainly rely on the first page of results to a search query. A study analyzing almost one billion queries on the AltaVista search engine showed that in 85 percent of the cases users only viewed the first screen of results (Silverstein et al., 1999). Web users' habits have not changed much over the years. Another study (Spink et al., 2002) compared data on the use of the Excite search engine from 1997, 1999, and 2001 and found that the mean number of results pages users looked at had decreased over time. The data in this study also show that the majority of users rely on simple queries without the use of advanced search features (e.g. use of multiple terms in a query, the use of Boolean operators or quotes around terms to limit results).

These findings suggest that users heavily rely on sites for presenting them with information rather than using sophisticated search techniques to fine-tune their queries. This implies that information prominently displayed on portal sites – whether selected because of high content value or for commercial reasons – has a good chance of being the destination of visitors. If users do not possess advanced know-how about how content is organized and presented to them online then they are especially at the mercy of what content sites decide to feature prominently and make easily accessible to them.

Sites spend significant resources on optimizing their content to show up as results. In fact, an entire industry has sprung up around "search engine optimization", offering advice on how companies and others can best ensure that their Web sites climb to the top of search engine results. In contrast, the sites with the most relevant content may be posted by a non-profit organization or an individual on his or her own initiative and only appear far down the results list because the owners of such sites do not necessarily have the resources to optimize for search engine positioning. In fact, free Web-hosting services which non-profits and individuals are more likely to use are known to be discriminated against in search engine listings (e.g. search engines place much less emphasis on large sites such as Geocities that provide free Web site space, rarely ranking them highly on results; moreover, users tend to question the reliability of content on these sites which leads to even less traffic). So the overall concern due to the prominence of commercial interests on the Web is not that users will unknowingly be roped into purchasing information they could otherwise obtain for free – although this may happen as well – but that they may not find what they are looking for or may miss the best available information because those resources are crowded out by the profit-seeking ventures.

Commercial sites will often rise to the top of result lists despite not having the relevant information. A search on Overture – which is an openly pay-for-placement search engine – for something as specific and non-commercial as the "museum of modern art" will yield eight commercial results before listing http://www.moma.org which is the museum's own site (this search was performed in January, 2003). And although Overture may not be a widely used search engine, it has deals with several of the most popular search engines to feature its results on their pages (e.g. in 2003, Yahoo!, MSN, AltaVista, Dogpile, and Lycos all featured Overture results prominently on their results pages with varying levels of disclosure about this partnership). This example shows that financial incentives do play an important role in what content users see prominently on the most popular Web sites.

Undoubtedly, the evolution of search engines and portal sites continues. Like other media (Piirto, 1994), Web sites also evolve over time as use patterns and the media landscape change. Content aggregators develop new strategies to remain important players in the industry. Google was a relatively late entrant into the search engine market yet gradually gained a sizable share of users with as many as 30 percent of searchers turning to its services five years into the company's inception (Sullivan, 2003). As of this writing, Google does not allow commercial considerations to affect its main search engine results. Nonetheless, Google also showcases ad-supported content on its results pages. Moreover, portal sites which contract with Google for their searches – such as Yahoo! and MyWay – display Google's ads from its AdWords program in ways different from those on Google's own site. For example, on MyWay, the results show up right above the regular results and the words signaling that these are "sponsored listings" are in very small font and unobtrusive.

So although Google's own site may not engage in some of the practices that raise concerns outlined earlier, a large number of users still depend on sites that feature ad-supported content before information that may be more relevant to their needs. Moreover, Google – like any other search engine – does have the ability to censor certain sites without users knowing about it. Local versions of Google in countries other than the US have been shown to engage in such content exclusion (Zittrain and Edelman, 2002) and some such cases have been documented for its American version as well. To be fair, Google has engaged in these exclusionary practices due to legal pressures and has developed a method to document and make public such legal reasons for censorship (Gallagher, 2002). Nonetheless, these are additional examples of ways in which search engines may manipulate to what content users have access.

Strategies for non-profits

Given the many ways in which commercial sites have advantages in the online landscape when it comes to gaining an audience – from the ability to employ search engine optimization experts to having the resources for paid search engine placements – non-profit content creators are faced with a challenge when seeking to reach a user base. This section outlines some strategies that do not require large monetary resources yet do contribute to visibility and encourage exposure.

First, it is important to recognize that having a large number of visitors may not be the primary goal. In many cases it is likely more important to reach relevant users instead of numerous Web surfers who are not interested in the site's content; thus it may be best to focus on the quality of the visitors instead of the quantity. If the site is for the online presence of an offline organization than there must be some information about membership and interested parties. If the site is a stand-alone enterprise then the site creators need to judge from their content and from gathering information about initial users to figure out the target population.

Second, it is important to figure out what other resources exist on the Web that would cater to similar users. This is important for two reasons. On the one hand, it is probably not advisable to spend large amounts of resources to replicate content that already exists. On the other hand, it is important to identify potential allies. Some search engines include in their algorithms information about how many and what types of other sites link to a Web page (e.g. Google's search algorithm works this way (Brin and Page, 1998)). The more links a Web page gets and from the higher-profile sites, the higher it gets ranked on some search results listings (Walker, 2002). So it is in the interest of like-minded non-profit content providers to join forces and cross-link, thereby contributing to the prominence of all involved in the linking. Once site owners identify other sites of interest, it may be a good idea to contact their maintainers and establish cross-links whereby each site points to the other. It may also be beneficial to include a link to the welcome page of the site from every other page on the site. In addition to the importance of this to search engine rankings, such clear navigational hints on pages aid the usability of the Web site.

Third, the organization or group must make sure that the content on the site is regularly updated. There are two separate reasons for this. On the one hand, visitors will be more likely to keep coming back if they know they can expect fresh content. On the other hand, providing up-to-date materials boosts the frequency with which search engines will index a site. Search engines have programs – often referred to as robots or spiders – that crawl the Web's content to update their databases with what is available online. These robots tend to pass by sites that are frequently updated more often than other sites (Hiler, 2002). Ideal in this case would be to include a blog or Weblog on the site with nearly daily updates. A blog is a frequently updated site with entries most often presented in chronological order (Stone, 2002). Various software programs exist to automate much of the process, requiring very little to no technical expertise. The entries on blogs do not have to be lengthy additions, they can be no more than simply pointers to other content online. The advantage of a blog is that it is relatively easy to maintain, it can have an interactive component, it does not have to include the addition of much content at any one time, and it can boost the rankings of a site if frequently updated (Hiler, 2002).

Fourth, allowing users to become actively engaged with site content can boost popularity and encourage loyalty as users become more directly involved. An interactive section on a site in the form of a Web forum can allow for this. However, such an interactive component may be complicated or expensive to launch and maintain. A viable alternative is to start an electronic discussion list. Users can sign up and receive emails from other participants. The site creators can make sure that they post periodic updates about site content on such a list, prompting people to visit the site for updated materials. Such lists are especially crucial for groups and organizations whose main mission lies in connecting people on an ongoing basis. For those users who are not interested in such frequent communication, it is also a good idea to offer the option of an announcement mailing list. On such lists only the list owner or list manager has rights to post a message. Such a list can be used strictly to update subscribers of upcoming or recent events, additions to the Web site and other related services.

Finally, it is important to recognize the power of word-of-mouth recommendations in spreading information about sites and online communities. If users receive periodic updates that include content potentially relevant to non-members they should be encouraged to forward the messages and draw in new users. To this end, it is important to identify clearly the Web site in every message that is sent out. Moreover, it is also worth investing in a personalized domain name, which are now available for a small fee. (Domain names are the .com, .org, etc. names used on the Web to easily identify Web sites.) The information about a site can be communicated easily and quickly, preventing spelling mistakes and mistyped characters that would result in dead ends for those seeking to reach a site. Moreover, the Web site address should be prominently featured on all communication materials of the group or organization (whether weekly email updates or hard-copy print resources).

At the organizational level, a possible strategy to sidestep commercial influence would be to create a non-profit portal or search engine where commercial interests do not play a part in determining content (Hargittai, 2000; Schuler, 2001 and 2002). In addition to keeping it commercial-free, it would be important to make the search algorithms openly accessible and transparent. One problem with existing search engines is that the algorithms they use are proprietary, leaving users in the dark about what rules guide the selection of the content they see (including possible exclusions as noted earlier). Unfortunately, there is a considerable limitation to these proposed avenues: even if such non-profit services did exist, there is no guarantee that anybody would know about them given the difficulty in attracting attention to a Web site, especially one without commercial backing.

Conclusion

Although seemingly neutral, search engines and directories systematically exclude certain sites in favor of others either by design or by accident (Introna and Nissenbaum, 2000). Commercial interests underlie the most popular Web sites and those to which users turn to find their way to online content. Non-profits lack many of the resources that nowadays seem essential to obtaining the necessary exposure for reaching users. The implications of this for diversity of content online is that sites presented by non-profits and individuals lacking resources will have less of a chance to reach audiences and users may not find the most relevant information in response to their needs.

Given the current state of online content organization and presentation, users must be educated about the myriad of commercial incentives that influence search result listings and directory placements. They have to be conscious of the fact that the most prominent results are not necessarily the most – or the only – possible sources online in response to their query. Users also have to learn how to do more refined searches and how to turn to a more diverse set of resources online in order to avoid the sidetracks that result from commercial interests. Although the Web does offer all users the ability to contribute to online content, all content is not created equal when it comes to reaching users. It is essential to keep this in mind when considering the Web's potential for giving voice to marginalized groups and its ability to bring together people into effective communities.

Snapshots of community practice

Part II

Snapshots of community
practice

Chapter 6

ICTs for health promotion in the community

A participative approach

Audrey Marshall

Health promotion and community

In 1948, the World Health Organization (WHO) issued a definition of health, which emphasised well-being: "a state of complete physical, mental and social well-being, not merely the absence of disease and infirmity." While this definition may not seem extraordinary to us today, it indicates an alternative, positive, and holistic approach to health, which contrasts with the more negative Western concept of health as an absence of illness, related solely to the condition of the body. The emphasis on well-being encouraged the growth of the health promotion movement, which started to explore ways of promoting and sustaining health not only for individuals but also for communities. Most readers will be familiar with health promotion messages, which urge us to stop smoking, moderate our alcohol intake or eat more fresh fruit and vegetables and very few would argue with such advice. However, advocating sensible behaviour on an individual level is only part of the story: the communities in which people live or work play an equally important role. For example, people may live in areas where sub-standard housing conditions lead to health problems, or where there is inadequate public transport and few shops, making it difficult to get access to fresh food – or they may not earn enough to afford a regular supply of fruit and vegetables. Individual health and health behaviours are influenced by social structures and the nature of the communities in which people live and work. Furthermore, the concept of the healthy community is more than the aggregate of the health of individuals living in a locality. It is a multi-layered concept, in which the physical and social environments where people live or work and the community resources they have access to combine to enable mutual support.

Policy-makers in health promotion have been linking the concepts of health and community since the 1980s, when a statement from WHO, known as the Ottawa Charter, defined health promotion as a community process. Health promotion is "the process of enabling people to increase control over, and to improve, their health . . . At the heart of this process is the empowerment of communities – their ownership and control of their own endeavours and destinies" (World Health Organization, 1986). The Ottawa Charter was key in making explicit the idea that health is not only a matter of individual responsibility and behaviour, but also a community activity and subsequent policy statements have reinforced this idea. In recent years health promotion practitioners and researchers have engaged in debate around the concept of social capital and how it might link to community health. Social capital emphasises trust, reciprocity, local democracy, citizenship, civic engagement, social relationships and social support. The idea that high levels of trust, civic engagement and social support in a community will foster individual good health, a sense of well-being and self-esteem seems logical. Providing the evidence that those same attributes contribute to health at community level is more difficult and initial results suggest that certain aspects of social capital may be more health-enhancing for communities than others (Campbell *et al.*, 1999). Campbell *et al.* go on to argue that the main attraction of using a construct such as social capital is that it enables public health and health promotion professionals to progress the debate and discussion about social, as opposed to individual, approaches to health. At the level of practice, social capital has the potential to provide a framework for the design and evaluation of community level health promotion interventions, and the Health Development Agency has recently produced a toolkit to help researchers capture "attitudinal data relevant to the measurement of social capital in neighbourhoods" (Health Development Agency, 2002).

Health promotion professionals are key players in community health. They are the bridges between statutory services such as health, education or social services and communities – whether these are geographical, interest-based or socially defined. They act as a link between policy and practice, often working with established community groups on health-related issues. The health promotion practitioners interviewed for the research which informs this chapter spent a significant amount of time working with health and social services staff, with community development workers and with communities themselves to bring health and well-being on to local agendas. They saw themselves as key to the building of healthy communities, involved – as facilitators – in projects such as community cafes, cooking groups and food box schemes.

The idea of building healthy communities has come to the fore in UK policy circles since the Labour government came to power in 1997, partly through a renewed interest in revitalising democracy but also because of an emphasis on tackling health issues through partnership and community involvement. One of the key issues is that of health inequalities, and tackling this problem is a core strand of the government's health policy.

Inequalities in health and the digital divide

Generally speaking, the health of a nation or society is dependent to a large extent on the economic prosperity of that nation or society. People in poorer countries tend not to live as long or enjoy such good levels of health as those in more prosperous countries. What is perhaps more surprising is the fact that within societies, even relatively affluent societies, there are wide discrepancies in levels of health. This phenomenon, known as health inequality, was recognised as a problem by the UK government in 1977, when they established a Working Group to investigate it. The resulting report (Department of Health and Social Security, 1980) analysed the trends in health inequalities during the 1960s and 1970s and made policy recommendations aimed at improving the material conditions of poorer groups of people and reorienting health and social services. Despite this report, the last decades of the twentieth century saw a marked increase in prosperity and health improvements to the population of England as a whole but a widening gap in health between those at the top and bottom of the social scales. In other words, the better off became healthier, while the poorer became unhealthier.

The role of health promotion in the health inequality debate is ambiguous since it has been effectively argued that the better off take more notice of health education campaigns and change their behaviour faster than the less well off. The net effect is therefore to widen inequality. While some would argue with this contention, there is evidence to support it. To take smoking cessation as an example, it has been shown that media campaigns can encourage smoking cessation in up to 12 percent of the population, but the highest failure rates are amongst those who are least well off (Wakefield *et al., 1993*).

Unfortunately, using ICTs for health promotion purposes could exacerbate this problem and contribute further to health inequalities in much the same way, since using ICTs to communicate about health will mean that communication occurs between those with better access to ICTs. They are likely to be the same groups of people, who are better off, better educated, have better health and respond positively to health promotion campaigns. Thus, the accusation that health education campaigns tend to widen inequality could be made with even greater force. The fact that certain economic and social groups of people in our society have better access to ICTs than others is known as the digital divide and the debate has been explored in depth elsewhere (Haywood, 1995; Loader, 1998). The facts and arguments will not be repeated here, but it is worth noting the temptation amongst some policy-makers to assume that the access problem is one that is being steadily eroded as more and more people can afford computers or can use them in their local school or public library. In other words, there is a belief that technical access eliminates ICT disadvantage. Access, however, is more than the opportunity to use a computer and is a complex issue. Commentators such as Kling (1998) argue that the opportunities offered by ICTs will be lost if the main complexities are seen as technical and the social aspects under-estimated. Those social aspects include literacy, the skills needed to find and interpret information and the development of relevant and appropriate content. In a study of the health information practices of a group of mid-life women, Henwood *et al.* (2003) comment that while almost half of the women have used the Internet, few participants have the necessary computer or information literacy skills to use it in a critical way, thus reinforcing Kling's comments.

One way of approaching the dilemma that ICTs might contribute adversely to health outcomes is to examine more closely the issue of health inequality. While commentators analyse it in different ways,[1] most agree that individual behaviour is only a small part of the picture. Measures of health – such as life expectancy, infant mortality and people's sense of well-being – are significantly related to levels of wealth, occupation, social support, housing and education. In 1997, the UK government again commissioned an Independent Enquiry to investigate the evidence related to health inequality and to make recommendations for tackling the problem. The resulting report (Acheson, 1998) analysed the recent trends, arguing that "inequalities in health are of long standing and their determinants are deeply ingrained in our social structure". The report cites evidence that people with good social networks are less susceptible to infectious disease, less likely to report being depressed and more likely to live longer than those with poor networks, and it advocates policies to "reduce social inequalities and to promote social networks". The subsequent government White Paper *Saving Lives* (Department of Health, 1999) outlined how the government intended to tackle the problem, proposing an integrated approach. The key to this is "people improving their own health supported by communities working through local organisations against a backdrop of action by the government" (ibid.: xi). National policy along with the adoption of local measures to progress implementation, such as local Health Improvement Programmes, has given a new impetus to partnership working for community health. Local health authorities welcomed the challenge to "build on the work already started by the existing community-wide partnerships" (East Sussex, Brighton and Hove Health Authority, 1999: 13). Hand in hand with a renewed focus on community health went a recognition that top-down policies are not enough in themselves to tackle the problems and that local people must be involved: "Critical to [defining priorities] will be agreeing how best to include the views of local people in the programme" (ibid.).

Communities, therefore, are seen as key in the efforts to reduce health inequalities. ICTs are powerful communication tools and as such can be one of a raft of measures to support communities in those efforts. However, in order not to risk widening the health gap they must be developed in ways which are socially equitable, contribute to community development and involve local communities themselves. In order to identify how ICTs might be used as a tool for building healthy communities, a critical examination of their role in health information and communication is necessary.

Using ICTS in a health context

The fundamental question to ask is whether or not ICTs offer any communication advantages over more traditional media in a health context. At the level of the individual there is evidence that ICTs do offer unique learning and communication advantages, as will be explained shortly. There is also evidence that ICTs offer important therapeutic benefits at individual, group and community of interest level. However, very little work has been done with regard to ICTs and geographical communities and it is argued here that using ICTs to support and sustain community development can contribute to health improvement.

In a general educational context, it has been shown that the multimedia aspect of ICTs offers considerable potential for individual learning. Ordidge (1998) cites a study of multimedia and its effects on sixth-grade learners, which showed that a combination of text plus animations and captions resulted in the "greatest recall, inference and comprehension" (Ordidge, 1998: 9). The ability of multimedia tools to offer interactivity and allow learners to control their own learning has also been linked to "increased engagement and learning, more positive attitudes, greater motivation, and increased perceptions of personal control" (ibid.). New technology, which incorporates such interactivity, offers an alternative path to the one-way communication model used in many health education campaigns.

In 1998 the then Health Education Authority (now the Health Development Agency) produced an enhanced CD-ROM as part of a national drugs education campaign aimed at young people. Called *D-code* it used a mix of rap voice-over, music, pop visuals and an interactive quiz to explore the subject. Using *D-code* was a fully engaging experience, which stimulated users' visual and aural senses as well as inviting them to test their knowledge on the effects of various drugs on their minds and bodies. The prize for a high score on the quiz – which could be completed over a number of sessions – was access to music software. An evaluation of *D-code* (Cragg Ross Dawson, 1998) found that young people responded positively to it and reported themselves to be much better informed. It should be noted, however, that the impact of the CD-ROM on their behaviour with regard to drug use is unknown.

There are examples of the therapeutic role of ICTs in health, where content has been generated and published by people themselves. One of the projects in the current Economic and Social Research Council (ESRC)'s Innovative Health Technologies Programme is looking at the use of ICTs for people with communication difficulties. The researchers on the project worked with a group of people with aphasia on producing an information website. One of the aphasia sufferers writes that although the "main point of the project was to make a website to give people with aphasia more information . . . the whole process has also been therapeutic, especially making this homepage".[2]

Artimedia[3] worked with a local multiple sclerosis support group in the North-East of England to identify how images can communicate the emotional and spiritual response to being diagnosed with the disease. Some of the women involved in this project participated in a seminar at the Health Education Authority in June 1999 and spoke movingly of the opportunities and sense of empowerment that this project had given them. Their work is published on the Artimedia website.

A similar project, spearheaded by the Photographers' Gallery in London, resulted in the publication of images from deaf people, as a means of exploring and expressing ideas about language, learning and deaf culture. The images were published on a website called De@fsite[4] and involved five artists with teachers and deaf children from different cultural backgrounds. The project gave the children access to deaf adults, sometimes for the first time, and it instilled confidence and creativity in them. Amongst the key learning issues to emerge were that new technologies, particularly in the arts environment, can cancel out issues of "difference" and that "children can be seen as creative individuals first rather than a special needs group" (Robinson, 2000).

Outside the context of therapy or group support, the evidence that ICTs have a positive benefit for community health is much more slight – although early indications are that they may do. A survey of UK community-based ICT projects found that while not set up primarily for health purposes "most projects believed they were contributing to health" and that "developing social contact was seen by many projects as the most effective way of developing healthy communities" (SHM, 1999a: 28).

An innovative project called CityNet (SHM, 1999b) was established as one strand of a wider programme of social action research in Nottingham, initiated in 1997 by the Health Education Authority (now the HDA). The aim of CityNet was to tackle social exclusion issues through participatory approaches to ICTs. It was founded on two principles: that involving people in the design and development increases the likelihood of a sense of ownership and that involvement in such a process can deliver specific benefits to their health and well-being. Initial findings suggest that the first principle has been reinforced: "The commitment to participation and inclusion of individuals from the target groups at the heart of the project is already promoting sense of ownership and stake" (Burdsey, 2002). The second principle is more difficult to prove and, while an evaluation is currently underway, is likely only to be confirmed or refuted over a longer period of time. It could be argued, of course, that the process of participating as agents of change is in itself empowering and a positive contribution to healthy communities and that the fact that it was an ICT project which acted as the catalyst is purely coincidental. This phenomenon has been noted in other contexts, for example the role of local cable TV in encouraging democratic participation (Allen and Miller, 2002).

To summarise, if ICTs are used imaginatively, as in some of the above examples, they can be powerful tools of empowerment. However, there are two prime challenges to meeting this potential: (1) identifying ways of encouraging people in local communities to come up with their own ideas about how ICTs could be used to promote health in their own communities, and (2) identifying means of assessing the contribution of ICTs to health outcomes at community level. Identifying appropriate health assessment methods for challenge (2) is beyond the remit of this chapter but challenge (1) goes to its core. Studies such as that by Rifkin *et al.* (2000) show that people who have been involved in planning and implementing health projects are more likely to support and sustain those projects. Similarly, in the field of community informatics, Day (2002) argues that identifying community needs through participative methods can lead to a more inclusive and holistic approach to community policy and practice.

Participative approaches in health promotion and ICT planning

Participative approaches have indeed been used effectively, as both a tool for health promotion and for involving ordinary people in ICT policy development. Rifkin *et al.* (2000) review the literature on participative tools in health promotion and include illustrative case studies of how some tools have been employed, such as participatory action research and rapid appraisal. Sclove's (1995) participatory design model and his experimental use of participative tools for technology policy-making is also directly relevant, in particular his use of citizens panels (Sclove, 1997a, 1997b), which have also been used in health contexts (Stocking *et al.*, 1991). Other tools, such as scenario workshops, have been used to explore technology in the context of urban sustainability (Street, 1997), and could be adapted for health. Conversely, tools that are widely used in health promotion, such as rapid appraisal, could be adapted for involving people in ICT policy. The following section looks in more detail at three participative tools: citizens' panels, scenario workshops and rapid appraisal, and considers how they might be used to explore ICTs for health promotion.

Citizens' panels

Sometimes called a consensus conference, a citizens' panel consists of a workshop lasting several days, convened to consider a particular issue and during which a lay panel listens to expert testimonials. In the conventional model, the panel must reach a consensus and produce a report for public dissemination. Citizens' panels have been used in the health field to assess technology since the 1970s and in 1984 the King's Fund, the independent UK health services management and policy organisation, developed a programme of citizens' panels to address concerns arising from the over-use of technologies in healthcare (Stocking *et al.*, 1991). In 1997 in the United States, the citizens' panel was used to look at telecommunications and the future of democracy (Sclove, 1997a, 1997b). The aim was to emphasise citizen involvement in policy deliberation: "the goal . . . is to offer a diverse group of non-experts . . . an opportunity to develop and publicize informed judgements on emerging technologies and policies" (Sclove, 1997a).

The main strengths of citizens' panels are that they allow ordinary people to question and engage with experts in a way that is empowering. The process facilitates debate around complex issues and enables ordinary people to have a meaningful input into the debate. Criticisms levelled at the tool are that the number of people able to be involved in the panel is limited, the process tends to be formal in nature and the emphasis on consensus can make it seem inflexible. However, it is always possible to adapt tools to fit the circumstances – a skilful facilitator, for example, could make the process less formal, and the emphasis need not be on consensus. The citizens' panel offers great potential for involving local people in an informed discussion of health issues, information needs and technical possibilities.

Scenario workshops

The Danish Board of Technology developed the scenario workshop. It has been used mainly in the field of urban sustainability and comprises a workshop, lasting several days, with participants from the local community. The workshop members consider and discuss scenarios representing different visions of the future and the results are disseminated publicly.

The scenarios themselves are designed to stimulate discussion and tend, therefore, to be devised around opposing principles. In a health promotion context the opposing principles could be a top-down or expert-driven approach versus a bottom-up, community-driven one. To illustrate the principles of the workshops, an example of the bi-polar focus of scenarios is provided here. At one end of the scenario axis might be the issue of public access and training to use an existing health information service such as NHS Direct Online.[5] In this scenario, the service is top-down and there is no opportunity for the community to modify or produce health information at local level. At the opposite end of the scenario axis might be community access to the tools, skills and training necessary to build an application that would address local issues and enable people to generate local content. The CityNet example cited earlier would provide a useful template for such a scenario. The purpose of using scenarios is not to have one "right" and one "wrong" but to encourage debate amongst participants and to instil confidence to take that debate into new territory.

The scenario workshop is a much more recent tool than the citizens' panel, being developed in the early 1990s, and has had less time for critical evaluation, although Street (1997) offers a useful commentary. Its main strengths appear to be that it facilitates the participation of a wide range of people on an equal footing and that the use of scenarios, which can be grounded in reality and tailored according to local need and context, make it attractive for tackling socially oriented subjects such as community health.

The Danish Board of Technology has looked at the feasibility of the scenario workshop in subject areas other than urban sustainability, including the development of ICT applications to meet the future needs and visions of local people. In particular they considered the provision of information and communication tools and facilities for citizens in local communities and explored the kind of ICT applications which could be used to promote democratic participation and prevent social polarisation in the information society (Andersen, 1995). This work provides a highly relevant model and could be easily adapted to fit a health promotion agenda, exploring the kind of ICT applications which could be used to promote democratic participation in health issues and tackle health inequalities in the information society.

Rapid appraisal

Rapid appraisal, sometimes and more accurately called participatory appraisal, is less dependent than the other two methods on single events such as workshops and is seen more as a process than a tool. It originated in the context of overseas development work and was developed by the Institute of Development Studies at Sussex University in the UK.[6] Rapid appraisal has been described by Chambers (2002) as "a growing family of approaches, methods, attitudes and behaviours to enable and empower people to share, analyse and enhance their knowledge of life and conditions, and to plan, act, monitor, evaluate and reflect". It encourages local people to share information in innovative ways and to participate in the analysis of that information and in finding solutions to problems. For data-gathering, facilitators often use visualisation techniques such as pictures and diagrams in preference to methods which depend on written or verbal skills. The aim of this is to encourage input from those who might have poor literacy skills or who are alienated by officialdom and jargon. It also means that people contribute the information directly, rather than through intermediaries such as interviewers and has the added bonus that most people enjoy working with visual information.

The health promotion practitioners interviewed as part of the research for this chapter were involved in a project using rapid appraisal techniques. The initial stage of the project, a food audit, included a seminar at which participants used their own knowledge to mark on a local map all the initiatives and projects which had anything to do with food. They used colour coding to distinguish between growing and supply; distribution; cooking and education. A photograph in the report (Johnson and Webster, 2000: 17) shows the participants absorbed in this task in a way that is difficult to imagine in a verbal context and the resulting map is a rich source of community information. This type of visual data-gathering is flexible enough to be used in places where people go in their regular routines. The health promotion staff, for example, took flipcharts to shopping areas, parks, schools, bus stops and community festivals and successfully encouraged local people to contribute information about food, thereby building up a rich picture as seen by the people themselves.

Subsequently, groups and individuals from the community met to identify and discuss the issues arising from the data-gathering exercise, many of which revolved around difficulties with shopping and transport. This in turn enabled them to find solutions, some of which required action by the local authority or other statutory bodies while others could be implemented at local level, such as the establishment of a food-buying co-operative, schemes for sharing cooking equipment and cooking classes.

The food-mapping project was part of a larger programme organised by Sustain[7] and the evaluation report indicates some very positive outcomes for the use of rapid appraisal as a tool. It allowed facilitators to reach people who normally would not become engaged in local issues; provided a large amount of good-quality information; allowed people's problems to emerge; encouraged creative solutions and involved policy-makers alongside community members at various stages of the process (Johnson and Webster, 2000: 7). Rifkin *et al.* (2000) came to similar conclusions when they traced the emergence of rapid appraisal as a tool in health contexts from the early 1980s, and they identify many of the same characteristics as Johnson and Webster (2000) which make the approach attractive to those working in health.

Using rapid appraisal to involve people in considerations about ICTs for community health could be challenging, since the issues are more abstract than immediate health concerns such as access to food. However, a community-mapping exercise would be an excellent way to show existing communication channels and information networks as seen by members of the community themselves. The visualisation techniques could also be used to gather data about many health issues and the fact that the tool encourages creative solutions is a positive indicator of its potential value in ICT development.

All participative approaches require considerable commitment on the part of organisers, funders and participants and there is no absolute "right" method. The tools which have been examined here offer different methods of engaging with local communities and it would be possible to use any of those tools in some way or to use elements from them to fashion a new tool for engaging with communities about health and ICTs. In order to take it forward, however, there must be some sort of mechanism to contact and reach the community. Health promotion professionals, already working with communities on health issues, would seem to offer an appropriate access route. The question that then arises is how they would view such an initiative.

Health promotion professionals

Health promotion professionals are key players in community health. They are the bridges between statutory services such as health, education or social services and communities – whether these are geographical, interest-based or socially defined. They act as a link between policy and practice, often working with established community groups on health-related issues. For any participative work around health and ICTs in the community they are an obvious starting point. However, their awareness of and attitudes to participation and ICTs are likely to impact not only on any participative project but also on the communities they currently serve. Qualitative research to inform this chapter was carried out in the summer of 1999 (Marshall, 2000). The research consisted of interviews with a group of staff from East Sussex, Brighton and Hove Health Promotion Service and included a service manager, two community development workers with expertise in coronary disease prevention and food and low income, and an outreach worker – working with homeless people, drug users and sex workers – on HIV prevention. The interviews were structured to elicit some general views about health in the community and, more specifically, their experience of and attitudes to – first – information, communication and ICTs, and – second – community participation and the use of participative tools for health issues in the community. Although there was agreement on the idea that health is a community issue, the attitudes of this group of professionals to ICTs, participation and the meaning of community itself varied considerably and were closely related to the type of work each individual did.

Schuler's model (1996: 12) of six core network values for communities was used to elicit general views of health in the community. Interviewees were encouraged to consider whether Schuler's values, which included health and well-being, information and communication and strong democracy were relevant to their real life situations. All participants spent considerable time studying the model and all saw relevance and resonance: "this is really good. Everything we're trying to do"; "some of these things are what we're trying to provide . . . this is a lot of our work." There was less agreement when the interviews moved on to more specific issues.

Experience of ICTs was limited and attitudes towards them were consequently cautious. They were very aware of access and inequalities issues, citing, for example, older people not having access to computers or lacking the skills and confidence to use them, and poorer families being unable to afford computers. There was a sense of having to defend traditional means of communicating against the threat of new technology and concern about a perceived dehumanising effect, with loss of human contact and interaction. The following comments illustrate this defensiveness and levels of concern: "Communication is meeting, talking, listening, then newsletters and shared opportunities to meet"; "[Communication is] mainly about talking – I do use leaflets but I don't give a lot out. The real value is in one-to-one, the human element"; "I'm worried about [technology] replacing contact . . . I have this picture of people gazing into screens, pressing buttons."

With reference to marginalised groups, there was a sense that ICTs were not relevant, other than as a backup to keep staff informed. There was general enthusiasm, however, for what other groups of people could do with new technology. There was praise, for example, for the design team's use of computer graphics to produce better-quality paper-based information products and for the newly created website.

Participation proved to be more familiar territory. Some of those interviewed had heard about citizens' juries, partly because one of the King's Fund pilots – referred to earlier – took place in Brighton and Hove in 1997 and a member of staff had been involved. [8] None of the group interviewed had heard of scenario workshops but all were interested in the concept. Those working with local communities were committed to the concept underlying participatory design, expressing the belief that local communities themselves hold the key to improving their own health, and they saw themselves working in partnership with the community to bring about change. Two of those interviewed were involved in the rapid appraisal project described earlier in the chapter and they were enthusiastic about the empowering aspect of the approach: "It's a tool to get people involved, in their own patch . . . we work from the premiss that people themselves have the information they need to take things forward."

Working with marginalised groups, on the other hand, gives a different perspective on participation. The outreach worker described the lives of the people he came into contact with as all about daily survival, in an environment where the concepts of community and participation are problematic: "You see it's a dog eat dog thing. And there are hierarchies. And it's ruthless . . . they have to look after number one."

The research interview concluded by asking the participants' views on using participative approaches to explore ICTs for health in the community. The reactions ranged from "what are you waiting for" to a more guarded "it would need a lot more thought". Reactions correlated with the level of community interaction they experienced in their current work, rather than with attitudes towards ICTs.

It was felt that a local participative exercise would contribute to professional learning as well as engaging many ordinary people in the process of technology development. There was some willingness on the part of those interviewed to consider such an exercise and considerable levels of expertise in participative techniques. The amount of preparatory groundwork and the level of funds needed were cited as barriers, although it was also felt that a project around health could be integrated with other community-participative exercises.

This study is a snapshot in time illustrating the views and attitudes of a group of health promotion professionals towards community health, the use of ICTs in their work with communities and participative methods. It shows that the professionals were cautious about using ICTs for health, expressing views which portray ICTs as barriers rather than aids to communication and displaying deep concern about the effects of ICTs on inequality. They were open, in varying degrees, to the suggestion of using participative tools to explore the issues and they had considerable practical experience in using such tools in and with communities. The outreach worker, working with homeless people, posed some additional questions and it is more difficult to see how the participative tools examined here could apply to such marginal groups. Further research on this aspect of the work is required, building on the growing literature on alternative methods for reaching homeless and marginalised people (Power et al., 1999; Power and Hunter, 2001).

The study showed that health promotion professionals could be effective gateways into communities, where their experiences of community work and participative methods would be invaluable.

Conclusion

There is evidence to indicate that ICTs can be effective as tools for health promotion. The examples of *D-code* and the websites developed by deaf people and aphasia sufferers are cited to show this. There is also evidence that involving people in the design and development of community ICT initiatives can contribute to health outcomes, as is shown by the CityNet example. However, the problem of health inequalities is deeply rooted in our society and using ICTs as a health promotion tool could exacerbate the problem. Current policy approaches to tackling health inequalities are cross-sectoral and intended to be inclusive of communities. ICTs can play a part in this process but to do so they must meet community needs and be developed so that local communities are involved in their design and development. Participatory tools, some of which have been discussed here, have been used widely in health promotion contexts and have also been used to explore a more socially responsible and inclusive approach to ICTs. There is therefore a strong theoretical foundation for using participative methods to involve local communities in developing ICTs for health gain. The study of health promotion professionals indicates that such methods could be used effectively on the ground and their experience of community work and community participation would be a valuable asset. The use of participatory tools has the potential to engage local communities in the development of ICT applications as a way of promoting health and addressing health inequality.

Notes

1   See for example Macintyre (1997) and Wilkinson (1996).
2   The Aphasia Help website address is http://www.aphasiahelp.org.uk/
3   Artimedia. The website address is www.artimedia.org.uk
4   The website is no longer live but the project is available as a CD-ROM from the Photographers' Gallery. Details are on their website at http://www.photonet.org.uk/programme/projects.html
5   NHS Direct Online. Launched in 1999, this is a UK government service aimed at the general public, giving information about common diseases and conditions, self-help advice on a range of common symptoms, tips on healthy living and an online enquiry facility. The website address is http://www.nhsdirect.nhs.uk
6   The Institute of Development Studies researches and develops participation methods. Further information is available on their website at http://www.ids.ac.uk/ids/particip/information/index.html
7   Sustain is the UK-based alliance for better food and farming. The website address is http://www.sustainweb.org
8   Unfortunately, she was on maternity leave at the time of the research.

Chapter 7

Cybercafés and national elites
Constraints on community networking in Latin America

Scott S. Robinson

What characterizes a Community Networking/Community Informatics (CN/CI) approach to public computing is a commitment to universality of technology-enabled opportunity including for the disadvantaged; a recognition that the "lived physical community" is at the very center of individual and family well-being – economic, political, and cultural; a belief that this lived community can be enhanced through the judicious use of ICTs; a sophisticated user-focused understanding of Information technology; and applied social leadership, entrepreneurship and creativity.

(Gurstein, 2003)

Introduction

What follows is an exercise in inductive thinking whereby some simple facts, a few strategic omissions in Mexico's Internet public policies, and experience with telecenters allow me to profile a larger scenario challenging the current design and prospects for Latin American community networking and digital inclusion projects. Community networking refers to locally anchored and driven information and communication services. The argument is straightforward: a survey of cybercafés and their clients in Mexico in relation to a new publicly funded connectivity program, scarce, useful online content, and qualitative data from this horizon elsewhere in the region suggest Latin American social and political elites share no significant commitment to digital inclusion policies in their respective national spaces. At the same time, traditional cultural parameters and economic conditions discriminate against extensive public community networking, although the emergence of networking in indigenous organizations and amidst migrants' kin groups are notable exceptions. The overall pattern has dramatic implications for IT public policy and community networking initiatives, their proponents and sponsors in the region, and their opponents both now and in the immediate future.

A regional overview

The regional horizon of digital services being currently rolled out, beyond the urban, national capitals and major cities, throughout Latin America reveals a number of interesting issues worthy of discussion. For example, the region is a mosaic of national connectivity programs with very distinct cost structures for digital services, and only four legislated universal access funds tapping private IT company profits (Brazil, Chile, Peru, and Colombia). Additionally, limitations on adopting new technologies, and lots of hemming and hawing among regulatory agencies, politicians, and the vested carriers (fiber and satellite), as well as hardware and software companies operating in every country combine to restrain policy development and implementation. While there has been a limited, but concerted attempt to create pilot telecenters in many places, usually funded by foreign foundations or development agencies, only a few Brazilian states, Chile, Colombia, and Venezuela as a whole have implemented scaleable official programs with sizeable resources. Such telecenter pilots must be distinguished from their commercial cybercafé cousins, which can be found everywhere today. A telecenter is a cybercafé that offers training in the digital tools and information usage, content development (web pages), is locally anchored, and actively recruits links to community activities, institutions and needs, public and private. While many telecenters aspire to this optimal combination of focus and priorities, most cannot mobilize local initiatives that scale and compete with the simple, fee for service cybercafés. These projects often end up limiting their initial service offerings while looking more like their cousins as time passes (Robinson, 2004). A failed telecenter initiative can easily become just another cybercafé in town, and many have.

Any discussion of telecenters and cybercafés in Latin America today must necessarily engage with larger issues regarding the role of national elites in determining public policy. Issues such as the lack of efficacy of the current neoliberal development model, decapitalized rural economies and extensive emigration, electronic media discourse and influence, political parties, non-governmental organizations, post-Zapatista rebellion, native organizations, emergent social movements, and public policies to achieve what has come to be generically labeled as "digital inclusion" all play a significant role. There is a need to analyze the process whereby these groups and their legitimizing ideas and rhetoric, historical heirs to privilege and power, feed the contemporary process of negotiating power alignments in what are, still, very traditional, hierarchical societies. The observable, yet surprisingly rapid rate of cybercafé expansion and presence (without government subsidies or marked regulatory support), throughout the region, has modified the prescribed medicine for the current affliction known to some as "The Digital Divide." Others, myself included, judge the growing polarization amongst rich and poor as another manifestation of an older concept, known simply in outmoded language as the neocolonial class struggle. This is, of course, a social process, rooted in regional and national history, and has profound implications on its own. The upshot of this complex flow of actors, conceptual paradigms, rules and interests, old and new, plus digital tools and social demands generates a rich *bricolage* with several dimensions in the region. These include the current model of Internet expansion, expensive digital inclusion programs, complacent elites, recent mass media adoption of the web and email for audience interaction, growing privatization of quality university educations, national diasporas, an increasing number of native groups' offices online, an enormous population of cyber semi-literates weaned on the basic skills at their local cyber shop without the will nor the incentives to seek information more useful for their daily wherewithal, together with public educational systems languishing in bureaucratic wrangling, mediocre results, and the growing hegemony of decision-makers weaned in private schools. This essay is a broad-brush sketch of these multicolored thematic tiles that form a backdrop mosaic for the local scenarios of community networking in the region, today and probably tomorrow.

Policy constraints

While Mexico is the second largest economy in the region, behind Brazil, and its political economy is entwined with the United States and Canada as a result of the North American Free Trade Agreement (NAFTA), there is to date no universal access fund sponsoring Internet connectivity throughout the land (to be found among its major trading partners). The telecommunications regulatory authority, COFETEL, remains subservient to the executive branch of the federal government, and the influence of the "dominant carriers" therein is readily apparent. It was only in mid-2002 that long distance charges were eliminated from calls within the same dialing area code. As a consequence, since about 1999 cybercafés began sprouting at a growing rate. Prior to this date Internet access for people in many small towns and villages was very expensive; in effect this *laissez-faire* policy discriminated against widespread cost effective access to the network of networks. Those independent ISPs who competed with the dominant carrier Telmex (Teléfonos de México, with 98 percent of the local telephony market), jousted with the dragon on unequal terms, obliged to use their lines and digital exchanges. In an interview conducted in Cuernavaca, Morelos in June 2002, an independent ISP client suggested that open Telmex lines were being disconnected every ten minutes, forcing ISPs and their customers to place repeat calls for which they were billed. Many small ISPs went under in this climate. The government's public policy seems to be non-existent, allowing the dominant players (competition in long distance and commercial networking services began in 1996) and the "market" to determine the rate of expansion of Internet access beyond urban centers. At the same time, the universal access fund stipulated in the current legislation (1996) was never created nor funded by the COFETEL, no doubt influenced by the reluctant major players whose profits would have been taxed as per the rules elsewhere in the region.

Nevertheless, demand for Internet access increased dramatically, assisted by significant media hype and advertising campaigns plus the pervasive insistence upon email use among radio and television personalities and during talk shows. Secondary school teachers began demanding homework to be digitally printed, using local computer rentals and increasingly, Internet resources (although the teachers remained non-users). In a hopscotch fashion, cybercafés (usually without the coffee) began to appear in small towns, even villages, a room with a few computers for rent, rustic places where one can use the Internet for a modest fee per hour, print some homework, perhaps scan a photograph or two, chat with friends. These are small, mom and pop businesses, often opened next door to or in the back of an ongoing family establishment and operated by young kin who studied computing somewhere, at a commercial training institute with a six-month program in a nearby market town, or perhaps even a few years at a public university or technology school.

The national universe of cybercafés, however, was ignored completely when the Fox regime designed its eMEXICO program in 2001, and finally began to field projects in late 2002. This strategic omission was the latest in this string of non-policies, and quite frankly, was the proverbial last straw, provoking me to conduct a survey of 259 of these establishments in four Mexican states together with a profile of their young digital consumers as well. The overall objective of this exercise was to understand this burgeoning universe of connectivity in previously unsuspecting places and to try to come to grips with the reasons for the evident string of omissions in public policies, in Mexico and elsewhere in the region. What follows are some reflections on these omissions, analysis of the cybercafé profile and user surveys, and their implications.

Institutional stagnation

To my mind, there is a fundamental contradiction between the economies of scale the connectivity technology today permits, and the reluctance of national elites, who largely control content and media regulation in their respective national spaces. Likewise, there is a noteworthy policy stalemate regarding what is to be done given the current stagnation in economic growth in the South, the dot.com slump, reduced international co-operation budgets, emerging low cost connectivity options (WiFi), and bellicose gestures in the North. This policy stalemate is to be found among the international financial institutions (IFIs), the UN agencies (remember the Dot Force?) including the World Bank (whose expensive Development Gateway has failed to catalyze widespread support), major foundation donors, the dot.com players with their philanthropic façades, even within the fledgling NGO-based telecenter movement. The IFIs are trapped inside their 1944 BrettonWoods *modus operandi* whereby, in the name of national sovereignty, they are unwilling or technically unable to oblige their shareholder members to adopt policies on a regional basis, with the corresponding economies of scale and impact. Consequently, the growing levels of poverty have made the earlier "Internet for All" declarations seem ingenuous and self-serving.

The model for Internet expansion in Latin America is strictly based on market demand. While the Latin elites were at first slow or reluctant to embrace the virtues of digital services and products, the pace has quickened since the late 1990s. Today, national and now regional elites, a mixture of intermarried families inheriting colonial privileges and a *nouvelle bourgeoisie* – the product of intelligence mixed with savvy deals with foreign companies, their products and marketing networks – are increasingly articulated by regional common market agreements and the corresponding joint ventures these permit and impose. By now they have incorporated the full range of digital tools and services permitted by their respective commercial, financial, media, and political domains. The Internet is here to stay, but, I will argue, as a new, additional instrument of political control by a privileged few. Beyond this small minority not many can afford basic much less broadband services that tap the potential of the technology and its increasingly rich content. From the lower middle class down to the base of the socio-economic pyramid – the poor, semi-literate and disenfranchised – remain without the means nor perhaps the incentives to get online and find scarce, appropriate content for their personal, family, and community welfare.

Zero growth and dual economies

The current stagnation in the Latin American economies reveals a pattern of de facto zero growth more than two years in the making. This translates into national and regional scenarios of massive out-migration; more and more people, women included, from rural areas whose products are worth less in the market, often due to dumping of subsidized agricultural products in the North, are heading out, with or more probably without papers to the United States and Europe, via Spain and Italy. Ecuador is the prime example. Food security is becoming an issue as population growth outpaces subsistence staples and environmental degradation is a threat in many places. Public institutions, under international pressure to privatize key public services, are taxed beyond limit to deliver education and health care for all citizens, including the migrants' families whose remittances increasingly resolve balance of payments problems and feed those remaining at home, in the villages and urban slums. The return or consolidation of a neocolonial dual economy is evident: a minority control financial services and oligopolistic markets while the vast majority live in poverty and families plan their emigration strategies in the widespread exodus currently underway. One market system sells products to and for the rich, including Internet services, and another, the one economists call the informal sector, provides a subsistence living for the vast majority who buy from the oligopolies and sell whatever they can in the way of products and services to each other. Remittances are now financing the survival of a good share of the non-banking informal sector, urban and rural, in many countries. To date, the Internet is *not* an instrument of communication and commerce for those immersed in this predigital system of exchanges.

Other processes have also altered the panorama in regard to the new digital tools. The tools themselves have matured while the former national telecommunications monopolies, recently privatized, have skillfully manipulated the regulatory frameworks, most often to their advantage, and laid fiber optic cables to serve their until now protected markets of corporate and government customers. Residential customers pay much more for dialup services in the South than their consumer cousins in the North. Mobile wireless telephony now outnumbers fixed line customers almost everywhere, but the providers tend to be the same companies; their challenge now is how to get their customers to pay for more services, including short messages. Some competitors now offer broadband connections via satellite, an expensive novelty in the region, therefore assuring access for all those with the ability to pay, at best 3 percent of the national populations. Connectivity has become the handmaiden of elite-controlled commerce, banking, media, and private education, and as a consequence the Internet has been absorbed as another instrument of social and political control. The promotion of e-government may be a shrewd substitute for e-governance.

Perhaps to offset this predictable (in hindsight) state of affairs, the international community has been preaching digital inclusion, but the rhetoric has focused on the Digital Divide, i.e. between those online (and hence metaphorically inserted in the information and knowledge networks that connectivity purportedly instigates) and those whose lives remain untouched by digital access to information. Little has been said in the official documents – generated at numerous UN agency-sponsored conferences – about the link between this Divide and the neoliberal developmental model that currently exacerbates poverty while permitting the growing enrichment of a powerful few, a situation elegantly argued by attendees at successive World Social Fora in Porto Alegre, Brazil. Class polarization among rich and poor is not addressed as a root cause of the "so-called" Digital Divide among the established institutional players who reject state-led solutions. Rather, the official Newspeak insinuates that computers and access are necessary antecedents for learning and poverty reduction, ignoring the structural constraints that digital inclusion projects are designed to conceal or mitigate.

The regional mass media have embraced the Internet as a marketing tool – often for their own investments in parallel Internet services – and to create an illusion of potential audience interaction with newscasters, cultural commentary programs, occasional government officials, and more importantly, pop music stars and their fan clubs. The advertising for brands and shops in the upscale shopping malls that serve the elites and the minority middle class wannabees in every Latin American city has become over time a mixture of traditional print media and web-based promotions keyed to television merchandising. The amount of traffic on the MTV en Español web server is an indicator of the recent articulation between programming geared to a youth market with the ability to pay and their probable Internet access. Mexico, for example, is a dual economy of limited, if not zero, growth, comprising regional monopolies, thousands of micro-enterprises, and millions living from remittances sent home by migrant kin.

Beyond political parties

Another process of growing significance has been the rapid spread of citizen-based Non-Governmental Organizations over the past decade or more. These NGOs are now engaged in low-intensity conflict with traditional political parties, themselves beholden to old guard elites who seldom represent any political interests other than their own and who consider electoral politics to be their rightful monopoly point of action and *raison d'être*. Many Latin American political parties languish in the age of politics where media is open to the highest bidder. A subtle crisis in governance is underway. Charismatic colonels can now win elections with the aid of incongruous coalitions of political interests united around platforms that fail to make connectivity and relevant content for the people a priority, although the campaign rhetoric may occasionally offer succulent promises of such goals. On many issues and in many countries, the NGOs have eclipsed the political parties on a range of contemporary issues including human rights, environmental concerns, and nowadays, digital inclusion. At the same time, their increasing sophistication has propelled them into public policy debates where their grasp of the issues and technical details often surpasses that of the political parties and their leadership. At the fringe, native organizations struggle to learn the use of ICT tools while building coalitions and weaving expanding networks of sympathizers. However, the old-line parties who still control the electoral and parliamentary machinery, including those that used to be considered to be on the Left, distrust the NGOs and native groups seeking "autonomy," effectively blocking digital public policy innovations they cannot control and do not understand. This impasse among the parties and NGOs is in effect a crisis in the system of political representation, and has stagnated substantive public policy debates in many countries.

A networked society is anathema to traditional patterns of patronage and political controls, and this plays out in many ways. The blatant ignorance of many members of relevant parliamentary telecoms commissions points to an ostrich in the sand approach; there are disturbing signs of Luddite attitudes among some progressives, distrustful perhaps of transparency and more fluid information flows. Meanwhile, the NGOs remain outside the orthodox political playing field, often fragmented, haggling about strategies while competing for foreign donor funding and performing on the few international venues the UN and other agencies patronizingly offer from time to time. On balance, the mainline instruments of political representation have refrained from embracing digital inclusion as a platform priority. The question of connectivity and public access to the digital tools is, to my mind, a key issue where opinions and political commitments vary dramatically, and where the ignorance of the issues re digital inclusion has led to a remarkable degree of negligence on the part of the traditional political parties whose platforms seldom, if ever, make bold gestures in this direction or reflect an understanding of the stakes at risk. These old guard actors resist becoming digital stakeholders, perhaps fearful that the process will compromise their power and sovereignty.

The observed rush to connectivity for the ruling minority has been accompanied by shrewd manipulations of the regulatory framework. Access to the regulatory commissioners in each national market is dominated by the same group of hardware, software, and carrier megaplayers we all know: IBM, Hewlett Packard, Sun, Dell, Microsoft, Oracle, Global Crossing, Cable and Wireless, Hughes, Gilat, PanAmSat, New Skies and others. In effect, their subsidiaries and lawyers in each national space are writing the de facto rules for entering markets with new technology that may or may not threaten legacy players with their first-to-market products. The subsequent closed system of rules and regulations is not conducive to technological innovation and might be put to the test very soon given the perfection and consumer roll out of the Wireless Fidelity (WiFi) technology using the 802.11g technical specs operating on the unlicensed (not everywhere) 2.4GHz spectrum.

Some companies may invest more resources in fighting rule changes that affect their market share than they spend on the development or offerings of better and lower-cost products and services in the Latin American markets. One forthcoming battle could see the more recent broadband carriers, including some satellite firms, all with unsold overcapacity on their fiber and transponders, teaming with local WiFi entrepreneurs anxious to reduce the market share and hence, power of the legacy players. But the challenge remains the limited purchasing power (and IT skills) of the urban lower middle class who could entertain the options in the name of greater educational opportunities for their children who are not finding the anticipated level of access at school nor appropriate content with incentives at the local cybercafés. To date, rural constituencies appear to be beyond the focus of policy-makers and local organizations have priorities other than building community IT networks and learning online.

Elite complacency

In this period of zero growth and dual economies, elite complacency with their recently acquired connectivity in their upscale market is a worrisome new factor to be considered. History suggests the neocolonial elites in Latin America are a voracious lot, intent on retaining their hereditary control of banking, commerce, media, and politics – in short, the reins of power in their respective territories – at all costs. Despite evidence of factionalism, these elites are now partners or business associates with transnational interests, especially in the digital tele-communications services market, and enjoy the privileges of membership in the dominant class of their national space. These privileges include a private educational system that guarantees elite reproduction, and the care and feeding of the Internet is one aspect of this pedagogical challenge. There is no question these national elites have incorporated the technology into their system of private schools and universities and it is the first generation of graduates from these institutions that has largely fueled the Internet rollout in all the countries of the region, and staff the regulatory commissions and the few extant digital inclusion programs as well. But it should be clearly stated this has become a self-serving procedure, and whereas these groups have integrated the digital tools into their domains and instruments of control, we must question their commitment to offering the tools and information access to the vast majority of their impoverished national populations. It is my contention this commitment is non-existent or very limited, especially in times of zero growth, and as a consequence, this is one of the factors contributing to the Internet stagnation scenario found throughout the region today and bodes ill for the immediate future.

Legacy players

The magical thinking (or is it thinking magic?) behind the now standard formulas for offering Internet services to the public in the geographically and culturally diverse Latin American states is both confusing and stagnant. The current pattern of national connectivity programs suggests they are in fact designed to protect and expand legacy markets for legacy players. Witness the design of the eMEXICO project wherein the bidding procedures are crafted so only the major players with large-scale systems and proprietary software may participate. In the case of Mexico, there is no commitment – on the part of either the political parties or the identifiable elites presently in power – to sacrifice a degree of revenues from the national budget to subsidize a national connectivity program which focuses on content and the incentives to use the tools and available information. Rather, the current design calls for state subsidies for market expansions and protection of the established players. This is not my brand of universal access; on the contrary, it is another way these firms can externalize costs while securing their oligopolistic markets for the near future. This is risk management at the people's expense, with the ruse that state-subsidized mass connectivity will lead to some murky degree of integration into the Information Society.

While the ramping up of national connectivity programs progresses in many countries – under the modality of market protection – the *New Washington Consensus* pervades the philanthropic and telecommunications policy atmosphere and networks. The United States appears eager to aggressively defend its perceived national interests, markets, and access to strategic resources wherever it chooses and no matter what. This unfortunate post 9/11 policy shift coincides with the telecommunications oversupply glut in Latin America and elsewhere, the growing realization that market-driven development strategies to reduce poverty in the region are not working, and, I fear, a perceptible move to giving more priority to policies and instruments of social control using the fear of terrorism as a device for mobilizing support and legitimacy for this strategic realignment. Granting more access to information may be less a priority under this shifting strategic framework than before 9/11, wherein the antiterrorism rhetoric justifies shackling innovation lest the radicals get their hands on powerful new tools, a probable ex post facto fret. At the same time a dynamic class polarization is underway, whereby the poor are increasing in number and the rich are fewer and even richer. As noted, national elites in Latin America, now in firm control of their recently privatized state apparatus, are a good example of this pattern, and their interests are to be seen in the design of national connectivity programs such as eMEXICO, Compartel (Colombia), and those being proposed (Ecuador). These projects are not about digital inclusion, as purported, rather they are designed, as noted, to expand and protect markets controlled by incumbent hardware, software and telecommunication players. Similarly, the highly touted e-government programs may be a synonym for social control wherein the citizen is conceived as a mere consumer of information while facilitating minor administrative chores. At this juncture, it appears policies are focused on helping business and solving practical problems of political control, downplaying issues of public domain information, rather than reinforcing the digital commons and providing useful, culturally appropriate content for novice digital consumers.

Digital *foquismo*

At the same time, many, myself included, are awakening from a lengthy slumber, a "digital *foquismo* fantasy," wherein we believed, analogous to the ingenuous guerrilla movements' strategy of the 1960s and beyond, that people will rise up, demand, and use online information in novel ways, if only we will bring a community telecenter near them! The "*foco*" was/is the locus of action outsiders may set in motion, and "*foquismo*" is the frame of mind that believes this will happen. Experience suggests there is no guarantee this will occur as a magical act of will. Many NGOs, with generous international funding, have spent the last three years or more, and considerable personal energy and resources, creating these micro institutions offering connectivity and training in periurban slums and rural places; but when the new cybercafé, or whatever it may be called, opens down the street or across the plaza, the telecenter is no longer financially sustainable. It cannot compete offering training and content creation services that are in fact under-priced and that few are able and even willing to pay for. Most often, the value-added dimension (mixed with the "information and digital skills will make you free" litany) is insufficient to generate loyal customers and satisfied users in impoverished places, often living off Diaspora remittances. Today, I wager there are very few community telecenters worthy of rigorous certification under this label. And all this occurs in a political climate where the elites (and the companies they represent) are delighted that others may invest their scarce resources in generating future demand for their products and services. On balance, there are few commitments at the level of national governments to invest in social capital, subsidizing telecenter connectivity, training program costs, and culturally appropriate content. For this reason, community telecenters cannot remain open for long once the original funding has been exhausted, and nearby commercial cybercafés offer a lower cost point of access. The issue of telecenter sustainability is linked to this overarching political ambience wherein the State and its managers ignore community initiatives: in fact may even scorn them as illegitimate meddling in their traditionally hegemonic space. At the same time, there is little value or political virtue attached to distributing what should be public information in the public domain. The Information Commons is a concept far afield of shrewd neocolonial elites, including the political parties, intent on maintaining their power and influence in spite of the new digital tools.

Cybercafé survey

The question of the legitimacy and sustainability of community telecenters has been on my agenda for some time. The experience of creating and managing three such facilities in northern Morelos State, in central Mexico, provided ample opportunity to learn some lessons the hard way and face the studied indifference of local officials, political parties, and even government digital connectivity programs. At the same time, the influx of small cybercafés in the small towns and villages served by the Morelos pilot telecenter project created a challenge to telecenter sustainability, a new situation that merited study and analysis. However, a small sample in three rural towns clearly would be insufficient to generate a pattern of behavior of the small cyber shops and their young customers, so a larger survey was in order. This opportunity presented itself in the middle of the year 2002, when it became clear, as noted above, that the government's eMEXICO initiative was getting underway without any mention whatsoever, much less taking into account, of the growing number of cybercafés spread throughout the land (and now distributed throughout all Latin American countries). A decision was made to attempt to survey the universe of cybercafés in four, small Mexican states: Aguascalientes, Colima, Morelos, and Tlaxcala. A subset of another 20 cybercafés was also included from a rural region of the State of Mexico adjacent to Morelos. Two survey questionnaires were developed, one to profile each cybercafé in the sample and another to profile what their customers do in these micro businesses. A total of 259 cybercafés were included in the sample and the series charts, available online, exhibit a profile of these small shops (de la Paz Sylva and Robinson, 2000). The variety of variables compared merit further discussion.

What stands out immediately is the number of these cybercafés in the four, small single-city states surveyed. This is also an indication of the demand for digital services on the part of those who cannot afford the equipment and monthly service charges from home and do not have access at school or at work, and all before the government's digital inclusion program rollout. This distribution profile reflects the relative lack of access for most, and at the same time indicates the tardiness of universal service public policy initiatives in Mexico. Only two state governments have connectivity programs, Guanajuato and Puebla, and neither co-operate with their universe of in state cybercafes. The only community telecenter project *per se* is the one operating in northern Morelos for which I am in part responsible (Robinson, 2002). This is an uncanny situation for a nation of 100 million people and, allegedly, the world's twelfth economy. The federal government's eMEXICO initiative faces an uphill battle, against both the universe of small, undercapitalized, and fragile mom and pop cyber shops, and the poor accountability of the bureaucratic culture extant in the public secondary schools and municipal offices where the program is beginning to install equipment with Internet connectivity.

The results from this research project indicate that most digital consumers are young, students, and are often sent by teachers to use the cybercafés during the school year. Occasionally, some teachers also use cybercafé facilities. However, the fact that very few school teachers are cyber-shop users today bodes ill for a rapid expansion of users in the school system, as government policy-makers plan. That 83 percent of users are younger than 25 bespeaks a budding culture of consumption in this age group. It also implies a growing polarization between young cyber-literates and the rest of the population.

Some alarming implications

The survey illustrates that the provision of training and local content develop-ment provides a clear distinction between community telecenters and commercial cybercafés. Only a third of commercial cybercafés offer training courses, and where training is provided it focuses on tool usage rather than information-processing or management. The cost of connectivity is not cheap – given average incomes in rural places – and users average less than an hour of online time per session, which is not much in terms of the immense amount of online resources available.

The research offers an interesting profile of the true pattern of digital consumption, and no doubt close to the mark for young people of both sexes in most Internet café users throughout the region. With 43 percent of online time devoted to chatting and email, we can surmise this is, on balance, playful behavior, having fun while interacting, often with sexual overtones and intent, with others. The interviewers confirmed this in private conversations, after the questionnaires were administered to users in each cybercafé during the survey. As a teacher in a public university, I find it distressing that only 26 percent of users' time, the last priority, is spent with homework. It should also be noted that the nature of this "homework" requires some scrutiny: the value of cut and paste homework papers, printed on lovely color printers, is rather limited, compared to reading texts, finding data, and synthesizing this information into a text draft of one's own authorship.

This situation of constrained digital tool usage in a context of few incentives for learning is worrisome. In fact, this may be the key factor that points to a digital consumption syndrome based on games, play, reinforcement of sports fetishism, and virtual sex that leaves the learning function far behind. If the young consumers are playing and complying with cut and paste homework assignments, can we then assume this *habitus* is here to stay and will be difficult to transform? I fear this is the case, and should be a premise for digital public policy planning in Latin America from here on out. The observed pattern of digital consumption in the cybercafé survey is alarming especially as national connectivity plans do not appear to recognize the need to generate useful research about ongoing digital consumption behavior. Similarly, programs are not designed to address the limitations of cyber-shop profiles, or what cyber-shop users are doing or need. The research reveals data suggesting users, in fragile businesses without community buy-in or official support, are less interested in learning, and much more motivated to what is playful and entertaining. It appears online behavior may simply be a continuation of media consumption patterns already well established by radio and television; the well-prophesized media-induced social control syndrome may have arrived full tilt.

Postmodern breaks

The cybercafé survey data suggest what we may call a "postmodern break" at work in traditional places. I would argue this rupture or break in tradition is to be found in the chat and pornography consultation behavior in the commercial cybercafés, where the youthful consumers are largely free to do whatever they want, with some exceptions. The contrast between this pattern of private consumption of online delights and what is permissible at home and in the village public square is indeed dramatic. Cybercafés in traditional cultural spaces are provoking a schizoid syndrome whereby young digital consumers are observing taboo images, and enjoying access to realms of sexual and other information they are prohibited to even discuss at home or in school. With a public education system in perpetual crisis, underfunded by governments beholden to elite interests, reluctant to channel more fiscal resources to public schools, sex education programs hampered by Catholic Church pressures, and "modernizing" initiatives managed by technocrats from private schools (including eMEXICO) that are culturally distant from their "subjects," it may well be that cybercafés in remittance economies are de facto training grounds for tomorrow's migrants. An absence of knowledge seeking is remarkable throughout the survey of cybercafé users and, to my imagination, forebodes a deepening of the crisis in public education where the infrastructure is rustic, teachers are underpaid and therefore not well motivated to innovate, rules of discipline are slack, and no one is expelled under normal circumstances (at least not in Mexico). Why should one continue in school if there are no jobs to be found?

Meanwhile, the Diaspora economies of the South are living and eating thanks to remittances from kin in the North. Whereas multilaterals sponsor research about the expansion of the remittance economies, there are few official efforts to lower today's usurious transfer costs, although increased competition has halved the rates in two years. The use of telecenters and cybercafés for families communicating with migrant kin is limited, not for lack of trying, but simply because migrants inside the United States, for example, do not, paradoxically, have ready access to connectivity, much less training to use the tools, nor share information-seeking values. There are notable exceptions, but free Internet service is only available in public libraries, which are not friendly places for illegal *latino* migrants inside USA.

Where are the action proposals making available digital tools that can lead to the reduction of transaction costs, allowing local, micro finance organizations to manage savings and credit in novel modes for those whose sacrifices lead to foreign exchange equilibria for the national elites? The political will to exercise available instruments of power to enable migrant communities to invest in digital instruments that lower communication and remittance sending costs and increase the resources available at home is absent. The hometown associations of migrants could pay for digital inclusion projects, if the national policy environments were friendly.

Skewed community networking

As a consequence of the above factors and argument, we are now at a turning point re the use of digital tools for social development in the context of the evolving political economy of IT in the dual Latin American societies. It is fair to assert that community networking in fact never arrived in the region, because it was unwelcome or lacked the policy and cultural incentives to seed and thrive beyond the elites. The networking to be found reflects the polarized social hierarchy of rich and poor. This kind of networking cannot be catalyzed with the young users in cybercafés who are largely poor and disenfranchised and more focused on online play plus personal and family survival issues rather than commitments to their community. My experience tells me that local political leadership, at the community level, ignores these questions, and may even fear the technology. While tradition rules at home, it may limit initiatives in the cybercafés in rural spaces as well. Thus while the elites have taken care of themselves, a stilted form of community networking to be sure, the poor may be destined to limited access and few incentives to use the available tools and information. This does not mean that community networking is absent among the indigenous and rural communities of the region, most of whom are immersed in traditional forms of exchange They are, however, increasingly dependent upon remittances from diasporic community members for their wherewithal nowadays and as a consequence are open to pragmatic innovations that reduce their communication and money transfer costs.

The current design of publicly funded digital inclusion programs in the region suggest the issue is not so much about money any more, rather about the political will to design cost-effective projects that offer services with culturally appropriate content and impetus among those groups already networking the old fashioned way. These options are now available with the legacy digital tools and those emerging from the ever present and dynamic innovation pipeline (e.g. Wireless Fidelity linked to the Internet by satellite connections). To my mind these programs are not attuned to the needs of presently unconnected potential users. It is evident the current digital culture created and supported by the consumption patterns of the Latin elite will continue to grow – albeit slowly – while vain attempts are made to expand these offerings to a mass market that does not exist. The recent history of bankrupt dot.coms in Latin America and elsewhere, plus the ongoing consolidation of today's most profitable enterprises, together with media convergence, all point to a merger fest that reinforces elite control of the dual economy at hand.

The few remaining pilot telecenters will struggle with user-focused learning and community networking stimulae in scarce supply. The limited extent of Internet penetration in most countries combined with government digital inclusion programs skewed to favor business not citizens mean that elites – and those that aspire to emulate their lifestyle and cultural consumption – dominate the consumption of digital resources. To my mind, this is a betrayal of the potential for greater democracy that can be achieved through community networking and more open access to online public information – processes that are wanting in the region.

This chapter does not paint an optimistic portrait. However, there is hope: perhaps two key groups, the diaspora and indigenous networks which often overlap will provide demand, some capital, and the will to innovate, adding digital tools to their extant transnational community circuits. This will require new forms of thinking, technical expertise, partnerships, and negotiating skills. While presently poorly equipped, these two constituencies are ripe for new forms of community networking.

Chapter 8

"Informationalizing" El Salvador

Participatory design of a national information and ICT strategy

Christina Courtright

Introduction

In the context of the worldwide information revolution, development agencies and policymakers have sought ways to help low-income nations take advantage of the benefits of information and communication technologies (ICTs) in order to overcome their historical disadvantages (e.g. Accenture *et al.*, 2001; World Bank, 1998). As the industrialized world widens its development lead with the help of global markets and the Internet, a significant proportion of the world's population continues to lack adequate food, housing, sanitation, education, income, or human rights (UNDP, 2001). Many influential opinions hold that the lack of digital technology is crucial in maintaining these "digital divides," and that therefore digitally focused strategies can lead the way toward their eventual mitigation (e.g. Analysys Consulting, 2000). Although it may be true that the failure to adopt information and communication technologies (ICT) is likely to worsen a nation's development prospects (Mansell and Wehn, 1998), no systematic, reliable evidence exists to explain *how* introducing ICT will in fact help bridge existing divides (Heeks, 1999; Menou, 1999). In addressing this challenge, it may be more useful to shift attention from ICT-led analyses and strategies to a broader development perspective that seeks to leverage the digital potential within each context:

> The central point in the debate about the digital divide should not be what is the best way to bring ICT to the poor, but what is the best way for the poor to take advantage of ICT in order to improve their lot.
>
> (Menou, 2001: 6)

In this view, then, strategies to help nations leverage information and ICTs for development should address traditional development problems in search of innovative ways to weave ICT appropriately into solution efforts, rather than start with ICT as an assumption. Using concrete development problems as a starting point will, in turn, shed light on *whether* ICT is even useful in a given context, and if so, *how*. This chapter will provide an illustration of this approach as it was implemented through a participatory action exercise in El Salvador, the smallest nation in Central America.

Background on El Salvador

Official statistics for El Salvador provide partial insights into the extent of its development challenges.[1] There are 6.2 million Salvadorans in a nation the size of Massachusetts (21,000 km^2). Over one-third of the population are under the age of 15; almost half live in urban centers, primarily in the capital and its outlying settlements; and one-third work in agriculture. The average income per capita is US$4,344, but its distribution is severely skewed: the wealthiest 10 percent receive 39.3 percent of national income, while the poorest 10 percent receive only 1.4 percent, and 26 percent earn less than US$1 per day. Life expectancy is 69.1 years; infant mortality is 35 per 1,000, and 26 percent of Salvadorans lack access to safe water.

The government spends 16 percent of its national budget on education, compared with, for example, 23 percent in Mexico and Costa Rica. Net primary school enrollment is 78 percent, and net secondary school enrollment is 22 percent. Adult literacy for women is 75.6 percent, and 81.3 percent for men. In all, El Salvador ranks 95 out of 162 in the UNDP Human Development Index (2001), and has shown a gradual improvement over the past 20 years in comparison with other countries.

The nation's civil war (1980–92), Hurricane Mitch (1998), and a series of severe earthquakes (2001) have not only widened disparities but also produced a net outflow of migrants. Approximately one-fifth of all Salvadorans have left the country over the past two decades (Landolt et al., 1999), and their family remittances totaled $1.75 billion dollars in 2000 – equivalent to 60 percent of export income, and covering 90 percent of the trade deficit (Banco Central de Reserva, 2001).

In terms of connectivity, El Salvador had approximately 7.6 telephone lines per 100 inhabitants and 25 lines per 100 households in 1999 (International Telecommunication Union, 1999). The national telephone company was privatized the previous year, and competition among land-line, cellular, and wireless service providers has only recently begun to flourish. By year's end there were 16 Internet service providers, with bandwidths ranging from 128 KBps to 4.5 MBps, yet with no interconnection among them, so that messages between local ISPs are routed through other countries (Ibarra, 2000). In 2001, the UNDP ranked El Salvador 54th of 72 countries in its Technological Achievement Index, which measures human skills and infrastructural development. This places the nation below the list of "leaders" or "potential leaders," primarily in Europe and North America, but above "marginalized" nations, most of which are located in Africa (UNDP, 2001: 45).

In terms of information distribution, in 1999 there were only 13 public libraries and approximately 125 "cultural centers" containing small collections of books, supplemented by dozens of specialized libraries in government and international agencies throughout the nation's capital.[2] There are five daily newspapers with a combined circulation of 48 per thousand inhabitants, 465 radio sets per thousand, and 677 television sets per thousand (United Nations Economic, Scientific and Cultural Organization, 1999). A network of 20 community radio stations struggles to preserve its FM frequencies despite legislation that favors commercial interests.[3]

Development strategy for a digital world: the case of El Salvador

Statistics provide only a partial sketch of the challenges El Salvador must overcome in order to adequately leverage ICTs for development, and they do not illuminate the best path to achieve this. A combination of history, culture, institutions, infrastructure, government type, and goals generate the context within which each country forges its own development path (Castells, 1996). Thus, a national stock-taking and strategy-building exercise was implemented recently in El Salvador in order to identify and analyze trends that favored or impeded the use of ICTs and information for development, and to propose an improved development path. The exercise included participatory analysis of traditional development problems, re-framing of the problems as information-related challenges, and project formulation.

In 1997, the World Bank and the government of El Salvador agreed to explore possible strategies that could help the nation position itself to take advantage of the worldwide information revolution, and a small grant was allocated to undertake a nationwide study. This effort, a prelude to a future loan, was meant to complement an existing World Bank-sponsored program for enhancing El Salvador's competitiveness in today's global, interconnected marketplace. It also accompanied an incipient educational reform process, launched soon after the country emerged from a 12-year civil war that was settled by negotiations and democratic reforms. Two local co-ordinators and one external consultant were hired to conduct the study, with oversight by the two sponsoring institutions but with broad discretion in terms of possible directions to take toward meeting that general goal.

The co-ordinators based their approach on two key assumptions: (1) changes in development agendas do not only occur through government and inter-national development aid, but also require a considerable "investment" by stakeholders at all levels affected by policy; and (2) the challenge El Salvador faced was not a priori one of adding technology, but was instead a broader question of how information and knowledge could be created, retrieved, shared, assimilated, and utilized more advantageously in everyday activities.[4] Thus, the team designed a broad-based participatory method (cf. Sanoff, 1990; Schuler and Namioka, 1993) to guide a program of nationwide discussions and studies. The goal was to explore the real and potential uses of information and knowledge in the context of existing socio-economic relations, culture, structures, and practices. The program was given an organizing name: Conectándonos al Futuro de El Salvador.

Program design

After weeks of preparatory discussions with a broad range of policymakers and development practitioners, six areas were chosen in which a better utilization of information and knowledge might lead to significant improvement in El Salvador's development prospects: education, relations with emigrants, community and municipal development, rural development, small- and micro-enterprise, and public and private large-scale organizations. For each area, program co-ordinators invited between ten and twelve stakeholders from a variety of organizations, institutions, and perspectives to join focus groups, or "learning circles," led by an outside moderator and one of the two co-ordinators. The goal of each circle was to envision what a "learning society" might look like in that area or sector, identify and analyze critical obstacles to that vision, and propose small-scale, innovative projects to leverage strengths and overcome weaknesses. Although the worldwide digital revolution and its implications for El Salvador were taken as the general context in which the discussions took place (Courtright, 1997), ICT was not the leading focus; instead, the role of ICT was located within a broader strategy of "informationalizing" development, that is, improving the creation, exchange, and usage of knowledge and information within broad development activities (cf. Castells, 1996; Menou, 1991).

The work of the learning circles was complemented by concurrent action and research projects. The action projects were focused on designing sample ICT services that related to learning circle discussions, to serve as points of reference. In one example, stakeholders in El Salvador called on telecenter pioneers in Peru to help lay out the blueprint for a national telecenter network that would respond to the issues and goals raised in the six learning circles. To this end, dozens of meetings were held with Salvadorans from all walks of life to discuss the concept of telecenters and their potential use in a variety of settings. Each meeting brought together a mix of sectors to ensure varying opinions and stimulate broader discussion. In another effort, the co-ordinator of the community-development learning circle led workshops in two different towns, in which stakeholders conceptualized and designed the elements of a local Web site, based on their assessment of its purpose and intended audience.

The research studies were commissioned on topics that would flesh out many of the problems identified in the learning circles: telephone density and Internet connectivity, government information policy and accessibility of its information resources, government ICT infrastructure and training, international migrant networking practices, technology transfer practices in local agriculture, environmental information resources, and institutional and legislative constraints on e-commerce. In addition, case studies of knowledge management practices in three important institutions (one bank and two ministries) were conducted to illustrate the challenges facing large organizations in El Salvador. Finally, once each learning circle had identified the critical issues in its area, and before they proceeded to the project proposal stage, an international e-conference was held to solicit "best practices" used in other countries to address similar critical issues (Conectándonos al Futuro de El Salvador, 1999).

The results of the diverse activities were collated and drafted into a proposed strategy and specific projects, after which they were discussed further in an open assembly and finalized in a document presented to the government, the nation, and the World Bank (Courtright *et al.*, 1999). Although Conectándonos al Futuro was officially concluded, many of its members continued their involvement in the issues it raised by participating in the incipient national network of telecenters, Asociación Infocentros.

Summary of principal outcomes

Instead of issuing sweeping recommendations, each learning circle devised one or more information-centered projects that could be piloted, evaluated, and scaled up accordingly. Each project was expected to have a demonstration effect and show how innovative ways of conceiving and addressing information flows and knowledge problems could re-channel development efforts with a minimum of funding. Many of the projects – but not all – were predicated upon the success of a telecenter network. In addition, several of the studies commissioned during the research program pointed to the need for broader policy recommendations at the level of the central government. The following are summaries of each group's diagnostics, including the new approaches and policies they proposed on the basis of their analysis.

The education group found that the postwar educational reform, while highly consistent with "learning society" goals, has not gone beyond administrative changes; teachers have neither the incentive nor the means to learn new ways of teaching. The considerable foreign assistance allocated for building multimedia centers in secondary schools will be ineffective if teachers are not encouraged to become flexible learners, with or without technology. In response, participants analyzed and proposed projects that favored localized learning circles among teachers, preferably with mechanisms to encourage sharing outcomes more broadly, as well as a policy to build target telecenters in communities whose secondary schools have multimedia centers, so that both students and teachers could reinforce learning.

The learning circle on migrants concluded that Salvadorans who emigrate acquire new skills and knowledge that can assist businesses, communities, and national-level projects; evidence shows they are anxious to maintain both cultural and economic ties while making a contribution to development. Yet an almost-exclusive focus on capturing remittances overlooks the multiplying potential of such non-monetary contributions. Participants proposed policies to encourage both migrants and locals to share knowledge and create information that would be valuable and interesting to both, by promoting commercial and cultural exchanges; involving skilled expatriates in academic, science, and technology programs; and hiring Salvadorans abroad to assist in internationally funded development projects, among others. In particular, the group stressed the need to document and disseminate the skills, interests, and talents of Salvadorans around the world.

El Salvador's 262 municipalities are relatively weak, yet opportunities can be found in recent tendencies toward administrative decentralization, organization and solidarity among mayors, and increases in mandated funds from the national budget. Although international organizations have often documented local conditions in great detail, this information has not been returned to local residents to help in planning. Members of the local development learning circle identified a critical need for inter-municipal programs to help local coalitions inventory their own communities and utilize this information in planning, together with data already collected by international organizations. In addition, they proposed co-ordination and exchange activities among municipalities nationwide, with or without electronic networking. A facilitator worked with two rural towns to conceptualize and design Web sites that reflected the type of information each town felt was necessary for both local and international use.

The rural sector is characterized by excruciating poverty and lack of education, declining agricultural activities, deterioration of the environment, and depletion of natural resources. Two key components in this vicious downward spiral are the lack of critical information and the lack of adequate methods of knowledge and technology transfer. Funding programs have not managed to reverse any of these trends due to institutional weaknesses and failure to target deeper problems. The rural development group proposed projects that focus on knowledge creation and transfer within rural sectors, independent of ICT use. A related project stressed the participatory creation of economic, social, and cultural information products by and for rural residents, to reinforce local identity and retain population.

Small and micro-enterprises are still largely informal in nature, lacking the legal, institutional, or financial resources to grow and expand. Furthermore, they tend to "swarm" to commercial trends, such as dry-cleaners or car-washes, until local markets become saturated. Profit margins are extremely low. Small-scale entrepreneurs face severe administrative obstacles to formalization, as well as low skills levels and difficulty in obtaining credit. Their assets include creativity, adaptability, and persistence. Similar to the rural sector, the learning circle for the small-enterprise sector proposed a training and support program to encourage knowledge-sharing among micro- and small-business owners, in the form of small-scale franchise operations. A crucial policy measure for their development is to reduce or eliminate the legal and bureaucratic obstacles to operating as a formal business.

Knowledge management in large organizations – both public and private – is poor, and this sector is characterized by rigid, bureaucratic, or family-run structures that are highly resistant to change; technology is often adopted yet not truly appropriated for more efficient use of resources. Participants in this learning circle proposed incentive, matching grant, and competitive programs to reward risk-taking, innovation, and knowledge management in both public and private sectors, along with the creation of an "innovation club" to facilitate social learning.

Broader issue: connectivity, content, and training

Despite high levels of growth and competition since the recent privatization of the state-run telecommunications company, relatively low telephone density and widespread poverty make Internet connections a rarity, and not feasible for the majority of the population in the foreseeable future. But connections alone will not resolve further obstacles posed by the lack of relevant content and user skills. Even if Internet access becomes cost-effective, a chicken-and-egg situation develops in that few Salvadorans will find crucial information, and few will take the trouble to create that information based on the assumption that few are online. Informationalizing socio-economic activity in El Salvador will require the massive creation of relevant online content and transactional capabilities (e-commerce, government paperwork), as well as skill-building. Participants agreed that a large-scale effort to combine Internet access with content creation and training could break through this logjam.

To this end, they proposed the gradual roll-out of a network of telecenters, with a focus on information creation and community outreach in order to build a critical mass of useful content, as well as the skills to create and utilize it. A franchise model was adopted in which individual operators obtain standardized training, equipment, support, and logos in exchange for a monthly fee, in order to ensure quality of service and the benefits of an economy of scale in both infrastructure acquisition and Web content production. After much discussion of governance models, participants agreed that the network should be owned by a national coalition of non-profit, educational, and government organizations, so that it would be responsive to the public interest. A long-term, interest-free loan was obtained from part of the proceeds that the government received from the privatization of its telecommunications network.

Broader issue: government information and ICT policy

Researchers who examined government information management and internal ICT policy recommended measures to encourage the government to become a "best practice" for the rest of the nation in technology and knowledge management, as well as to build greater efficiency and transparency into its operations: (1) design and publicize a national information policy; (2) promote electronic government transactions and publications, in concert with the network of telecenters; (3) develop internal knowledge and information management practices; (4) rationalize ICT distribution, maintenance, training, and use in public administration; and (5) promote information policies at local government levels.

Conectándonos al Futuro also suggested that the government's role in promoting the adequate use of ICT in development be one of leadership, not ownership:

> . . . reduced responsibility for direct management in many areas of society, transferring those functions to civil society and private enterprise when and if they are capable of taking charge of them more efficiently; in exchange, focus efforts on correcting market imperfections, and eventually creating those incentives necessary to generate capacity instead of dependence.
>
> (Courtright *et al.*, 1999: 86)

Short-term program outcomes

A newly elected government took office at the same time that the above recommendations were issued. Although many of its members had participated enthusiastically in the learning circles and telecenter project, and had even incorporated many of the program's ideas into their electoral platforms, they found their best intentions frustrated once in office. Political infighting, severe budget limitations and competing priorities, and bureaucratic inertia combined to make it impossible for the new government to commit to an overall program to implement the Conectándonos projects through a World Bank loan, although it would have been a comparatively small investment.[5]

Despite this setback, the momentum and interest built up during the course of the 18-month participatory research program helped many of its participants to take up the challenge of informationalizing the activities of their own organizations. Informal discussions, held over the past three years with former program participants, show continuing concern with this challenge, and a willingness to link with the telecenter network to create synergies between its goals and their programs. Particularly encouraging is the creation of a new government office to forge ties with Salvadoran emigrant organizations around the world, staffed by a former Conectándonos member. The initiative, originally proposed by the migrant learning circle, has resulted in an electronic newsletter with thousands of subscribers worldwide, as well as an online global database of Salvadoran individuals and groups abroad that facilitates commercial, intellectual, and artistic ties.[6]

Due to similar bureaucratic difficulties, the promised funding for the telecenter network did not materialize until mid-2000, over a year after the Conectándonos program ended, and the first telecenters did not open until September of that year.[7] Two years later, only 40 of the projected 100 telecenters have opened for business, and Web site production has been slower than expected. Despite the original conception of the network as a member association run by a broad array of civil society organizations, the Board of Directors has a restricted, high-profile membership, and has recast the association as more élite than originally intended. Spending on advanced technology has consumed a greater-than-expected chunk of the organization's budget, and individual telecenters tend to resemble trendy cybercafés more than community information centers. Although most of the network's substantial seed loan has already been spent, few of the centers are self-sustaining and there is little hope for additional sources of investment.

Nevertheless, there has been a significant growth of useful Salvadoran information on the .SV domain server, which by late 1999 had registered over 800 sub-domains and over 25,000 Web pages (Ibarra, 2000); figures for today are undoubtedly much higher. A brief review of Web pages indexed on the Asociación Infocentros portal (Asociación Infocentros, 2002) shows, for example, dozens of how-to sites for accomplishing government-related transactions, daily market prices for agricultural products, an extensive cultural and artistic directory and calendar, news, and other useful sites directly accessible from the home page.

Long-term reflections and lessons learned

Although the Conectándonos al Futuro research program helped spark new trends in development patterns in El Salvador, the failure of follow-through programs and the lack of broad-based participation in the telecenter network has meant considerable missed opportunities and a loss of initial momentum. A "culture of the Internet" appears to have grown significantly in El Salvador since the Conectándonos al Futuro program began, but trends to date certainly do not point to a reduction in national inequalities, which is what the program set out to achieve. Although the most obvious reasons for these shortcomings have been mentioned cursorily and tentatively, a thorough evaluation program would be necessary to propose long-term remedies.

Still, the participatory nature of the Conectándonos al Futuro program did generate insights into key trends and processes that would have been largely invisible to an expert commission or research by external consultants. The careful mix of stakeholders representing many facets of development challenges ensured that assumptions were questioned, contradictory considerations were weighed, and visionary goals were carefully measured against constraints. We believe this approach and methodology can be fruitfully applied to other national contexts, as the perspectives obtained through its multi-sector, action-oriented methods shed light on approaches to ICT and development in general as well. The following are examples of broader lessons learned in El Salvador that might serve in other contexts:

Within-country and between-country challenges

Analysts of the "digital divide" have noted that disparities tend to exist both within countries and between countries (cf. Kagan, 2000). These two dimensions should be kept analytically separate when assessing problems and progress alike (Accenture et al., 2001). It is also crucial to assess the implications of favoring one strategy over the other. The case of El Salvador provides an example of the complexities involved in attempting to address both sets of disparities in an integrated fashion.

In the context of a globalized economy, with the growth of regional trading blocs and the disappearance of protectionism, the economic activities that traditionally ensure a country its particular market share (in El Salvador: coffee, cotton, sugar) become increasingly precarious. "Retooling" a national economy to meet these new challenges is a slow and painful process, provoking controversy and conflict among sectors, as job markets shift, traditional producers are overrun by duty-free imports, and inequalities deepen. Thus, a country that seeks to compete on a new footing in the world market faces internal struggles over how to ensure short-term gains while attempting to make long-term investments in both human and economic capital. The digital revolution may appear to offer solutions to both the long- and short-term requirements of globalization, particularly when new trading partners increasingly rely on ICT for efficiency. A "between-country" approach to an ICT and development strategy involves pressing for technology adoption in certain leading sectors, training high-level workers, changing laws to facilitate international electronic transactions, and perhaps even attracting investment in information industry activities. Many in El Salvador favored this approach.

But what effect will such a priority have on those who do not participate directly in internationally focused activities? Do national inequalities deepen proportionately, or is there a "trickle-down" effect that benefits all? Since developing countries have strictly limited public investment resources, a decision to favor a between-country approach may undermine the possibility of devoting equal or greater attention to internal inequalities that could be mitigated – with and without ICT – by better education, health care, production techniques, public administration, and environmental management. In what might be considered a "trickle-up" philosophy, Conectándonos al Futuro clearly favored a "within-country" approach, with its emphasis on local knowledge management and information creation, although many of the proposed projects also had favorable implications for overcoming between-country divides.

Technology-driven development

No matter how much emphasis is placed on the many aspects of development that are involved in efforts to meet the challenges of globalization, it is perpetually tempting to fall back upon an "ICT fetish" (Heeks, 1999) and lead with technology. Aware of this temptation, the leaders of the El Salvador exercise persisted in analyzing problems of information and knowledge management within the context of existing development areas, and its approach to technology was always either hypothetical (what-if scenarios) or carefully situated within this broader context. Nevertheless, during the program's tenure, not a week went by without the leaders receiving a technology-driven proposal from a technology leader, a grassroots activist, a government policymaker, or an international consultant.

In retrospect, however, the telecenter network appears to have succumbed to this temptation. Although great care was taken during the Conectándonos program to frame it as "more than just an ICT project," its subsequent roll-out appears to be hampered by a technology-led vision that has become disconnected from grassroots development efforts, at the expense of socially grounded, content-rich centers. From the policy standpoint, it is not unusual to prefer high-profile, visible outcomes over gradual, process-based trajectories, and thus technology easily becomes the centerpiece of telecenter efforts (see, for example, Gómez and Ospina, 2001; Roman and Colle, 2002). In the case of El Salvador, it is likely that the predominance of government-linked policy specialists on the staff and Board of Directors of the telecenter network, and their subsequent neglect of broad-based participation, contributed to this focus.

Development-as-process

Development is a never-ending process, marked by milestones instead of endpoints. In order to put into motion a process of change, the Conectándonos al Futuro program focused on obtaining an assessment of development trends rather than a statistics-based snapshot. The projects proposed by the focus groups targeted those trends, in an effort to create positive dynamics by identifying weaknesses and leveraging strengths. Outcomes are, of course, extremely difficult to assess. To that end, the proposed projects were located within a general evaluation framework that included ground-zero assessments, on-the-fly corrections, stakeholder involvement, and replication and dissemination of partial successes. Nevertheless, it is always easier to measure, for example, numbers of households with running water than it is to assess social learning processes, with or without technologies (cf. Menou, 1993, 1995a, b; Menou and Potvin, 2000). An end-product approach to development is simpler to assess, but it sidesteps the complexity inherent in ongoing processes of change.

Local and national information content

In the introduction to its 1998 report, the World Bank stated that developing nations "differ from rich ones not only because they have less capital but because they have less knowledge" (World Bank, 1998: 1). The solution proposed in the report has two principal components: help developing nations access knowledge from industrialized nations, and promote more science and technology. The El Salvador exercise, however, came to a different conclusion, more in accordance with Cronin and Davenport's (1991) proposition:

> It is not simply that less developed countries have fewer and poorer quality information assets at their disposal; rather that so much potentially useful information . . . is not recorded, and often even when formally or systematically recorded, may only be available for local use and accessible within a controlled or restricted environment.
>
> (Cronin and Davenport, 1991: 3)

All the focus groups and case studies in Conectándonos al Futuro identified a grievous lack of available, useful information to resolve both simple and complex needs; thus, the creation and management of local informational content became a central theme of proposed solutions. Of course, obtaining and interpreting international information was also seen as important, but participants in Conectándonos al Futuro – even in the "large organizations" focus group – placed a premium on building the capacity to transform and manage local knowledge as a foundation for the productive use of externally generated information resources. In other words, the *production and organization* of Salvadoran information was seen as more empowering for both national and international development purposes than merely the *consumption* of international information, no matter how useful. As mentioned above, this concern was a driving force behind the creation of the national telecenter network.

Resolving the content deficit is even more imperative for low-income groups, who spend a disproportionate share of their time and resources attempting to obtain crucial information. In this sense, the findings in El Salvador complement the conclusions of a landmark study published recently in the United States on the lack of relevant, accessible content for the poor (Lazarus and Mora, 2000). To counter critics who cite low literacy as an obstacle to fruitful use of content, program participants stressed the traditionally co-operative nature of information use among the poor, many of whom rely on family members, friends, and local organizations to assist them in interpreting printed information, if it is available in the first place (cf. Heath, 1980; McConnell, 2000).

Conclusion

The case of El Salvador illustrates a participatory and process-oriented approach to strategizing for change in an "informationalized" world. Salvadorans from many sectors worked together for 18 months to understand critical problems in traditional development areas, and designed ways in which information creation, knowledge management, and ICT use could help leverage new processes. Although the plans were not adopted in a comprehensive program, a national network of telecenters was created and continues to grow, and the themes widely discussed throughout the exercise continue to appear on many agendas. It remains to be seen in what ways the telecenters and related initiatives are contributing to development in El Salvador, and how their benefits are distributed. Although the lack of ongoing assessment makes it difficult to analyze the types of progress that have occurred since the program's end, the participatory analytical and action-oriented methodology ensured that key questions were thoroughly debated. The central issues raised and lessons learned during this exercise should not be overlooked in future strategy exercises of this type.

Acknowledgments

The author wishes to thank Michel Menou, Clemente San Sebastián, Pierre-Olivier Colleye, Rafael Ibarra, Ana Patricia Silva, Mario Roger Hernández, and many other participants in Conectándonos al Futuro, for continuing to discuss and assess the process and outcomes of this innovative exercise. Thanks also to the editors of this volume for their encouragement and suggestions.

Notes

1 Statistics primarily from the United Nations Development Programme (2001) based on 1998–9 figures, with additional figures from the World Bank (2000) and Central Intelligence Agency (2000).
2 Author's conversations with Salvadoran librarians, 1991–9.
3 Author's conversations with radio network leaders, 1999.
4 These assumptions were primarily grounded in the experiences of the two co-ordinators, with strategic direction and assistance from Michel Menou, an external consultant (cf. Menou, 1991, 1993, 1995a, b).
5 In addition, the series of earthquakes that took place in 2001 severely undermined El Salvador's infrastructure and economy, exacerbated budget constraints, and left the nation on a long-term crisis footing that overshadows the usual discourse of development challenges (World Bank and International Monetary Fund, 2001).
6 Personal interview with program director, 23 July 2002.
7 Data and assessments contained in this paragraph were collected during two visits to El Salvador, in 2000 and 2002, that included interviews with key participants and visits to several telecenters.

Chapter 9

Social cyberpower in the everyday life of an African American community

A report on action-research in Toledo, Ohio[1]

Abdul Alkalimat

Introduction

What will the experience of the African American community be in the information age? This is a critical question as it appears more and more that the social transformation underway utilizing information technology is permanent, and increasingly redefining standards for social life: literacy, job readiness, upward social mobility, and social power. Most African Americans were not among the early adopters of this new technology and therefore appear to be beginning the twenty-first century in much the same way as the twentieth century, not at the cutting edge of economic development. This reality can be changed.

This chapter reports on an action-research project designed to explore the ways in which the everyday life of a community can become the content of its virtual community identity, and by so doing create a bridge over the digital divide. The project is based in Toledo, Ohio (USA) and is a joint effort by the Africana Studies Program at the University of Toledo and the Murchison Community Center. The field-work for much of the research reported here was done by the first master's degree graduates in eBlack Studies, Africana Studies based on information technology. They continue to work together in the Murchison Center as executive director, Americorps VISTA volunteer, and volunteer teacher.

The Murchison Center began in 1992 as a program of the St James Baptist Church. It has become a full service community technology center, with 20 networked workstations, cable Internet connection, and capacity for printing and multimedia. The program includes after-school tutoring and adult classes four nights a week. The annual budget of the Murchison Center has been about $30,000, not including VISTA funding, which pays several volunteers just under $800 per month. There have been stages when the decisive influence on the center was the church, the government, and then the university. Each stage was cumulative, so that previous influence and contributions were not lost. Current transformations appear to be towards greater community influence and inputs to the Murchison Center (Alkalimat and Williams, 2001).

The local community is the kind of neighborhood where people are usually locked out of the access and training needed to be an active part of the information society. As master's student, center co-founder and executive director Deborah Hamilton described the area,

> It is located in central city Toledo where the community . . . is 70 percent poor or near poor. Ninety-seven percent are African American in the immediate area (census tracts 25 and 26, Toledo, Ohio). The 1990 median income is $12,400 and $15,400 respectively in both census tracts. Single mothers head more than 60 percent of the households. One fourth of the residents are under 13 years of age.
>
> (Hamilton, 2002: 13)

Overall, Toledo is a metropolitan area of over 500,000 people, 20 percent of whom are African American. It has a shrinking manufacturing base historically linked to the auto industry headquartered in Detroit 50 miles to the north. Its irony in the global economy is that Toledo produced the classic World War II Jeep that was vital in the war against Germany. Now today Daimler-Benz owns the plant, which produces the Jeep Cherokee. Toledo's capital used to be local, community-based, and big enough to finance local projects like building a major art museum (1901), university (1872), and manufacturing, especially glass and auto components. Now most of the big capital is absentee-owned.

Toledo has had considerable effort put into developing community level technology resources. Two 1996 initiatives led to the formation of a local organization called Coalition to Access Technology and Networking in Toledo or CATNeT.[2] A local housing manager got a Housing and Urban Development grant to build and staff several computer labs in private apartment complexes, and a local academic researcher got involved with a State of Ohio initiative, the Urban University Neighborhood Network. The network started with 9 labs and now has a membership of 34 labs (Stoecker and Stuber, 1997). A recent survey to locate all of the public computing in Toledo found over 250 public access sites including schools and libraries (Williams and Alkalimat, 2004). In addition, the Toledo labs are active in a statewide organization (Ohio Community Computing Network)[3] and a national organization (Community Technology Centers Network).[4]

The Toledo model shown in Figure 9.1 proposes how a socially excluded community can be transformed into a networked community, able to mobilize cyberpower to advance its interests. In the model, the transformation from a historical community to a networked community is catalyzed by cyberorganizers and by the organizing and mobilizing impact of the content and interactivity of cyberspace. This is how the actual social organization of the community can create or co-operate with cyberorganizers to build an existence in cyberspace. The process intensifies as the community becomes more engaged in using information technology and dependent on the new opportunities of an entire community sharing a virtual collectivity. It is precisely this collective that will learn how to act, first in cyberspace like sending mass emails or signing a petition,

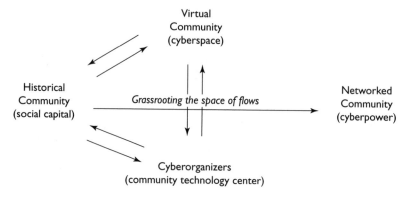

Figure 9.1 The Toledo Model

or swarming emails, then by leaving cyberspace and taking action in the real world. Both of these actions, virtual and actual, can be called cyberpower, as the key staging area for the collective action was in cyberspace.

We will now use this framework to report on four of the cyberpower projects. Cyberfamilies is a project to utilize the existing practice of research for family genealogy to build a database beginning with individual extended families to network and link-up an entire community. Cyberhair is a project based on databases of beauty salons, combs, and information resources about hair care and design. Cyberchurch is a project to build a dynamic database of church websites, and extend that into a comprehensive virtual community of individual churches and the entire religious community. Cyberschools is a project to use cyberspace

Table 9.1 The historical community: the actual experience and its virtual representation (the Toledo Model)

Actual experience	Virtual experience	URL
Neighborhood	Virtual Dorr Street	http://www.murchisoncenter.org/dorrstreet/
Family	Cyberfamily	http://www.murchisoncenter.org/cyberfamilies/
Church	Cyberchurch	http://www.cyber-church.us
School	Cyberschool	http://www.murchisoncenter.org/cyberschools
	First Saturday	http://www.murchisoncenter.org/firstsaturday/
Business	Cyberhair	http://www.murchisoncenter.org/cyberhair
CTC	Murchison Center	http://www.murchisoncenter.org

in two ways, as a directory of individual school web pages, and a site for a community wide campaign to pass a state mandated proficiency test. This is a work in process.

Cyberfamilies

Historical community

The family is generally regarded as a core institution of every society. It has been the vehicle for procreation and social reproduction – people have babies to replenish the community by creating a family, and then in turn rely on the family to socialize the children to become members of society. The research focus on the Black family, especially on changes in Black family organization, has charted the Black family from its origins in Africa through the destructive terror of slavery, sharecropping tenancy, and industrial city life. Within this, the most persistent debate has been over the relative importance of slavery in understanding the persistence of family disorganization today.

This leads to one of the main obstacles in building a family database. There are limited records of biological parenting under slavery. Although a slave culture did emerge and provide a counterweight to the system, official records regarding family continuity were based on the slave owner and not the slave. In addition, family relations without formal legal marriage, and generally without documentation, present a problem for anyone researching family history. On the other hand, it is precisely these problems that lead people to value the successful attempt to reconstruct family networks.

Cyberfamilies pointed up a big difference between lineage as tracing one's origins versus family history as tracing one's socio-biological network, inclusive of all its many branches and hubs. A lineage network will include the shortest available distance between two points in a family network, but a social network includes all available branches. Some family members seek historical meaning by linking with a particular ancestor, others by linking with broad social forces in society and the world. In my own family, the progenitor is Free Frank, a slave who bought himself and 19 other family members. The family points to him as the main frame of reference. The question is – "How are you related to Free Frank?" On the other hand, during family gatherings people might have spoken of the role the family played in different wars, of the different professions and industries people worked in, cities where different family hubs were located, and so on (Simpson, 1981; Walker, 1983).

The family has been a hot topic in cyberspace, even for African Americans who are not online to the same extent as other ethnic groups. We identified two main kinds of genealogical sites designed for African Americans: general genealogical sites on African Americans, and research databases such as the census, government records and so on, including a great deal of information on specific families.[5] In addition, many personal websites have some kind of reference or link to family content. The people who make up the content in most of these sites often do not know that information about them is available in cyberspace. This is public information.

Cyberorganizer

The cyberorganizer for this project is Pauline Kynard. Ms Kynard completed her undergraduate degree in Africana Studies while working as Director of the Art Tatum Resource Center in African American Culture of the Toledo-Lucas County Public Library, Kent Branch. She developed the Cyberfamilies project as her undergraduate thesis project. The project is now a formal collaboration between Africana Studies at the University of Toledo and the Art Tatum Center.

The first stage was to identify one or more families who met three criteria: basic research materials have been collected, a family member is willing to work with the project as liaison with the family, and the family agrees to have this information freely available on the cyber families website. Working with her on their respective families are another undergraduate major in Africana Studies representing the Jaynes family, and my sister who had started a web project on our McWorter family. The three families were different in their approach to family history, but each already had completed a great deal of research. The Kynard and Jaynes families are large families settled in Toledo for three generations. The McWorter family is part of the official record of African Americans in the state of Illinois from the 1830s.

Cyberspace

Ms Kynard worked with each family to organize available material and assist in additional research. When discussing the digitization aspect of the project it was necessary to discuss continuing research on the family. Once she has gathered and codified the information the task was for the Africana Studies Media Lab to write software for a database to express the full branching of a family social network. The working model enables every person in the network to become the center of an investigation that can follow every branch of the network that we have information for. It is a matter of statistical calculation to determine how many links we are away from each other. The most celebrated finding is that people are no more than six connections away from each other in actual reality, but the way that cyberspace has been constructed any given web page is 19 clicks from any other, but this finding only applies to the 24 percent of cyberspace that is available via simple surfing (Barabasi, 2002: 25–40, 165). Clearly our actual social lives are more connected than our representations in cyberspace. But this need not be the case.

Each individual in a family network has a page. This places them at the center of kinship links to the broader network, through their parents and their children. Each individual is at the same time at the center and the periphery of an expanding network of humanity, going back into history and forward into the future. Stable communities will be more closely connected, but over generations most groups are likely to be much closer than people think.

Networked community

The first outcome from the pilot stage of this project is that Ms Kynard was asked to prepare a CD for the Jaynes family reunion. This project has now become an organizing activity in the family to digitize their history and current make-up. Second, she is preparing a slide-lecture presentation on the project for community groups interested in genealogy. And, the library is considering expanding its uploading functions such as is required by the cyberfamilies project, i.e., giving more importance to creating digital libraries of local content.

The project is moving to an institutional process that will create a new generation of family cyberarchivists, e.g. students in school. Plans have been developed to implement a module for graduating seniors at the local Black high school to develop digital family history. They will have the option to contribute their family information to the database of cyberfamilies. As the families interconnect then the identity of the network will shift from family in a narrow sense to community in a broad sense. We will discover as never before the logic of kinship and be able to transform it as a network into a communications channel for cyber activity. The latent social cyberpower of this dormant network will be activated. This will be its digital awakening and engagement.

Cyberhair

Historical community

Taken together, hair care and hair design are an important part of social life, culture, and identity in every society. In the Black community they are especially critical because African hair has unique qualities for hair sculpture and because there is a long tradition of African American cultural excellence in this activity. The hair salons are centers of economic, cultural, and social action. Doing hair is rooted in deep cultural economics, encompassing family labor, barter with friends, or doing it by oneself.

The beauty salon was created to provide a service in the urban Black community, especially in the twentieth century. As a result of proletarianization, African American families became smaller, family networks were de-territorialized, and many services became commodified. The salons became centers of cultural production and economic exchange as well as "third places," sites of public discourse that form a hub serving across a dense network of families, friends, and acquaintances. Transgenerational interlocking networks of families and churches are vehicles for discourse. Beauty salons are a vital part of the African American public sphere.

The main icon of the Black woman as entrepreneur is Madame C.J. Walker (1867–1919), founding leader of the Black hair care industry. She invented a new chemical process for hair care and design. But her impact went way beyond this. She recruited and trained a corps of hair care workers and, in so doing, gave beauticians a greater professional profile. This was the most stable form of independent business ownership for Black women in the twentieth century. She provided significant financial and moral support to the writers, artists, and institution-builders who became known as the "Harlem Renaissance." She also did so with the political militants of the "New Negro" movement.

However, today the political economy of the Black hair care industry is changing. One major example is the retailing and wholesaling of Black hair care products. In Toledo there is one Black hair products distribution company over 40 years old. Over the last ten years Asian business interests have opened at least four megastores, each with more than ten times the floor space and product selection than are found in a Black-owned store. Salons located in the major malls and department stores now include Black people in their market. This has led to a tension between the traditionally more networked, "conversation-intense," and slower beauty parlor in the community and doing hair as a commodity in a time-driven, mass market, mall environment.

The beauty salon in the Black community has historical roots but is in a state of crisis. There is some hope for the future, however, as the main Black high school has a growing cosmetology program. Enrollment there is greater than that in many of the more high tech areas that lead to a college major in engineering and computer science. Enrolling in cosmetology is also evidence of a desire to get a skill and possibly be self-employed and able to support oneself and a family.

Cyberorganizing

The Cyberhair project emerged in three stages: a conference, a class project, and a MA thesis project. The conference defined the project, the class began the enumeration of salons, and the thesis work built the Cyberhair website, "Black People's Hair."

A symposium – "Black People's Hair: A Symposium on the Political Culture of Everyday Life"[6] – was held during the first year of the UT Africana Studies program on March 6–7, 1997. This brought Black studies to life for UT students, many of whom were first in their families to attend college. It was a day when art historians who focus on African hair, hair braiders, and students could bring their knowledge together. The conference was scholarly, with presentations on the mutual influence of African and African American hairstyles over the last five centuries. It was practical, with hair braiders demonstrating their work on volunteers. And it was emotional and personal, with participants sharing stories of their struggles with their hair and their identity.

The conference set the framework for the Cyberhair project in three ways. The project would focus on cultural production rather than cultural performance. It would advocate Panafricanism as a cultural approach. And it would advocate the adoption of information technology as a technological foundation.

The Africana Studies program then organized an undergraduate course called "Cyberspace and the Black Experience" (*Chronicle of Higher Education*, May 19, 2000: A18). Along with readings and seminar discussions, the course initiated a practical research project to build a database of Toledo's African American beauty salons. Here a debate emerged over whether it was a "politically correct" action to study places that were hostile to a positive Black identity, meaning places that did anything other than natural hairstyles. The one sister in the class with "trendy locks" was opposed to going to the beauty salons for this reason, but the others who all wore styles more in the mainstream of Black Toledo agreed that this project would make a big impact on the overall Black community. They were responding to the design of the assignment, to build a cyber resource that might motivate people to become computer literate and cross over the digital divide.

The one young man in the class took up the task of completing the database as his masters project in Africana Studies. In his thesis, Brian Zelip explains his situation:

> I am a white male. Every salon I went to was a Black salon. 78 percent of the salons were owned by women. All of the salon owners were in their mid-30's or older, whereas at the time of the research I was 24 years old. . . . It was anticipated that the research being carried out by me would be faced with some degree of resistance and non-cooperation.
>
> (Zelip, 2002: 88)

He bases this on the social meaning of color, gender, hair, and age. However, he then attributes his success to how these barriers were overcome: the salon owners' respect for the research sponsors (UT Africana Studies and the Murchison Center) and for his knowledge of the African American community and culture. Zelip had been the hip-hop deejay on the campus radio station.

Cyberspace

The website was built around the 1997 hair conference, the database of beauty salons, and a collection of images of Afro combs. This anchored the digital identity of virtual Black hair in the actual space of cultural production rather than cultural performance. Beauty magazines stress cultural performance – gorgeous women, lots of documentation of spectacular events, product ads, and celebrities. The magazines are like dream books to guide stylist and the customer. In contrast, Cyberhair's emphasis on cultural production targeted the universal experience of everyday life.

The Africana Studies Media Lab digitized a collection of combs from the US and elsewhere that the author gathered over a 35-year period. The process of organizing the digitized images facilitated our discovery that the Afro comb has passed through four historical stages: traditional, industrial, Panafrican, and global. The combs began in traditional society (made of wood), underwent further development in industrial society (metal), took new forms during the struggles for national liberation (wood, metal, and plastic), and now reflect the reality of globalization (extruded plastic).

Networked community

In the project, students become cyberorganizers, relying on the historical community of salon owners, stylists, and customers to help build the site and determine its future evolution. Out of 50 salons, seven owners were found to have active email addresses, but none of the shops had a computer in the salon for business or the public. But as a result of contact with our project several salon owners and stylists have taken computer classes at the Murchison Center.

Zelip went on a study tour of South Africa and took the opportunity to document hair care practices. On one occasion he found a beauty salon next to a cybercafé. The hair stylists had never been online. He gathered them in the cybercafé to view Black People's Hair on the web. When he returned to Toledo, he showed slides of the South African experience to the stylists who were in the site. This is a small example of cyberspace creating a Panafrican experience at the grass roots in the twenty-first century.

Survey data collected by students identified a small number of salon owners who are interested in making efforts to use computers and the Internet. The Murchison Center set aside computers to place in salons, and a masters student from the University of Michigan School of Information joined the project as cyberorganizer to carry out the installation and support of the PCs. This will enable the project to support the use of software for the salon as business, and the Internet and the World Wide Web for customers. In the future we will investigate the possibility of uniting an intensely individualistic group of entrepreneurs into a collectivity to serve common interests.

Cyberchurch

Historical community

The church is the most comprehensive social institution in the African American community. It provides a total experience based on its embodiment of culture, ideology, social organization, economic development, leadership, ritual, and a moral order. It is important among the social cyberpower projects because it also has had a long history of adopting new advances in communications technology. Today one can experience the Black church in person, on the radio, on television, in print, on video, CD, DVD, the Internet and the World Wide Web. The actual church takes up regular time each week and provides host space for many community activities. It seems only a matter of time before the church in cyberspace will rival the traditional gathering of a congregation.

Our survey suggests that there are at least 300 churches that primarily serve African Americans in Toledo. This constitutes the most powerful set of leaders, real estate interests, ideological consensus, and mass mobilization in the Black community. However, the church has to adapt to the new technology if it is to serve youth as they become cyberactivists. When we began our project less than ten churches had their own web page reflecting the community-wide impact of the digital divide. When the church adopts a new technology it also has the role of infusing it into other community activities as well. It is in this sense that Cyberchurch is a pivotal project.

Cyberorganizing

Cyberchurch began as a research assignment in an Africana Studies course on the Black church. Reverend Al Reed, a local minister with a social activist background, was recruited to teach the course once a week every Saturday morning. This schedule was set to allow for non-traditional working students to enroll in the course. Each student was assigned to gather church information for a web page. We began without much computer literacy. However, the majority of students became comfortable and fluent with basic computer software and aspects of the web. In fact, out of this course, a couple of students even became teachers at the Murchison Center and leaders of the Cyberchurch project.

A second process was outreach to church leadership to attend free computer literacy orientation sessions offered weekly by the Africana Studies program. The main result of this has been a greater interest in the project. Many of the participants in the early morning outreach sessions also began attending evening workshop sessions. The process of building a virtual community was itself becoming a meaningful social group meeting on a face-to-face basis. These discussions were important for several reasons: they became focus groups to get community feedback on the project, they educated people about the project and got them to buy into the plan, and it allowed students to emerge and make the transitions from student to community worker.

The project plans four progressive levels in the expansion of the Black church into cyberchurch. Level one is a church in the online church directory, with a web page containing publicly available information about the church, including a photo. Level two is a church that has supplied information about its staff, organization, calendar, and program and that has at least ten of its members with email signed up to a Cyberchurch electronic discussion list. Level three is a church website with sound files, and/or video of at least one sermon and one song by the choir. Level four is a church with its own community technology center.

An action-research team called the Toledo Spiders carried out the data collection for level one. This team was made up of undergraduates and led by a graduate student in Africana Studies, all paid with federal work-study funds. The team used digital cameras and tape recorders to document conferences and churches as part of the Cyberchurch project. The project began to take off as people were motivated to get their own church online, and community organizers began to see this as a positive organizing project. The Murchison Center staff is currently organizing to visit each church to make direct contact with the church leadership. Unless a church member has participated in Cyberchurch classes, this visit is generally the first notice the congregation has of the project, which is usually followed by a regular announcement in the printed church bulletin distributed every Sunday.

There are five main lessons from this work: first, standardization of a main template for the project solved problems created by first trying to use freeware and free web hosting with people with low computer literacy. Second, emphasis on email seems a more democratic way to build a networked community while building a main web location as a virtual base of operations. Third, early adopters of this program were church seniors, but the critical mass for the church to become a networked community will be the youth. Fifth, student workers have to be mentored in terms of technical skill, attitude, and time management. Lastly, the greatest resource in building a cyberorganizing project is the bonding social capital that sustains participation.

Cyberspace

The general plan for the page is to combine the feature of a general portal with a database of individual church web pages. Again, our emphasis is on cultural production. We are approaching the church in terms of sites of cultural production (churches, seminaries, and publications) and tools of production (holy texts, hymns, and theologians). Linking all of this together can create an environment embracing all organized religious activity. One sister attending a Cyberchurch session responded to this design with a smile on her face saying, "My Lord, if we can all get together like this in cyberspace then we can all be in the same church."

On the site, each church's web page is based on a standardized template. The page allows for voluntary submission of information to start the process of a church being added to the database. Confirmation by the Cyberchurch team is necessary before any information is posted.

The logic of this structure follows an intervention by cyberorganizers into the internal organization of the church resulting in the church becoming itself a cyberorganizing force within the community. The cyberorganizer can join the church or just work with it, but also there will be church members who have or gain the skill who become cyberorganizers as well. In fact it is not too early to see the emergence of a new field for church professionals, cyberministry. The digital archive of the Black church experience will constitute its historical identity, and digital interaction will become a major vehicle for collectivizing religious experience.

Networked community

The church as a networked community can come into existence as each of the four levels of the Cyberchurch project is achieved. The key is level two, when church members join the electronic discussion list. With more than 250 churches at level one now, level two may result in more than 2,500 people on an emailing list. We are currently in the process of building level two and the mailing list. The Cyberchurch team meets in a working session once a week. They will constitute the editorial collective for a newsletter based on a unified church calendar. This will be sent out as an email message, while the annual calendar will be archived on the website. The role of cyberorganizing in this case is to build a discussion list although it is starting out as a mailing list.

A community organization in Chicago has also joined Cyberchurch, adding Chicago churches to the site. On a national level, the project has been joined by the National Society of Black Engineers[7] with more than 300 local college chapters of African American students in engineering and computer science.

The project is also networking the existing resources in the community. Five women who have become cyberorganizers in the Cyberchurch project are also now the webmasters for their respective churches. Several churches have started labs on their own, and have affiliated with CATNeT.

Cyberschools

Historical community

The school as a social institution and a site for social change has always been an important part of the African American community. Free Black communities established schools before the Civil War in the eighteenth century, and then universal public education was established during the Reconstruction in the South in the nineteenth century. A third level was reached in the 1950s and 1960s, when the school became a key battleground in the twentieth century. Throughout these high points were critical shifts in the political orientation of the Black public sphere. There were different great debates that dominated public discourse: the emancipation debate (including the abolitionists, the Civil War, and the Reconstruction), the self-determination debate (the alternative views of people such as Marcus Garvey, Booker T. Washington, and W.E.B. DuBois), and the Black liberation debate (especially the alternative perspectives of Malcolm X, Martin Luther King).

Schools are vehicles for socialization. Each school level with a simultaneous experience (for example, the students in one high school at one time) constitutes a generation. This same group will share social experience throughout their life cycle. The schools in Toledo had a functional fit with the economy when industrial mass production required lots of workers with general skills. People graduated from high school into the factories and got good, often lifelong, jobs.

In the 1960s, Black youth were overcoming lower rates of success, but by the twenty-first century the process has been reversed. At this stage of deindustrialization, the Toledo schools have become dysfunctional, falling far short of expected levels of achievement. The teachers are mainly white, and the students are mainly Black. The economic interests of the union are discussed independent from the quality of education facing the children and their parents. The school is the primary battleground over whether the future of the current generation of Black youth is to be part of the information society or delinked in isolated lower-income inner city "forbidden zones."

Cyberorganizing

There have been three stages to this project:

1   The Community Math Academy: a two-year long initiative at the Martin Luther King Elementary School focusing on "parent power" and information technology;
2   Cyberschools: a networking from the base of one school to create a web portal for a group of schools;
3   Online practice proficiency test: a web page with new practice math tests every month from September to March.

The core group of the CMA included eight people, four cyberorganizers based in the university (one faculty and three graduate students) and four grandmothers based at the Murchison Center and the surrounding community. Every person in the group had a computer or was provided a refurbished one through a program of the Murchison Center. The CMA established a discussion list. We knew it was working when one of the grandmothers used the list to organize a community barbeque. Michelene McGreevy was the student cyberorganizer on this project and she based her master's thesis in Africana Studies on her work (McGreevy, 2002).

Our first initiative of after-school tutoring in the Murchison Center led to meeting with parents and grandparents with a concern for school reform. Their focus was on the school where everything seemed to be going wrong. The parents had long since stopped attending meetings and the teachers' union did not have a positive relationship with the community. The CMA became active in building the local Parent-Teachers Organization. When we joined, the meetings were called and attended by a husband and wife team of parents with little or no support. CMA's involvement led to increased attendance by parents at meetings. A consequence of this was that conflict arose, prompting the need for a contested election. During this period, the appointment of a new principal precipitated a change in school administration. Parent involvement in these meetings was not encouraged as the new regime sought to gain control.

In response to this the project shifted focus from the actual to the virtual, to building web pages for schools to recruit parents, teachers, and students to unite in an effort to take virtual control of their schools by defining them in cyberspace. The initial focus was on building web pages for each school, going well beyond the administrative page on the main website of the Toledo Public Schools. This was aimed at making the school a transparent user-friendly seeming place. We also wanted to demonstrate the power of machine-assisted community memory. One example of this is that when the local Black high school won the city championship in basketball it was in the newspapers for one day and that was the end of it. We put up a web page on it and it remains there today as fresh as ever to bolster the local spirit of excellence.

This second stage shifted from a focus on a high school and its nine feeder schools to a focus on the high school alone. There was positive recognition of each new page of local content, but as the school and the local community leadership did not promote the necessity of building a virtual identity this was a good but not very utilized community resource. Our attempt to digitize the bonding social capital was a highly valued but seldom used resource. The missing element was support from the local school culture, especially the legitimacy of support from parents and teachers.

The third phase of this project focused on the crisis of poor academic achievement as measured by low scores on state-mandated proficiency tests. These annual tests cover five subject areas, and are given to three grade levels (4th, 6th, and 9th). It is now necessary to pass these tests or be held back to repeat the grade level until you pass the test.

We began giving practice proficiency tests in math every first Saturday. The project grew from nine students to 400 students. The tests are based on official state guidelines by a student community teacher work team, and the tests are monitored and graded by a collective of college student volunteers. Now the first Saturday practice tests are online and available for access to everyone.[8] The tests are a major battlefront in education, as the state is requiring more testing. Our project is designed to mobilize people in the struggle for good test scores. Some people will be helped in the short run and their children will get higher scores. In the longer run we are building a social process that can be linked to other efforts for school reform.

Cyberspace

Each stage of this project has had a corresponding representation in cyberspace. A webliography of links served as a resource for the tutoring activity. Cyberschools was a portal with a common template for web pages about each of the ten schools. The tests online are for printing and administering, with a separate answer sheet for immediate review and study. Each of these cyberspaces is useful: global, local, struggle for good test scores.

Networked community

We have positioned two paths to networking in this project, the digitization of local school culture and the digitization of test preparation. One is a focus on the local, the particular differences of each school, while the other is global, and points to the universal struggle faced by all students. As computer literacy becomes universal in the high schools then both paths will be used, but under these circumstances the use of the online tests has had the greatest result as it maximizes the potential of a small group to meet the needs of a very large group. The proficiency test is a state level law hence our project online is of immediate use to everyone in Ohio.

The greatest potential for new cyberinitiatives lies within the high schools in the USA. There is widespread availability of computers and high-speed Internet access. The youth are wellsprings of creative energy. Our work is but a prelude to the revolution being born among the hackers, gamers, texters, and all the other smart mobs that Howard Rheingold (2002) has helped bring to our attention.

Conclusions

Just as there are many bridges across the digital divide, there are alternative ways for a community to become networked. There are at least five models: (1) early utopian community free-net projects, (2) experimental communities like Netville, (3) dot-coms built for mass participation like eBay, (4) social movements and political campaigns, and (5) public computing for social cyberpower. We have reported on action-research in Toledo, Ohio involving a project to implement and study the public computing model, based at the Murchison Community Center.

Our approach focuses on four factors: historical community, cyberorganizers, cyberspace, and the networked community.

1   The historical community: We have found the content of the historical community in the institutional structures that sustain and reproduce the community. We have concentrated on the family, the church, the school, and the beauty salon as key institutional contexts. In addition to digitizing the content of institutional life, two other points of focus emerged. The first is to pay attention to the antagonisms that the community faces because these struggles create the social future of the community; and the second is the recruitment of emerging cyberorganizers from the indigenous activists that keep these institutions going. The search is for the ways in which social cyberpower contributes to the sustainability of an institution and the overall community.

2   The cyberorganizer: Social cyberpower is associated with public computing, especially the school, the library, and the community technology center.

Organizing forces for actual social struggle in this way is emerging as a new field for research and curriculum development as there is a growing need for the kind of work reported in this article. We anticipate that information technology will induce changes in the fundamental methods of social research and social activism alike. The challenge is for academic programs to learn how to link research and practical experience. The land grant college system did it for agriculture and mass production industry, and now we need to do it again in terms of information technology.

3   Cyberspace: The work thus far has emphasized collecting and uploading content into dynamic databases that are configured to assist poor communities in organizing efforts for their own behalf. In addition, all of our databases must be configured to interface with each other so we will in fact be reaching higher and higher levels of collectivity.

4   Networked community: We have merely put basic ingredients together for the virtual reincarnation of a community. The magic of cyberspace's future will be created as more of humanity gets online. It is in this context that the virtual struggle for the future is on. In general what is at stake is the fundamental social structure of cyberspace, and that is one of the most critical factors that will be influencing democracy and quality of life. We have the polar opposite choices of the corporation or the community. Our action-research is to learn about and work for the community paradigm as the future of the information age.

Notes

1   Partial support for this project came from the Urban Affairs Center and the College of Arts and Sciences at the University of Toledo.
2   http://uac.utoledo.edu/metronet/catnet/
3   http://www.occcn.org
4   http://www.ctcnet.org
5   See the following: http://www.afrigeneas.com, http://www.prairiebluff.com/aacemetery, and http://freedmensbureau.com
6   http://www.murchisoncenter.org/cyberhair/conference.htm
7   http://www.nsbe.org
8   http://www.murchisoncenter.org/firstsaturday/

Part III

An emerging community technology research agenda

Chapter 10

Citizenship and public access Internet use

Beyond the field of dreams[1]

Ellen Balka and Brian J. Peterson

Introduction

A "New Partnership Between Government and Citizens" was outlined in the Speech from the Throne to Open the Second Session of the 37th Parliament of Canada, read by the Governor-General of Canada on September 30, 2002, in the Senate Chamber on Parliament Hill in Ottawa. It reflected the existing government's views of citizenship and social cohesion:

> Canada has a unique model of citizenship, based simultaneously on diversity and mutual responsibility. This model requires deliberate efforts to connect Canadians across their differences, to link them to their history and to enable their diverse voices to participate in choosing the Canada we want.
>
> (Governor-General of Canada, 2002)

Such views have been central to the development of numerous programs that together comprise the Connecting Canadians program, which reflects the federal government's "vision and plan to make Canada the most connected country in the world" (Connecting Canadians, 2002).

The Canadian government has embarked on developing an ambitious range of programs designed to improve the quality of Canadian's lives through increased use of the Internet. Programs such as the Community Access and Voluntary Sector Network Support Programs, LibraryNet, the Smart Communities Program and Health Promotion Online have helped Canada gain an international reputation as a leader in government use of information and communication technologies.

Discourse about access to the information highway in Canada is built upon and reflects all too frequently unexamined claims that access to the Internet will lead (among other things) to better-informed citizens and greater participation in civil society. The information highway is frequently presented as the primary mechanism through which citizens will gain access to information that will enhance their ability to function in, and contribute to, civil society – the Internet is seen as a keystone of citizenship in the twenty-first century.

As representatives of all sectors of society from social change groups to elected officials turn their attention towards securing access to the information highway, important issues have remained unexamined (Gorgeç, *et al.*, 1999). Emphasis on securing access to the information highway has obfuscated questions about how new information technologies in general, and the Internet in particular, are being used. In this chapter, we contrast the Canadian government's views of Internet use with use patterns we observed in a local library in Vancouver, British Columbia, Canada's westernmost province. We consider whether or not the Canadian government's Internet access strategy is meeting stated goals, and particularly those pertaining to social cohesion and citizenship.

We address these issues by reviewing the goals of the Canadian government's access strategy, which include the promotion of citizenship and social cohesion. This sets the context for discussion of findings from an observationally based pilot study of Internet use conducted at a local public library. During a week in the Renfrew Branch of the Vancouver Public Library, we conducted detailed observations of two of eight Internet terminals, during all hours the library was open.[2] In addition, we administered a brief questionnaire to library patrons at the conclusion of their Internet sessions. Willingness to answer the survey was high.[3] Only 18 patrons (10.9 percent) refused to respond to our survey. We obtained a response rate of 89 percent (see note 4 for detailed explanation).

After providing an overview of our study site and briefly presenting some of our quantitative findings (reported extensively in Balka and Peterson, 1999 and 2002), we consider whether or not library-based Internet access is supporting the goals of citizenship and social cohesion, through discussion of our qualitative data. Our findings suggest that, to date, the goal of supporting citizenship via library-based public access to the Internet has not been achieved. Our observations also suggest that some degree of social cohesion has been achieved in relation to publicly accessible Internet sites, however, the mechanisms through which social cohesion is being realized in relation to publicly accessible Internet use varies markedly from the vision put forth by the Canadian government.

Citizenship and the Internet in the information age

In recent years, many claims have been made about the potential of new communication technologies to enhance public participation in democratic society. Popular writers and government officials alike have equated access to the Internet with new possibilities of citizenship, and organizations such as the Washington DC-based Center for Democracy and Technology work to advance "democratic values in new computer and communications technologies" (Balas, 1998). Libraries, historically seen as an important institution within democracy (Schiller and Schiller, 1988) have been targeted as an institution that can deliver equitable access to online information (Gutstien, 1999), which is increasingly seen as essential to emerging forms of cyber-democracy.

Libraries are to play an important role in Canada's strategy to provide citizens with Internet access. For example, Recommendation 13.12 of the Information Highway Advisory Committee (IHAC) report (1995) suggested that because Canadians are comfortable with public libraries, "in the new information age, libraries can play a new role in the provision of sophisticated technical assistance and mediated access to ever-expanding sources of electronic information and services." The IHAC called upon government to "develop and support pilot projects aimed at promoting libraries as public access points."

The federal government embarked on an ambitious plan to give all Canadians access to the Internet by 2000 (Kilgour, 1998). The placement of Internet terminals in Canada's public libraries reflects the goals of LibraryNet, which "aims to provide Canadians with affordable access to the Internet through our public libraries and to promote the use of the Internet in libraries for lifelong learning, community, and economic development" (Canada's SchoolNet, 1999: 1–2). In addition, the Internet is seen increasingly as "a way to access federal, provincial and municipal information services" (Connecting Canadians, 1999).

The Internet as infrastructure for new forms of citizen involvement with governments

The Internet is seen as a new vehicle for serving citizens and exercising influence throughout the world. "The KBS [knowledge-based society] poses important issues of governance, challenging the capacity of nation states to regulate on the one hand, but providing new vehicles to serve citizens and to exercise influence in the world community on the other" (Policy Research Initiative, 1999). The Internet is seen as a major vehicle through which citizens can be served. For example, "the Government of Canada has recognized a growing desire among Canadian citizens to be more involved in their country's governance." In the *Fifth Report to the Prime Minister on the Public Service of Canada* (April 1998), the Clerk of the Privy Council identified citizen engagement as "the next big challenge" the Canadian government must address, and suggested the government "explore ways to give citizens a greater voice in developing government policy" and to "give a fuller, richer meaning to the relationship between government and citizens" (OECD, 1998: 5).

Programs such as Canadian Governments Online have been developed with the explicit purpose of increasing the connection between citizens and government. Bourgon (1997: 2) wrote that "on the verge of the 21st century, technology is allowing us to imagine new ways of connecting citizens, of eliminating the disadvantage of physical distance – and of giving a fuller, richer meaning to democracy and citizenship." She suggests that "during the coming years, we will be called upon to redefine the relationship between governments and citizens" (ibid.: 5).

The Internet is seen as a way to deliver more client-centered services. It enables the provision of responsive, client-centered government to citizens. One vision is that of "triple A government" – anytime, anywhere, anything. This concept, which is taking root in several parts of the world, implies that service is provided to the public from any location at any time, work is performed from any location at any time, and cross-government solutions emerge naturally without the client being aware of the structures.

(Policy Research Initiative, 1999: 5)

The Internet is seen by the government as a way to provide Canadian citizens with "new opportunities to engage citizens in participatory democracy, be it through electronic townhalls or teledemocracy" (Policy Research Initiative, 1999: 5).

The Internet as a catalyst for social cohesion

The Internet is seen as a mechanism for increasing the connectedness of Canadians, which in turn is seen as an important step in the maintenance of social cohesion and citizenship. The Senate of Canada has defined social cohesion as "The capacity to live together in harmony with a sense of mutual commitment among citizens of different social or economic circumstances" (cited in CIRCLE/CCRN, 2000: n.p.). It refers to elements of people's day-to-day relationships which are conditioned and constrained by economic and political practices, that are important determinants of the quality of their lives, and of communities' healthy functioning (Labonte and Laverack, 2001).

Advances in telecommunications are seen as making decisions faced by citizens more complicated, while making citizen participation more important:

Citizen participation and engagement are becoming increasingly crucial as citizens become more sophisticated and governments face more and more complex choices. The rapid pace of technological development, and particularly communication and information technology, increase the complexity of choices that face citizens and governments.

(Canadian Heritage, 1999: 2)

The assumed connection between access to the technology, social cohesion, and citizenship is further articulated by Heritage Canada, which had as one of its goals the development of "a strategy to encourage community, civic and citizen participation" (ibid.: 1). It is hoped that, through support of initiatives that will allow Canadians access to the information highway, Canadians will become increasingly "involved in nation-building as a key strategy to enhance social cohesion and encourage full participation in Canada's future" (ibid.: 2).

Citizenship and access to the Internet

The need for policies to address a potentially widening gap between those with access to the Internet and those who lack access to the Internet has been articulated by Heritage Canada:

> There is a distinct risk that not every segment of the population will be equally able to make the transition to the emerging, knowledge-based world. As a result, government policies may well be needed to ease the transition, to compensate for disadvantage, and to insure basic access and rights be maintained.
>
> (Ibid.: 2)

The realization that not all Canadians have access to computer-mediated communications at a time when increasingly the Canadian government is communicating with its citizens electronically and encouraging the use of the Internet as a strategy for building social cohesion has contributed to the development of a range of programs aimed at extending access to the Internet to all Canadians.

The possibility that increased use of the Internet will contribute to disparities rather than reduce them has been acknowledged at senior levels of the Canadian government. For example, in *Canada 2005: Global Challenges and Opportunities* (Policy Research Initiative, 1997: 8), it is acknowledged that

> For this potential [of the Internet] to be realized universal access must become a reality . . . Concern is mounting therefore about the need for universal access to new information technologies and the information networks which link them together, as the first vital step towards promoting social cohesion in the knowledge-based society.

Programs such as the Community Access Program (CAP, which provides residents of rural areas with access to computers) and LibraryNet (aimed at putting Internet-ready computers in all Canadian libraries) were designed to mitigate differences in access to computers and the Internet. The desire to make the Internet accessible to all Canadians, combined with a demand for access to the Internet by marginalized groups, has fuelled the rapid introduction of Internet-ready terminals within libraries throughout the country, including the Vancouver Public Library system. However, in spite of the claims made about the Internet as a vehicle for the delivery of new, more participatory forms of government and the role of the Internet in promoting social cohesion, little empirical investigation of Internet use in public libraries has taken place (Gorgeç *et al.*, 1999). Studies that have been conducted have typically focused on the use of the Internet by librarians rather than patrons. Although Gorgeç *et al.* analyzed a sampling of user log files in an effort to determine what library patrons use Internet terminals for, we know of no other observationally based study of

Internet use in public libraries. Our work, based on a week of observations at a branch of Vancouver Public Library, sheds light not only on use patterns, but also on how the Internet terminals at the public libraries fit into the patrons' everyday lives.

The research setting: the Renfrew Branch of the Vancouver Public Library

The Renfrew Branch of the Vancouver Public Library (VPL) is housed in one of VPL's newest buildings. Situated next to a community center that houses a pool and weight room in a park-like setting, the building was five years old at the time of the study. The Renfrew branch is in a quiet residential neighborhood, southeast of downtown Vancouver. The average family income in the neighborhood where the Renfrew Branch is located (Renfrew-Collingwood)[4] was, at $44,559, $13,061 less than the City of Vancouver average of $57,620 in 1996. Sixteen of Vancouver's 22 neighborhoods boast higher income levels than Renfrew-Collingwood; only five neighborhoods have annual family incomes lower than those in Renfrew-Collingwood, where the branch is located. Compared to other neighborhoods in Vancouver, the neighborhood where the Renfrew Branch is located is not affluent.

Like most of Vancouver's neighborhoods, Renfrew-Collingwood is ethnically diverse. Nearly 66 percent of the neighborhood's residents are visible minorities, compared to a visible minority population of 44.7 percent in the City of Vancouver. People of Chinese origin (43.8 percent of Renfrew-Collingwood residents) constitute the largest ethnic group in the Renfrew-Collingwood area. Only two of Vancouver's 22 neighborhoods – Oakridge (a very affluent neighborhood) and Strathcona (one of the city's poorest neighborhoods) – have a greater percentage of Chinese residents than Renfrew-Collingwood.

Caucasians make up the next largest group in Renfrew-Collingwood, representing 34.2 percent of the neighborhood population. The Caucasian population in Renfrew-Collingwood is considerably smaller than the City of Vancouver Caucasian population (55.3 percent). Only two other neighborhoods in Vancouver have proportionally smaller Caucasian populations – the Victoria-Fraserview neighborhood (just southwest of Renfrew-Collingwood), and the Sunset neighborhood, which is just west of Victoria-Fraserview.

The ethnic diversity of the neighborhood where the Renfrew Branch is located is evident not only from a quick look around at the patrons, but also in the linguistic diversity of material on the shelves. The library carries material in a range of languages including Chinese, French, Vietnamese, and English. Although a majority of residents in the Renfrew-Collingwood area understand English (83.3 percent), French (0.1 percent) or English and French (3.3 percent), 13 percent of the neighbourhood's residents speak neither English nor French. For less than a third of the neighborhood's residents, either English or French was their mother tongue.

Research findings

Equitable Internet access: precursor to citizenship

> We're just barely set up with our sign up [indicating we are observing] talking to staff when one of our first users come in (2 adolescent males, Asian), go to computers C and D, and one male Asian youth (8–10 years old) goes to computer E. As he signs on he reads a pile of *MAD* magazines . . . An older East Indian male goes to computer F at 10:15 (Ellen's Field Notes, June 4).

In the 45 minutes following the entry above, we observed a steady stream of young men and boys arriving to use the library's Internet terminals. Only one woman interrupted this flow of males. Although it is a school day and school is in session, the Internet terminals – with the exception of the one occupied by the lone adult woman who arrived at 10:45 – are being used by school-aged boys and young men. At 10:55, two adult men, who we later find out are a school principal and a district truancy officer, show up at the library and do a "sweep." They speak to each of the children and young adults using the Internet about how many classes he's missed that day and they get the kids to leave the library. The librarians later tell us this is not an average day (the truancy officers had never shown up before). Though perhaps the presence of the truancy officers is atypical, in the following week we determine that the presence of the truancy officers does not seem to deter other truant kids who skip school to use the library Internet terminals. We also determine that the predominance of boys and young men using the Internet terminals for things like seeking information about and playing online games and computer chatting is typical of any other day at the Renfrew Branch of VPL.

Gender

In our week of observations at the Renfrew Branch of VPL, we conducted detailed observations of two Internet terminals, and tracked the gender of users on the six other Internet terminals. Over the course of the week, we found that two-thirds of the users of the terminals we observed (62.7 percent) were men, and one-third of the Internet users (37.3 percent) were women. Internet users at the Renfrew Branch of the Vancouver Public library are twice as likely to be Jacques than Jill.

Age

During our week at VPL, we found that nearly 40 percent of Internet users were under 15 years old. An additional 23.7 percent of users were between the ages of 16 and 20, for a total of 62.7 percent of Internet users younger than age 20.

Only 8.5 percent of Internet users were age 36 or older. Clearly, the Internet terminals at the Renfrew Branch of VPL serves a largely male and largely adolescent and young adult population.

One of the assumptions underlying the ideal of equitable access is that access will be required in order for citizens to engage in new forms of cyber-democracy.

> Sneaker boy times out, now Malaysian girl logs on and at controls. Little boy moves to [terminal] E as soon as user previously at E leaves. I don't think he can log on [because he has no time left]. Little boy logs onto E successfully and Sneaker boy moves to E to be his partner. At the table behind Ellen, the regular with the bike helmet waits impatiently for a terminal (Brian's Field Notes, June 10).

Ethnicity

During our week of observations, 51.7 percent of Internet users were Chinese, and 18.6 percent of users were Caucasian with East Indians comprising 6.8 percent, and Filipinos 5.1 percent. Not all ethnic groups go to the library to use the Internet terminals. Use of the library Internet terminals was somewhat higher amongst the Chinese community than their representation within the neighborhood (43.8 percent) would suggest. In contrast, library Internet use by Caucasians was somewhat lower than their representation within the neighborhood (34.2 percent) would suggest. These patterns of use may reflect differences in the demographics of the Chinese and Caucasian residents in the neighborhood, as well as differences in life circumstances. More information (for example, about rates of home computer ownership and home Internet access based on ethnic origin) is required to understand why some groups do not make use of the Internet access provided by the library. In addition, it may be that different ethnic communities see – and in fact use – the library in different ways, and these differences, which we know little about, may influence patterns of library Internet use.

The age of patrons using the Internet terminals during our observation period also varied with ethnic origin, as Table 10.1 indicates. Particularly striking were differences in the youngest group of users, (under 10 years of age) which did not include any Caucasian patrons, and the comparatively large proportion of Caucasian users between the ages of 21 and 25. Although we speculate that a lack of access to day-care services amongst residents of Chinese origin in the Renfrew-Collingwood area may explain the greater percentage of young Chinese Internet users at the Renfrew branch (who may use the library as a surrogate form of after-school care in the absence of other services), further study is required to validate this assertion and develop explanations for other use patterns that vary in relation to ethnic origin.

Table 10.1 Age distribution of Chinese and Caucasian Internet users responding to post-use survey

Age	Under 10	11–15	16–20	21–25	26–30	31–35	Over 36
% of Chinese Internet users	14.8	23.0	23.0	4.9	9.8	14.8	9.8
% of Caucasian Internet users	0.0	22.7	22.7	18.2	13.6	9.1	13.6

Exercising influence in local and global communities

A frequently mentioned goal of the Canadian government's Internet access policies revolves around providing Canadians with opportunities to exercise their influence in local and global communities. In the context of Internet use, we suspect that desired outcomes of such a policy goal might include activities such as communicating with others locally and globally about issues of civic or civil importance (such as environmental issues, government policy, etc.) via the Internet, and engaging in other Internet-mediated communicative acts that might lead to democratic change. Given the demographics of the Internet users we observed, it is not surprising that exercising influence in local communities took on a somewhat different meaning.

> Note: I don't think the adult patron with the bike helmet (the primary user[5] at terminal E) is impressed with all these youths. Candyboy is trying to find out when E prime will be done. E prime does not appear impressed (Brian's Field Notes, June 10).

> At the table behind Ellen, the regular with the bike helmet waits impatiently for a terminal. Mom comes and collects Candyboy and Stars and Stripes at 6:18 (Brian's Field Notes, June 10).

> Aussyboy and his friend are back, they literally force the older users off of terminal G. They log onto terminal G at 6:38 (Brian's Field Notes, June 10).

> Patron at E complains to kids "hey there are only supposed to be 2 per station." They ignore him. One puts hands on his chair, he tells them to get off the chair; they leave for 10 seconds and come back, are now even louder (Ellen's Field Notes, June 10).

The library Internet terminals fit into library patrons' lives in many different ways. For some of the young (male) regulars (Aussyboy, Candyboy, and Stars and Stripes), the library was the place they went after school and on weekends, and the Internet terminals lay at the centre of their social worlds. One of the adult male patrons was involved in a cyber courtship; another adult male patron was searching for information about the temperament of various breeds of dogs. A young adult woman used the Internet to engage in regular cyber-chat sessions with her mother in Mexico. Other adult users checked foreign language news or financial information online, and occasionally an adult would engage in job seeking activities online.

Each of the uses to which the Internet was put engendered a different kind of culture of use. For Aussyboy, Candyboy, and Stars and Stripes, as well as their older peers who engaged in computer chatting as well as online games, the Internet terminals were literally a home away from home, and their use of the Internet for online games took on the raucousness of a basement recreation room. For some of the users engaged in research activities (such as the patron seeking information about dog breeds), a more sedate atmosphere was desired. The patron involved in the cyber-courtship sought an audience (excited about a scheduled first meeting with his cyber date, he felt compelled to share the details with all those around him); the woman who chatted online with her mother in Mexico sought a bit of privacy.

Varied users and varied uses combined with overcrowding (greater demand than could be met as well as large numbers of people in small spaces) sometimes resulted in clashes between users. A frequent outcome was that the younger, louder users were able to exercise their influence in the local community, leaving users who sought a bit of quiet or a bit of space as they used the Internet frustrated. These somewhat generational clashes may serve as a deterrent to those who wish to use public access Internet terminals for uses more in line with the government's stated goals – though it should be noted it remains unclear to what extent the Internet is used to pursue stated goals in general, and by those using public access Internet sites in particular.

It should be noted that the library had policies (such as a limit of two people per computer) designed to mitigate the kinds of clashes we observed. However, it was difficult for library staff to simultaneously enforce these policies, and perform their normal professional functions (e.g. assist patrons in locating materials); typically, they engaged in enforcing regulations only when a complaint was brought to them.

The patterns of Internet use we observed and the clashes that sometimes resulted caused us to think a great deal about the development of programs that might support various groups in developing social agency in relation to the Internet. For example, designating certain times as "family use" times might facilitate inter-generational skill transfer about computers, or designating some times as "adult times" (a common practice in community pools and ice rinks) might make it easier for some groups to gain access to the Internet. Although it is tempting to think that any policies aimed at ameliorating such clashes must occur within a fairly rigid framework with clear rules and enforcement, it must also be noted that managing local Internet use adds to the strain of librarians' jobs.

Cyber-democracy

As suggested above, ideas about using the Internet to support democracy are plentiful. Typically, notions of cyber democracy revolve around three related themes: (1) increasing access to government services via the Internet and supporting the relationship between governments and citizens through Internet-mediated contact; (2) stimulating citizen engagement and community and civic participation through the Internet, and (3) the possibility of using the Internet as a means of communicating with the government about a range of issues, which could include online voting.

During our study period at the Renfrew library, the use of Internet terminals for access to government information was conspicuously absent in the activities we observed. Although we observed library patrons using the Internet for a variety of tasks including game-playing, computer chatting, email and retrieving foreign language news, accessing government information was not one of them. Of course this does not mean that the Internet is not used for this purpose; only that it was not often used in the library for this purpose. Given the demographics of our users – a majority of whom were children and youths under 20 – this is not a surprising finding. Among those who did use the Internet to access government websites, by far the most commonly sought information was about employment.

As we have just noted, we saw no evidence that the Internet was stimulating citizen engagement and civil involvement in a traditional sense. However, we did observe an interesting phenomenon, namely online voting, that one can argue is a form of community and civic participation and that perhaps does reflect the government's stated objectives:

> The primary user at terminal F is at the hotmail main page. Replies to another message. The secondary user notices me, but again looks over at terminal F. The secondary user is sitting at terminal E again but is passive . . . A 4th person (an Asian girl) is standing really passively behind terminals E and F, looking around as if bored . . . The secondary user is involved, but only by talking to the primary user at terminal F. I can't tell whether she is involved in composing what is being typed or if she is just keeping him [the primary user] company. I think that he is on free vote. The secondary user is talking about how many votes someone got (Brian's Field Notes, June 9).

> 2 other young boys, (I recognize them from last week) come in. The Aussy kid kicks another boy off. They access free vote, and the youngest kid (smallest) over takes controls and navigates to free vote. I think to myself, 'aren't they too young to be interested in free vote?' (Brian's Field Notes, June 8).

Over the course of our study period, we began to develop some rapport with some of the "regulars" – library patrons who came into the library a few times a week or in many cases (such as the case of "Aussy boy," whom we will discuss in more detail below) daily, specifically to use the Internet. We learned that Free Vote (http://www.freevote.com) is an online program that allowed kids to vote for who the coolest (or uncoolest) person they knew was. Free Vote allows webmasters to create virtual "voting booths" where web surfers can come and cast their vote on any issue a member of the public wishes to poll others about, for instance, the possible uses for a derelict building.

Although voting for the coolest person in the class was probably not the original intention behind the application (which was originally designed as a free service for anyone to use), and one could argue about the merits of using Free Vote in the way those we observed were using it (to cast votes about their classmates, which could prove quite hurtful to some), the concept is interesting in that it is an example that illustrates how democratic agency can be exercised with the aid of Internet technology. Although the use of Free Vote that we observed could arguably be deemed frivolous, Free Vote could be used as a tool in the context of cyber democracy if issues about security and accessibility are adequately addressed. In the context of our observations, Free Vote was used in a manner that reflected the interests of a sub-set of the users we observed. Thus, within the broader context of exploring the potential of the Internet in the context of democracy, the use of software such as Free Vote may warrant further attention.

Social cohesion: new ways of connecting citizens

Our findings concerning the role of the Internet in promoting social cohesion reflect concerns raised that "the information revolution, many believe, has the potential to promote social cohesion both within societies as well as between. Yet there are also tendencies in the opposite direction" (Policy Research Initiative, 1997: 4).

During our study period, we observed several uses of the Internet (such as maintaining contact with family members (who were often abroad) via Internet chat and email) that can be understood as activities that might lead to or comprise social cohesion. Although stated policy objectives suggest that the Internet ought to play a role in promoting social cohesion by connecting Canadians in different locations, at the conclusion of our study we were struck by the extent to which the presence of the Internet contributed to the formation of social cohesion at a local level:

> On the computers behind me, two females appear to be working collabo-
> ratively together on a project. One appears to be a mother, the other a
> daughter. It's about 2:13 . . . The mother from the mother-daughter team
> has moved from terminal E to terminal F; was unsure how the system
> worked (e.g. didn't know that you can only log onto one computer at a
> time, under your own card). It appears as though this is her first time using

the Internet; she still has not logged on yet. She has logged on using her daughter's card (Brian's Field Notes, June 4).

Mother at E is also writing an e-mail and son is sitting behind her on the same chair. She is pushed right up to the edge of their chair. Now she takes the child and puts him on her knee. Just browsing through hotmail site and the 1st primary user is still explaining things like how to send a message and how to manage the account (Brian's Field Notes, June 9).

As the two excerpts from field notes above suggest, for some, the library Internet terminals seem to serve as a locus for familial social cohesion. On several occasions we observed inter-generational familial groups using the Internet terminals. Typically these groups were from a visible minority group, and one family member often took the lead in teaching other family members how to use the Internet. Although the stated library Internet use policies at the time of the study prohibited patrons from using the Internet to send and receive email or engage in computer chatting, this proved impossible to enforce. In reality, the lure of communicating with family members in other geographic locations often seemed to serve as a catalyst for skill transfer and learning (and provided an opportunity for younger people to teach parents or adults about technology). The Internet terminals clearly played a role in fostering relationships at a local level as well as for those communicating with distant friends and family.

They both are smiling and giggling. They are sharing the keyboard very strangely and inefficiently. A different girl comes and stands behind them, a brief exchange occurs and the girl leaves. There is constant dialogue between the two boys. The sister is watching passively, an interesting dynamic. They've met someone on the chat line (Brian's Field Notes, June 5).

The library Internet terminals also seemed to serve as a locus for peer group formation and social cohesion at a local level. We were quite surprised to learn, for example, that Aussyboy, a young Internet regular of Chinese origin who seemed to be at the centre of the under-10 social network, had moved with his family from Australia only a month before we met him. He seemed to spend all of his out-of-school time in the library, and when he wasn't the primary user of an Internet terminal in the library, he was typically scavenging for time on Internet terminals.[6] Although he had lived in Vancouver only a short time, he had carved a niche for himself as an Internet regular at the library, where he daily met his new friends with whom he played computer games, ate candy (supplied by Candyboy, who seemed to have a small business procuring candy from the local store, which he re-sold to less adventuresome (or more obedient) under 10 year olds, such as Stars and Stripes), and socialized.

At the conclusion of our study, we had become aware of a phenomenon well known to librarians: that the library is a place where parents felt they could leave their children while they were working (e.g. after school).The Internet terminals played an important role in occupying the "regulars," many of whom were in the library daily, including weekends. Some parents who came to the library to seek print material would deposit their children at the Internet terminals while they went to other parts of the library.The Internet terminals in the library not only contributed to a sense of local social cohesion, but use of the terminals in this manner also seemed to reflect a sense of community well-being or social cohesion.

Although the library Internet terminals were central to the creation of a sense of local community for many of the youths that we observed, for some of the adults we observed, use of the Internet terminals in a public setting was somewhat more problematic.

> Asian man sits at E. Gets pencil and paper, looks at the screen for a minute and leaves. It appears as though he didn't know what he was doing (Brian's Field Notes, June 4).

> Older women (adult) sits down at terminal. Starts doing something and a group arrives and youth assumes control over controls (Brian's Field Notes, June 9).

For those who did not regularly use the Internet, use of the library Internet terminals could be an isolating experience.An inexperienced adult Internet user who is not able to figure out how to browse the Web or log onto the terminal, and is surrounded by Internet-savvy youths, may get frustrated and end up not using the system at all.Although clearly public access terminals can serve multiple social functions, without attention to the social contexts of use, the terminals can contribute to social marginalization, rather than social cohesion.A range of social interventions (e.g. time dedicated to seniors), and the dedication of ample human resources to maintenance of the technical infrastructure of public access terminals, and the learning needs of users, will be required to support a reality of the Internet as a means of citizenship and social cohesion, rather than a field of dreams.

Conclusion

Our findings suggest that for women and members of some ethnic groups, the "Field of Dreams" philosophy (build it and they will come) does not translate into Internet use in the library setting we observed – or at least not in the ways that Canadian government discourse about the Internet has suggested. Our findings suggest that although in some respects current use of the Internet in libraries is inconsistent with the goals articulated in current public policies, some of the governments goals – of promoting social cohesion – may be met indirectly in relation to public access Internet terminals, largely because the Internet terminals became the locus for social interaction – both peer group and familial – for many users.

Vancouver Public Library staff have done an exemplary job in their attempts to make the library's Internet terminals accessible. For example, they regularly run Internet classes (including classes targeted towards specific groups, such as seniors), and they work hard to keep equipment that sees a high volume of use working well. Although we were able to imagine a range of social interventions (such as giving preference for terminals to certain groups at certain times), as well as some technical interventions (e.g. creating group use rooms where small groups could use the Internet without interrupting the quiet of the library), it was more difficult to imagine how such interventions could be implemented without adding to the already hectic workload of library staff. Clearly, in order for the government vision for the Internet to be realized, resources must be allocated for staffing and social programming, as well as technology.

Although the government may have developed a "triple A" program (anytime, anywhere, anything), the segment of population gaining access to the Internet through the public access terminals we observed seldom took advantage of these resources. Additional research that focuses on Internet use patterns of those with home Internet connections, combined with more extensive study of the activities Internet users engage in, will be required to determine to what extent online government resources are being used in meaningful ways by Canadians.

Notes

1   Material reflected here represents the authors' interpretation of the data and understanding of Internet use at Vancouver Public Library. The views expressed here do not necessarily reflect views of the Vancouver Public Library staff or administration.

2   Data were collected between June 4 and 10, during which time the library was on summer hours. The library was open from 10 to 9 Tuesday – Thursday; and 10 to 6 Friday and Saturday.

3   Out of 165 patrons that used the two terminals we conducted detailed observations of, 118 patrons (71.5 percent) answered our survey questions. An additional 18 patrons (10.9 percent) had responded to the survey earlier in the week, and were deemed repeats. Only 18 patrons (10.9 percent) refused to respond to our survey. If our repeats (all of whom answered the survey earlier in the week) are subtracted from our total number of patrons, our corrected response rate is 89 percent.

4   Unless otherwise noted, demographic data reported in this section were obtained from *Vancouver Local Areas, 1996: Data from the Canadian Census*, published by Community Services, City of Vancouver, March 1999.

5   In excerpts from our field notes, primary user refers to the person who is using the keyboard and/or mouse at a given terminal. The secondary user refers to an additional person (a friend or family member) who is with the primary user at the computer, and is engaged in the activity taking place on the Internet terminal, but who is not using the keyboard or mouse.

6   At the time of our study, patrons were allowed to use the Internet for two half-hour periods daily, separated by at least one half hour. Time limits were imposed by timer software. Often when the young users had used their daily time allotment

or were waiting for a half hour to pass so they could log on again, they would go to vacant terminals in hope that another patron had failed to sign off, or they would join another young user as a secondary – or perhaps primary user – during the other user's allotted time. We referred to these practices as scavenging for time. Regular users often engaged in a range of strategies to work around the timer software, such as using log-on IDs of multiple family members.

Chapter 11

A human rights perspective on the digital divide

A human right to communicate

William J. McIver, Jr.

Motivating a human rights approach to bridging the digital divide

Significant inequities exist in access to telecommunications technologies and services globally – including in the United States (Haywood, 1995: 114–126). A number of major studies in recent years have illustrated major disparities in access to the Internet for certain minorities, the poor, and people living in certain geographic areas (NTIA, 1995, 1998, 1999, 2000; Hoffman and Novak, 1999). This has become an increasingly critical issue as access to advanced tele-communications and information technologies becomes increasingly necessary to function in society.

Policy development toward bridging the so-called "digital divide" can and must include a human rights perspective, specifically in the context of a human right to communicate. The familiar amalgam of market-oriented and informal civil libertarian arguments around the digital divide are not sufficient for developing effective policies to address it.

Access to the Internet can be analyzed within formal and well-established human rights frameworks, primarily in the context of universal service. Human rights theories and acceptance of them have taken great strides over the past millennium, and universal service in telecommunications has been the subject of study and policy debates in international diplomatic and standards bodies for nearly 150 years. These legacies have contributed to the development of the concept of a human right to communicate. Yet reference to this legacy and use of its artifacts (i.e. frameworks, communiqués, declarations, and treaties) is, for the most part, absent in the cyber rights community.

The primary goals of this chapter are to: motivate the need to include a human rights perspective in addressing the digital divide, give a conceptual and historical overview of the development of applicable human rights concepts, and present human rights frameworks that might be used to implement and enforce these rights.

Defining universal service

Universal service is defined by the RAND corporation in its study *Universal Access to E-Mail* as facilities and services that are "available at modest individual effort and expense to everyone in a form that does not require highly specialized skills, or accessible in a manner analogous to the level, cost, and ease of use of telephone service or the US Postal Service" (Anderson *et al.*, 1995: 7).The sole criterion under which a communication modality should be considered for universal provisioning is taken in this chapter to be that it is consistent with public necessity, as defined by the standard set forth in Article 25 section 1 of the Universal Declaration of Human Rights, which states:

> Everyone has the right to a standard of living adequate for the health and well-being of himself and of his family, including food, clothing, housing and medical care and necessary social services, and the right to security in the event of unemployment, sickness, disability, widowhood, old age, or other lack of livelihood in circumstances beyond his control.
>
> (United Nations, 1997)

Communication modalities from the telegraph to the Internet have and will continue to play an important role all of the facets of living covered in Article 25.

Civil libertarian and market-oriented perspectives

A United States-centered discourse on cyber rights, including censorship, privacy, and universal service, began to emerge in the late 1980s within cyber rights, business, and governmental spheres. This was spurred on, in part, by: civil liberties cases, such as that of Steve Jackson, a game manufacturer who was targeted by the Secret Service (EFF, 1990); President Clinton's National Information Infrastructure initiative; a host of trials and planned deployments of advanced telephony, broadband, and wireless services, fuelled by the post-divestiture environment; and the evolution of the Internet from an elite communication medium for academic, military, and industrial research into a medium that has become more consumer-oriented. This discourse has largely failed to reference human rights concepts.

The 1990 announcement of the founding of the critically important Electronic Freedom Foundation (EFF, 1990) and John Perry Barlow's essay (1990) on the occasion of its founding, "Crime and Puzzlement," made no reference to human rights. They made, instead, brief or oblique references to (US) civil rights, although their mission is arguably of a global nature.

The popular "Magna Carta for the Knowledge Age" (Dyson *et al.*, 1994) declared cyberspace is "the latest American frontier" and surveyed a number of issues calling for such a declaration, including property and intellectual rights, social anxiety, and the role of government in cyberspace. It failed, however, to follow to a logical conclusion its identification of "the need to affirm the basic principles of freedom" by identifying with the human rights legacy set in motion by its namesake, the Magna Carta of 1215.

The US discourse on universal service has been based largely on market-oriented arguments, and informal or indirect references to civil liberties. The consequence of applying only a market-oriented focus is that fundamental human needs are usually overlooked. CPSR's *One Planet, One Net*, for example, characterized the use of the "Net" as "inherently an exercise of freedom of speech, to be restricted at great peril to human liberty," but offers only a business-oriented example as a negative consequence of restricted access, stating that "[t]he Net offers great promise as a means of increasing global commerce and collaboration among businesses, but restrictions on information exchange would eviscerate that promise."

Human desires – to play games, play the stock market, or express one's feelings – are often implicitly equated with and taken to represent the totality of human needs in this discourse; and human needs are seen as requirements which can be met through market forces. History continues to show, however, that markets and domestic civil rights are sometimes insufficient for providing remedy or protection of fundamental human needs (James, 1996: 238–242). Various communities have recognized this and as a result have sought interventions in their plights under human rights frameworks implemented by international bodies such as the United Nations.

Some requirements for access to the Internet fall within the domain of government. Recent work in the area of digital government, for example, has revealed the lack of appropriate access points to and integration of US government information systems, which hinders the provision of social services by forcing individuals – often the poor – to travel long distances between offices (Bouguettaya *et al.*, 2001 and 2002). Explicit mandates or incentives for business involvement in these areas are often not sufficient. For example, persistent resistance by telecommunications companies to honor the E-Rate requirement of the Telecommunications Act of 1996, which requires these companies to provide access lines for Internet access at special discounts to schools and libraries, has been well-documented (Hammond, 1997: 204; Rosenbaum, 1999).

The role of information technologies in numerous life and death struggles calls out for concretized and analytic uses of the notions of freedom of speech and liberty. For example, humans have been using information technologies to provide information to people in other countries to effect human rights interventions. Radio broadcasts and satellite transmissions were used in 1994 to report the beginning of the massacre in Rwanda. Electronic mail played a key role in disseminating information about the 1993 massacre of Yanomami in Brazil (see NICANET at www.igc.org). Facsimile technology was also a critical conduit for information during the Tiananmen Square massacre (Nye and Owens, 1996: 20–36).

Expression in these contexts can, thus, be seen as part of a specific life-critical process of exchanging information – the act of communication. A right to communicate is, arguably, more fundamental than freedom of expression. Communication is a basic human need because it is a fundamental social process necessary for expression and all social organization. Information, thus, has a social function. It should not be viewed only as propaganda or a commodity, nor should it be controlled only by the power structures of the market or the state.

The basis for the human right to communicate

The original basis for a human right to communicate derives from the Universal Declaration of Human Rights (UN, 1993), adopted in 1948. The centerpiece of the declaration with regard to communication is Article 19, which states:

> Everyone has the right to freedom of opinion and expression: this right includes freedom to hold opinions without interference and to seek, receive and impart information and ideas through any media and regardless of frontiers.
>
> (United Nations, 1997)

Article 19 is buttressed by two other articles. Article 27 section 1 states:

> Everyone has the right freely to participate in the cultural life of the community, to enjoy the arts and to share in scientific advancement and its benefits.
>
> (United Nations, 1997)

Scientific advancements that have enabled modern communication such as telephony, the Internet or other technologies that enable the World Wide Web can be seen in the context of Article 27, not as the exclusive domain of those who are able to negotiate the market place to acquire them, but as entitlements of people whose societies support their creation (e.g. through government research grants or a reallocation of resources). The rights set forth in Articles 19 and 27 imply that a society must maintain adequate literacy rates and basic infrastructure for their enforcement. Article 28 addresses this in principle, stating:

> Everyone is entitled to a social and international order in which the rights and freedoms set forth in this Declaration can be fully realized.
>
> (United Nations, 1997)

Articles 19 and 28 can be seen as complementary since it is argued that communication is a necessary component for maintaining a social and international order in which rights such as those set forth in the Universal Declaration of Human Rights are enforced.

Counter-arguments

A human rights approach to addressing the digital divide will likely be criticized for being inflexible and, therefore, incapable of accounting for the very real priorities that face communities attempting to provision service. Human rights (or originally natural rights) have been criticized at least since the late eighteenth century as being absolutist. Some might argue that to claim communication as a human right implies the requirement to carry out implementations of the right that are not in the best interest of some societies. It would be unreasonable, for example, to implement individual Internet access in societies where literacy rates are low and public health and other basic services are lacking.

The focus of this chapter, however, is not on specific technical implementations for universal service. Its purpose is, rather, to examine the concept of communication as a basic human right and to explore the possibility of policy development for bridging digital divides from the standpoint of the formal frameworks that have been developed around this right.

A human rights approach to addressing the digital divide is also not likely to be seen as compelling by those who criticize it on grounds that they are absolute and do not "trade off." The cost and complexity of the various technical solutions to a right to communicate as well as the levels of technical competence to use them might be used as evidence against a human rights claim. Following this logic, evidence for a human rights claim to communication take the form of the preconditions for the technical implementation of that communication: basic infrastructure, financial resources, and technical competence. The Universal Declaration of Human Rights recognizes this dilemma in its preamble by stating that it is:

> . . . a common standard of achievement for all peoples and all nations, to the end that every individual and every organ of society, keeping this Declaration constantly in mind, shall strive by teaching and education to promote respect for these rights and freedoms and by progressive measures, national and international, to secure their universal and effective recognition and observance . . .
>
> (United Nations, 1997)

What makes a right to communicate compelling are not the preconditions for its implementation, but the very fact that communication is a basic human need because it is a fundamental social process necessary for expression and all social organization. This need does not vary with respect to the level of economic development of a society. All humans need to receive and impart information to live. The urgency with which a right to communicate should be addressed varies with the level of development of a society. Lack of access to communication, for example, has been identified as a critical factor in public health crises around the world (see Garrett, 2000).

Advanced technologies such as the Internet must be considered only a part of a potential technical implementation of a right to communicate. The overriding concern should be in selecting technologies that are suitable and appropriate to a community. In this context, it is necessary to be open to the full range of communication modalities and technologies, including analog broadcast technologies, inter-personal communication methods, and institutional mechanisms such as libraries. It must also be realized that most telecommunications technologies can be deployed at granularities appropriate to a community's needs and resources, from community-level points of presence to individual access points. Garrett suggests that providing citizens of underdeveloped countries with community level points of access to health information would be a critical starting point for addressing health care crises such as AIDS epidemics in many of these underdeveloped countries. However, such access points should support more than one-way information flows from expert to patient, allowing people to both select and create communication flows they find useful and necessary to address life critical problems (e.g. between local health professionals and between patients).

Defining human rights

Human rights derive from human needs. A human right can be defined as a universally recognized legal right, which if not granted would cause the lives and livelihoods of human beings and communities to be impeded or harmed. Legal theorists define a legal right in norm-based jurisprudence as an entitlement with "a real, objective, juridical existence apart from [its] enforcement" (Dane, 1996: 216). A freedom differs from a right in that it is not imperative that the freedom be exercised in order to avoid impeding the lives and livelihoods of human beings. A freedom's exercise is subject to the will of the individual. The only requirement of a society is that it not allow the exercise of a freedom to be hindered.

The identification of human rights in a global context has historically been complicated by the existence of many different jurisdictions in the world, some based on very different norms (ibid.: 209). The corresponding existence of many different processes of adjudication complicates the identification of enforcement procedures and remedies for such rights when they are identified. The world community has, nevertheless, made critical strides in the past century toward the identification of universally accepted rights. The defining moment for this was the unanimous adoption of the Universal Declaration of Human Rights (UDHR) by the United Nations on December 10, 1948. This declaration was non-binding. Its adoption was followed by the creation of corresponding instruments that were meant to be binding and enforceable in international law by the states that ratify them: the International Covenant on Economic, Social and Cultural Rights; and the International Covenant on Civil and Political Rights and Optional Protocols, adopted by the UN in 1966 and 1976 respectively. These three documents constitute the International Bill of Human Rights (United Nations, 1993).

The passage and ratification of international human rights declarations and covenants is obviously no guarantee that they will be observed. It is also not certain that citizens of a country know the rights to which they are entitled under these agreements. This is not a reason to abandon human rights. They are critical because they provide, in the words of Hamelink, "[a] universally available set of standards for the dignity and integrity of all human beings" (1994: 58). These standards offer a common, well-established lexicon and framework – much like software standards – in which debate, identification, implementation, and enforcement of solutions to human problems can be conducted, hopefully in a more efficient and effective way. This has been seen in the implementation of the International Criminal Tribunal for the former Yugoslavia.

Development of a human right to communicate

Freedom of expression has long been regarded as a necessary component of democratic societies. Plato, *c.* 380 BCE, described people living in a hypothetical city where democracy had been established, saying: "first of all they are free, and the city becomes full of liberty and freedom of speech, and in it one can do anything one pleases" (Grube, 1974: 557b). Communication as a right distinct from that of expression is a relatively new concept, however.

Communication can be defined as a democratic and balanced dialogue between two or more parties. Freedom of expression can be seen as addressing the formulation and content of communication, whereas a right to communicate focuses on the means and processes required to form and convey expression. Individuals may enjoy freedom of expression, but face heavy restrictions on access to media necessary to disseminate it. Individuals may need to protest the violation of other rights or to seek information that could affect their standard of living. A right to communicate, thus, addresses both the critical day-to-day communications needs of people, and a requirement necessary for the protection of other rights. Many consider communication as a distinct human right because its absence would impede the lives and livelihoods of individuals, communities, and whole societies.

The trajectory from the European Enlightenment to the development of communication as a human right leads from support for universal service and then information rights, to recognition of the ability to communicate as individual and community entitlements. This has taken place along three dimensions: the evolution of human rights themselves; the development of world telecommunications policy; and the response of NGOs and developing and underdeveloped nations to the dominance of Western transnational media and the advent of new technologies such as direct broadcast satellites.

The evolution of human rights

Three generations of human rights have been identified: civil and political rights; economic, social and cultural rights; and the emerging area of collective rights (Marks, 1981;Vasak, 1990). The first generation of rights was articulated in such documents as the Magna Carta of 1215 and the United States Bill of Rights. Economic, social, and cultural rights evolved out of the Universal Declaration of Human Rights and are addressed in the International Covenant on Economic, Social, and Cultural Rights, adopted in 1966. Collective rights address self-determination, cultural preservation, and development of groups of people. The charter of the UN and the African Charter on Human and Peoples' Rights, adopted in 1981, articulate rights that are representative of third generation human rights (United Nations, 1997).

The development of communication rights has come about because of the shifts in the legal philosophy required to traverse these three generations of human rights. The recognition of rights within successive generations constitutes a shift from what may be described as a legal positivist perspective, which views laws only as policies which are developed and enforced in a unidirectional manner, from state to citizen; to a perspective embodied in modern natural law theory, which views laws as rules or forms of guidance that depend on co-operation and reciprocity between the state and its citizens for the system of guidance (i.e. the legal system) to function correctly. Identification and understanding of human rights from this latter perspective has required a progressive willingness to engage in moral evaluation of the conditions of humans and the societies in which they live (Bix, 1996: 231–232). This in itself is critical to the choice of a human rights perspective in discussing access to communications technologies.

The key artifacts from this evolution are those supporting freedom of expression such as the US Bill of Rights. The most significant of these is, arguably, Article 19 of the Universal Declaration of Human Rights (United Nations, 1993: 7), which embodies a much broader basis for the later and more explicit identification of communication as a human right.

Adoption of the UDHR was followed by the adoption of: the European Convention on Human Rights in 1950; the International Covenant on Civil and Political Rights (ICCPR), in which Article 19 of the UDHR is codified; the American Convention on Human Rights adopted by the Organization of American States in 1969; and the African Charter on Human and Peoples' Rights, in effect since 1986. All of these documents articulate in some way the freedom of communication and information. Most are not binding and the few that are have been characterized as weak and not complete in terms of articulating a right to communicate. The African Charter expresses only the "right to receive information," and section 3 of Article 19 in the International Covenant allows for "certain restrictions" to be applied by each state.

Some legal scholars argue, however, that a right to communicate may hold up as a principle of international law under the doctrine of estoppel (Malanczuk,

1991). The doctrine provides that a party cannot simultaneously accept and reject an instrument; or, in other words, having availed themselves of parts of it, defeat its provisions in any other part. It has been suggested that this doctrine can by extension provide that states signatory to an agreement must at least be bound by the consensus reflected in that agreement in interpreting human rights treaties.

Universal service

Early international standards bodies formed around the deployment of postal services, telegraphy, telephony, and radio to resolve realized and potential international political and technical conflicts that they raised. It was in this context that the notion of universal service first emerged. The International Telegraph Union's Convention of 1865 supported the availability of telecommunication services for all people (Hamelink, 1994: 66).

The original goal of universal telephone service for AT&T around 1907 was to establish a monopoly. Customers during this time often had to choose between competing telephone companies whose networks had disjointed coverage. Theodore Vail, the president of AT&T at the time, wanted to establish universal service, not as a way of meeting human needs, but as a way of reducing competition through the interconnection of competing networks (Anderson *et al.*, 1995: 117; Mueller, 1997).

The Communications Act of 1934 included the first provisions supporting universal telephone service. This contributed over time to changes in the United States in expected norms and standards for access to information, emergency services, and the performance of other life-critical tasks via the telephone. Today access to a telephone is considered a necessity, even in the most underdeveloped regions of the US. This norm, for example, has been more strongly codified following the 1934 Act in such legislation as California's Lifeline Bill, which stipulates that a minimum level of basic telephone service be made available to all (Moore, 1983).

A response to mass media

The evolution of human rights in general and the developments leading to the conception of universal service, such as the advent of telephony, provided catalysts for the evolution of the concept of a right to communicate. It was, however, the response by non-governmental organizations and developing nations to the unidirectional nature and undemocratic uses of mass media that ultimately motivated calls for more explicit declarations of a right to communicate.

Humans have historically been subjected to vertical, unidirectional forms of mass communication, which has produced negative consequences to public awareness of issues of importance to them, political participation, and policy-making (see Bagdikian, 1997; Chomsky and Herman, 1988; Schiller, 1996). McChesney chronicled in a seminal study (1993) the struggle between 1928 and 1935 to define the US radio broadcasting model and its aftermath. His study demonstrated that the resulting total victory of a corporate, for-profit model over that of a democratic, non-profit model stifled the development of public and community radio in the US for the next 30 years.

Calls to eliminate the imbalances and inequalities in communication in international law came primarily from the nations of the developing world, leading to a call in the 1970s for a New World Information and Communication Order (NWICO). The United States, it should be noted, eventually pulled out of UNESCO in 1983, partially out of disagreement with the NWICO advocated by the other member states (Malanczuk, 1991).

The concept of one-way data flow was developed in the 1950s as a characterization of the dominant news flows from the industrialized nations to developing and underdeveloped nations at the time (UNESCO, 1980a: 36). Freedom of information was seen as a one-way process of transmitting information from those in power to ordinary individuals. Hamelink points out that the imperialist nations began broadcasting to their colonies starting in the 1920s. Independence movements within the colonies and ultimately the independent states they would become had to contend with the political and cultural impacts of colonial media on their pre-revolutionary nationalists movements and the internal inter-ethnic conflicts they usually entailed. Such conflicts continue.

The Bandung Conference in 1955 at the advent of the non-aligned movement, and the United Nations Conference on Trade and Development in 1964 were forums in which issues of post-colonial communication and North–South communication imbalances were raised (Hamelink, 1994).

In 1961, the United Nations General Assembly adopted resolution 1721D (XVI), which supported the right of access to satellite communications by all countries on a non-discriminatory basis (Hamelink, 1994: 67). In 1969, Jean d'Arcy, Director of Radio and Visual Services in the UN Office of Public Information, introduced the concept of a right to communicate in response to developments in satellite technology. He recognized that new technological developments such as communications satellites were creating possibilities for communication that Article 19 did not adequately encompass. Article 19 was drafted mainly out of concern for mass communications media (Birdsall, 1998). The new technologies d'Arcy observed were beginning to enable greater access to two-way communication.

A number of efforts to develop a right to communicate have taken place over the decades since d'Arcy's observation. In 1969, the Organization of American States adopted the American Convention on Human Rights at San José, Costa Rica, which called for freedom from restrictions "to impede the communication and circulation of ideas and opinions" (OAS, 1969). The Canadian government began examining the concept of a right to communicate around this time. A Canadian Department of Communications task force called the Telecommission issued a report titled *Instant World*, which in its early drafts advocated a right to communicate (Birdsall and Rasmussen, 2000). UNESCO in 1974 began supporting a right to communicate, reiterating the language of the 1969 OAS document cited above (UNESCO, 1980). The MacBride Commission in UNESCO issued a report the same year, which recognized communication as a new right. In 1989, the Dag Hammarskjöld Foundation called for more work to guarantee humans a right to communicate, stating that citizens have the right "to inform and be informed about the facts of development, its inherent conflicts and the changes it will bring about." Global problems, they argued, cannot be solved without these guarantees. The strength of the third sector, comprised of people and organizations (e.g. NGOs), in counterbalancing state power and markets has been shown; however, communications must be democratized in order to sustain this strength.

By 1994, the drafting of a People's Communication Charter was underway in preparation for the fiftieth anniversary of the UDHR (Frederick, 1994). The charter was initiated through the work of the Center for Communication and Human Rights in Amsterdam, the Netherlands and the Third World Network in Penang, Malaysia (Hamelink, n.d.). The charter was motivated by a perceived need to address, in part, "insufficient channels [for people to communicate] ideas and opinions" (PCC, 2000). Other integral concerns include what are seen as "pervasive forms of censorship, distorted and misleading information, stereotyped images of gender and race, restricted access to knowledge." A consortium of organizations, which included the MacBride Roundtable on Communication, endorsed this effort. In 1996, the Platform for Communication Rights formed and in 2001 it initiated the Communication Rights in the Information Society (CRIS) Campaign.

Significant United Nations activity took place in the year 2000 with regard to addressing the digital divide within a human rights framework. Secretary-General Kofi Annan in his report to the Millennium Assembly of the United Nations (United Nations, March 2000) urged member nations to undertake a development agenda which includes "review [of] policies in order to remove regulatory and pricing impediments to Internet access, to make sure people are not denied the opportunities offered by the digital revolution." Responding to these recommendations, the declaration adopted by leaders of the member states at the Millennium Assembly of the United Nations included the following in its section on Development and Poverty Eradication:

> To ensure that the benefits of new technologies, especially information and communication technologies . . . are available to all.
> (United Nations, September 2000: Section III Article 20)

The most recent efforts around developing a right to communicate have taken place in the context of preparations for the UN-sponsored World Summit on the Information Society (WSIS) to be held in Geneva in 2003 and Tunis in 2005.

The CRIS Campaign has engaged in an effort to place a right to communicate on the WSIS agenda and a vigorous debate among supporters and opponents of a right communicate has commenced (see http://www.itu.int/wsis).

Opposition to a right to communicate

Opposition to a right to communicate has been varied. Western countries have generally opposed it on the grounds that it was part of the establishment of some information order. Other countries have opposed it because they saw it as justifying the importation of Western values (Hamelink, 1994: 300). The business sector in some countries has shown resistance to such a right on grounds that it would result in undesirable government interventions in the market (Birdsall and Rasmussen, 2000).

This opposition to a right to communicate is not supported by the realities facing civil society. Bagdikian (1997) and others have chronicled the increasing corporate dominance and concentration of ownership in the media and tele-communications industries with the complicity of governments over the past few decades. This trend has demonstrably reduced the ability of citizens to seek, receive, and impart information. In addition, this trend has arguably reinforced the ability of predominantly Western producers of content to continue the one-way information flows raised within the non-aligned movement in 1955. These realities provide added weight to claims for a right to communicate. If the importation of Western or, more generally, outside values is of concern, citizens would be empowered to respond through the implementation of their own rights to communicate.

NGOs representing the press community such as the World Press Freedom Committee and the Coordinating Committee of Press Freedom Organisations have viewed certain articulations of a right to communicate that go beyond Article 19 as allowing the subordination of press freedoms. For example, Article 10 of the People's Communication Charter, which states in part "All people have the right to participate in public decision-making about the provision of information; . . . and the structure and policies of media industries" is seen as enabling scenarios where governments or citizens are able to make legally binding demands on editors and media organizations to provide a means of commu-nication or to censor content (Bullen, 2001). Other NGOs such as Article 19 Global Campaign for Free Expression believe that a right to communicate is already embodied in established human rights frameworks and that such a right should be viewed as an "umbrella term" that covers relevant existing rights. Further, efforts to establish a new right to communicate are seen as potentially "[undermining] or directly [breaching] established rights" (Article 19, 2003). Many, particularly the press freedom community, simply call for the enforcement of Article 19 as being sufficient to bring about a right to communicate.

The concerns raised by Article 19 Global Campaign for Free Expression are legitimate and, in fact, many scholars and advocates of a right to communicate share them. The intent of a right to communicate is decidedly not to undermine existing human rights. A right to communicate has been defined by a number of scholars in relation to a collection of existing human rights (Le Duc, 1977; Harms, n.d.; McIver and Birdsall, 2002). Articles of the Universal Declaration of Humans Rights commonly cited as being under the "umbrella" that constitutes a right communicate include:

- Article 12 – Privacy;
- Article 18 – Freedom of thought, conscience, and religion;
- Article 19 – Freedom of expression and the right to seek, receive, and impart information through any media;
- Article 20 – Freedom of peaceful assembly;
- Article 26 – The right to education; and,
- Article 27 – The right to participate in the cultural life of the community as well as intellectual property rights.

The "potential for censorship" argument against a right to communicate is legitimate to the extent that articulations of a right to communicate depart from or undermine accepted human rights, whether they are actually enforced or not. This type of opposition reinforces the need for a right to communicate to be defined within an umbrella of existing rights. In addition, it should be pointed out that other provisions within existing human rights frameworks – if enforced – would provide protections against the scenario described above by the World Press Freedom Committee. These include rights to own property in Article 17; the very right to freedom against censorship implied by Article 19; and Article 30, which prohibits the abridgment of any rights in the declaration.

Other motives must therefore be called into question concerning the press freedom community's opposition to a right to communicate. It arguably mirrors the type of opposition from the business community cited previously. A newsletter published on March 6, 1997 by the World Press Freedom Committee, for example, chose to cite the following statement, among others, from a document issued by several countries that wanted to renew a discussion of NWICO: ". . . developed countries (are) employing their media to disseminate false and distorted information of events taking place in developing countries" (quoted from World Press Freedom Committee, 1997). The implication of this citation in the context of their newsletter is that the claim of media bias of this sort was false and that it, along with the other concerns they cited, do not constitute legitimate claims to communication rights by any entity other than the press. Convincing evidence supporting these governments' concerns can be found, as cited above, from many sources, including Chomsky and Herman (1988). In this context, a right to communicate, if properly enforced, would ensure democratic possibilities for communication for the press, nations, and citizens alike.

Finally, scholars of communication rights beginning with d'Arcy have stressed that Article 19 is not by itself sufficient to support a right to communicate.

Satellite, data communications, and other technologies continue to create possibilities for communication not anticipated by Article 19, including the potential for interactive transmission of content with global reach by nations, communities, and citizens. Article 19 was developed in the context of the mass communication medium of radio that was dominant in 1948. Its authors could not have anticipated the need for provisions addressing participation, interactivity, collectivity, and other principles that have come to be recognized by many advocates of a right to communicate.

Provisions of a right to communicate

Various proposals have been made concerning the provisions that should constitute the human right to communicate. The Dag Hammarskjöld Foundation (1981: 2–3) proposed that such a right should support the following principles:

1 *Pluralism*: the right to communicate should be available to all.
2 *Direct communication flows*: all entities in all sectors of a society should be able to communicate directly with each other without external control.
3 *Social function*: information has a social function. It should not be viewed as propaganda nor a commodity, nor should it be controlled by the power structures of the market or the state. Information should contribute to reducing ignorance and preconceptions.
4 *Media analysis*: it is important to analyze and report on the processes and meta-information which are transported across a medium.
5 *Communication versus information*: communication should occur through a horizontal mutually beneficial exchange of information, not through a vertical transfer from those who have control of a medium to passive receivers.
6 *Appropriate use of technology*: technologies should be reviewed as to their potential impact on a society and power structures within them.

Hamelink has proposed a comprehensive framework for supporting communication as a human right, which includes three components: norms, enforcement procedures, and implementation mechanisms (1994: 301–313).

Conclusion

Human rights frameworks can and must be used as part of the solution to addressing the digital divide, independent of specific communication modalities. Such an approach would bring with it the advantage of providing policy-makers with a universally available set of standards for addressing human needs and a common lexicon with which to debate, identify, and implement solutions.

Access to advanced communication modalities has become more of a fundamental human need as they are used increasingly to provide basic services necessary to maintain an adequate standard of living or, conversely, as their lack of use could result in a hindrance to lives and livelihoods. This human need can best be articulated as a human right to communicate.

Well-established human rights instruments and processes offer the best framework with which to guide the development of policies for bridging the digital divide. This includes norms, enforcement procedures, and implementation mechanisms. While critical components of a right to communicate, such as Article 19 of the International Covenant on Civil and Political Rights (United Nations, 1993: 28), have been established as international law within ratified treaties, a comprehensive human right to communicate has not itself been established in international law. However, activities over the past decade by non-governmental organizations such as the People's Communications Charter, the actions of the Millennium Assembly of the United Nations, and recent efforts by the CRIS Campaign around the World Summit on the Information Society are perhaps encouraging signs that a right to communicate will eventually be adopted by the world's nations.

Acknowledgment

This research was partially supported by a Rockefeller Foundation Bellagio Fellowship.

Chapter 12

An asset-based approach to community building and community technology

Nicol E. Turner-Lee and Randal D. Pinkett

Introduction

At the intersection between community building and community technology lies tremendous synergy. Each of these domains seeks to empower individuals and families and improve their overall environment. Surprisingly, approaches that combine these areas have received very little attention. In response to the "digital divide" (NTIA, 1995, 1997, 1999 and 2000) the challenge in many minority and low-income communities has been to identify strategies for engaging residents with technology, providing economical access to technology, and encouraging meaningful use of technology. These efforts have largely focused on establishing infrastructure and providing training. As computers and the Internet continue to penetrate these communities, it begs the question of what can be done to truly leverage the benefits of information and communications technology. From among the three models of community involvement with technology – community computing centers, community networks, and community content (Beamish, 1999) – there are a limited number of examples where technology has been used to promote community building by regarding residents and other community members as key stakeholders in the process. Conversely, from among the multitude of models for community revitalization, such as community organizing, community development, and community building (Hess, 1999), we are only beginning to witness the benefits that are afforded by incorporating technology into these approaches in a truly meaningful way. By combining the efforts of the community building and community technology movements, we can strengthen both domains and unleash their unifying and collective power to transform communities.

Our perspective on these issues is grounded in two theoretical and practical frameworks: asset-based community development and sociocultural constructionism. Asset-based community development (Kretzmann and McKnight, 1993) is an approach to community building that views community members as active change agents rather than passive beneficiaries or clients. Sociocultural constructionism (Pinkett, 2000; Hooper, 1998; Shaw, 1995) is an asset-based approach to community technology that sees community members as the active producers of community information and content rather than passive consumers or recipients. As community building and community technology initiatives move toward greater synergy, there is a great deal to be learned regarding how they can be mutually supportive, rather than mutually exclusive.

This chapter will share the results of two ongoing and comprehensive efforts to integrate asset-based community building and community technology. The first project is being conducted in a federally assisted, affordable housing development located in Chicago, Illinois. The objectives of this project are two-fold: first, to demonstrate how a community technology center (CTC) located on the first floor of the housing development can be relevant to resident capacity building through the development of online job readiness and community networking tools. Second, to demonstrate how appropriate online tools can support asset-mapping and mobilization within the designated community by strengthening its economic, human, and social capital. The second project is being conducted in a resident-owned, affordable housing development located in the Roxbury/South End section of Boston, Massachusetts. This project involves both a CTC located in the community center as well as new computers and high-speed Internet access made available for each family in their home. The goal here is to establish a model for other housing developments as to how individuals, families, and a community can make use of information and communications technology to support their interests and needs.

The methodology for both projects included: (1) one-on-one interviews with the residents; (2) an asset-mapping of neighborhood resources in the community within a specified radius of the building, such as businesses, schools, community organizations, churches, and voluntary associations, as well as residents' individual skills and abilities; and (3) the design and implementation of a comprehensive community web system, the Creating Community Connections (C3) system, to facilitate relationship building, information sharing, and resource brokering among the aforementioned constituencies. We begin by describing the theoretical framework underlying these efforts in greater detail. This is followed by an overview of each project, the methodology for implementing each project, and preliminary results. We conclude with lessons learned from both initiatives and recommendations for future community building and community technology initiatives.

Asset-based community development

Community revitalization can begin from one of two underlying paradigms: *needs-based* or *capacity-focused*. A needs-based paradigm focuses on a community's deficiencies and problems. Such an approach is often top-down, beginning with what is absent in the community; and outside-in, relying heavily on the efforts of external agents, such as technical assistants. Because needs-based approaches suggest that services are required to build local capacities, individuals are perceived as clients dependent upon social services. Needs-based community approaches, therefore, encourage both the residents and the professionals who service them to bypass local assets and resources. Capacity-focused paradigms, on the other hand, recognize the skills, talents, and gifts of local community members. This approach begins with what is present in the neighborhood and relies heavily on the efforts of internal agents, such as residents, associations, and institutions. A capacity-orientation lies at the heart of asset-based community building – a model for community revitalization that is focused on developing the capacities of residents, associations, and organizations to work towards sustainable neighborhood change.

Asset-based community development (Kretzmann and McKnight, 1993), a particular approach to community building, assumes that social and economic revitalization starts with what is already present within a community, specifically the existing commercial, associational, and institutional foundation. This involves pinpointing or mapping all of the available assets in the community, and connecting or mobilizing them in ways that multiply their power and effectiveness. An asset-based approach to community building perceives local residents and other community stakeholders as active change agents rather than passive beneficiaries or clients.

The focus on local assets redirects attention to the extensive social capital of communities. Putnam (1998), who popularized its application to political civic engagement, defines social capital as the norms and networks that encourage sustainable community action. In general, the social capital of local communities represents individuals and institutions that are mutually supportive and reliable (Temkin and Rohe, 1998). The individual capacities of residents are the basic building blocks of any community. As people exercise these capacities, they often find they need the talents of others in their enterprises. This leads them to join with other individuals who will work with them toward a common goal. When they do this, individuals combine their own talents with the capacities of others to form associations and support local institutions that can make extensive and valuable contributions to their community. For example, Stagner and Richman (1996) identified friends and extended family members as the main source of support in low-income families, emphasizing the need for strengthening these types of informal support networks. A significant premise of asset-based community development, therefore, is to involve as many community stakeholders in the creation of plans, visions, and projects that support community building.

Information and communication technologies can play a significant role in promoting community building by facilitating information, communication, and resource exchange between a host of community organizations and among a range of different activities. To this end, we advocate a new class of community-based technological tools that are consistent with principles of sociocultural constructionism (Pinkett, 2000) and are designed specifically to support asset-based community development.

Sociocultural constructionism and community technology

The digital divide (NTIA, 1995, 1997, 1999 and 2000) within society is well documented as many low- to moderate-income, rural and urban individuals and families continue to experience relatively lower levels of access to computers and online services than their mainstream counterparts. Disproportionate racial and ethnic access further deepens this divide. Furthermore, a closely related content divide has also emerged that is characterized by a lack of technology applications and relevant information that addresses the needs of low-income and underserved Internet users (The Children's Partnership, 2000).

Three primary models have emerged as solutions for addressing the disparities in computer and Internet access, use, and content (Beamish, 1999). The first model is community networks, or community-based electronic network services, provided at little or no cost to users. The second model is community computing centers or community technology centers (CTCs), which are publicly accessible facilities that provide computer access for people who can't afford a computer, as well as technical instruction and support. The third model involves community content, or the availability of material that is relevant and interesting to some target audience (e.g. low-income residents) to encourage and motivate the use of technology. These approaches can be classified according to what they provide: hardware, software, and training, infrastructure, online access, or content. They can also be classified according to the groups they target: individuals, schools, youth, community organizations, and the general public, or specific groups such as a neighborhood, racial or ethnic minorities, the homeless, and the elderly (ibid.).

Community technology is "a process to serve the local geographic community – to respond to the needs of that community and build solutions to its problems" (Morino, 1994). Our approach to community technology is rooted in the theory of sociocultural constructionism (Pinkett, 2000), a synthesis of the theories of cultural constructionism (Hooper, 1998) and social constructionism (Shaw, 1995). Sociocultural constructionism argues that individual and community development are reciprocally enhanced by independent and shared constructive activity that is resonant with both the social environment of a community of learners, as well as the culture of the learners themselves. Technologies that are consistent with this paradigm empower residents to express their cultural heritage, enable broad community information, communication, and resource exchange. Some examples include personalized web portals for residents, an online community newsletter, a community asset-mapping database, and customizable templates for residents, associations, and institutions to create their own web pages. Such an approach empowers residents, local associations and institutions, and neighborhood businesses to share information and resources that they deem important such as recipes or artwork, volunteer opportunities, and hiring needs. Sociocultural constructionism is an asset-based approach to community technology that sees community members as the active producers of community content rather than passive consumers or recipients.

The best practice of the asset-based model views community members as active change agents. The concept of sociocultural constructionism argues that community members can be active producers of community information and content. Combining these two perspectives in how we understand community technology can start to bridge both the digital and content divides. In the following section of this paper, we describe two projects in community technology centers (CTC) that are based on the paradigms of asset-based community development and sociocultural constructionism.

Northwest Tower Apartments, Chicago, Illinois

Northwest Tower Apartments is a predominantly African American, low- to moderate-income housing development located northwest of Chicago's downtown area. Of the approximately 500 residents, 65 percent are female and 42 percent are under the age of 18 years old. As this is a subsidized housing development, 30 percent of building residents receive public assistance and 36 percent receive some sort of government subsidy or pension. While the median income for Chicago is $31,000, 40 percent of the resident population is employed in wage-earning jobs that typically fall at or below 50 percent of the city's median income.

In 1996, Northwest Tower residents purchased the 150-unit development under the US Department of Housing and Urban Development's (HUD) Low-Income Housing Preservation and Reservation Act (LIHPRA) program to maintain affordable housing at the site. As part of this program, residents formed a non-profit organization called the Northwest Tower Resident Association (NTRA) to manage building operations. In 1998, the NTRA was provided seed money through the US Department of Housing and Urban Development's Neighborhood Networks program to develop an on-site community technology center. In 1999, the computer center was renamed the Neighborhood Technology Resource Center (NTRC) with the sole mission of creating, administering, and tracking educational, career development, and job placement initiatives in this multi-family housing development.

To demonstrate how a community technology center could be relevant to resident capacity building by integrating community building and community technology, three phases were completed at Northwest Tower: (1) individual capacity mapping, (2) neighborhood asset-mapping, and (3) design and implementation of a comprehensive web system, the Creating Community Connections (C3) system. The NTRC was used as the technology access point and residents were directly involved in the identification of neighborhood assets (steps 1–2), and influenced the design of the C3 system (step 3).

In Phase 1, a resident capacity inventory was conducted at the housing development. Five residents administered a pre-designed resident capacity survey instrument (Turner, 1999). Personal interviews were conducted over a three-week period with adult residents, aged between 18 and 55 years. In all, 72 of 105 adults completed the resident capacity survey. The survey addressed the following topics: community satisfaction and homeownership, employment experience, individual skills and abilities in a variety of employment categories, use of and interest in technology, community involvement, and purchasing patterns.

Overall, the results of the individual capacity mapping demonstrated that residents of this federally assisted housing development were rich in occupational skills and capacities that can significantly meet local and regional employment demands. By far the highest number of reported skills fell in the categories of office, creative, and educational training. Some of these skills were highly specialized, such as ordering office supplies and completing data entry, while others were more general, such as document filing or telephone reception. In all of the skill categories, there were also a number of individuals interested in learning a new skill or occupation. At least 10 percent of all respondents were interested in learning construction-related skills or moving into professional occupations, such as social services, accounting, or human resources. This apparent willingness to move into vocational or career-oriented jobs most likely reflects respondents' desires to obtain livable wage scales, as opposed to minimum wage jobs. While technology competency was low among respondents, their willingness to learn computers and computer-related fields was quite significant. An average of 25 percent of respondents was interested in acquiring some level of computer training. Survey results were subsequently adapted and entered into the C3 system that will be described more fully in Phase 3.

In Phase 2, surveyors identified neighborhood resources, inclusive of churches, community agencies, schools, municipal buildings, libraries, voluntary associations, and local businesses that existed within a 16-block radius of the housing development. Several methodologies ranging from the review of public data sources to field visits were used to locate resources. In all, 188 local businesses were identified within 16 blocks of the housing development. In addition to general contact data, additional information was gathered from businesses, including their hours of operation, number of employees, type of business (according to a defined typology) and Standard Industrial Classification (SIC) code and division. This information was subsequently adapted and entered into the C3 system. In addition to local businesses, 96 community organizations were also identified. Contact information, as well as the type of organization (e.g. childcare, educational, etc.), was recorded for entry into the C3 system.

Since one of the goals of the project was to understand how community technology facilitates information and resource exchange, the data obtained from Phases 1 and 2 were published in a database that could be accessed for local employment and volunteer opportunities and brokering between community organizations (Phase 3). The first instantiation of the database resided on a single computer at the on-site lab and included the resident database with a résumé creation function, local business database, and community organization database. The second instantiation resulted in a more holistic solution, the Creating Community Connections (C3) system, an online tool that is based on the principles of asset-based community development and sociocultural construc- tionism as shown in Figure 12.1. C3 is built using the ArsDigita Community System (ACS), a freely distributed, open-source software platform. Local stakeholders were involved in testing the C3 system for its functionality. C3 is designed to leverage and strengthen individuals' economic, human, and social capital for the purpose of community building.

The main features of this inaugural version of C3 include customizable web portals and interactive resident, business, and organization databases. The web portals provide users bookmarks for popular websites, and allow them to track their system activity. The interactive resident profile module allows users to enter, track, and update both their employment/volunteer skills and capacities, as well as create and print a contemporary résumé. The interactive local business database give users the ability to review, query, locate, and research goods, services and hiring needs within their immediate neighborhood and link to business websites and email addresses. Business administrators can also enter and update their capacity record in real time.

With similar capacities, the interactive community organization/association database grants users the ability to connect to neighborhood resources, such as

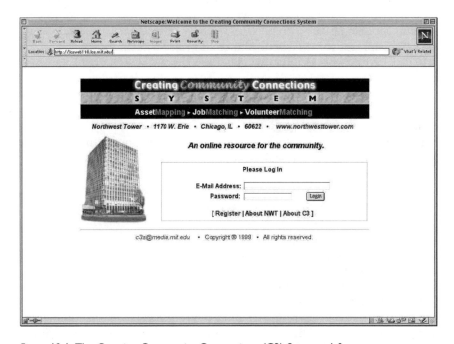

Figure 12.1 The Creating Community Connections (C3) System v1.0

schools, churches, social service agencies, libraries, neighborhood associations, and health care facilities. Users can also query organizational capacities, such as assets needed, assets willing to share, as well as link to organizations' web and/or email addresses. Like business administrators, organizations and associations can also enter and update their capacity record.

In addition to the valuable information provided on the C3 system, several brokering tools were built to facilitate local employment and volunteer placements. The job and volunteer posting boards offer up-to-date employment and volunteer opportunities and include automatic email notification of potential matches. Community organizations, associations, and businesses are able to post opportunities, track responses, and view résumés from any online location or via email notification. Version one of the C3 system also includes full search capabilities of resident, business, and organization capacity records for users to identify assets and resources within the community. Finally, a built-in case manager provides real-time statistics on system users and community resources.

The final phase of the Northwest Tower project, which is currently underway, is to begin populating the C3 system with more individual capacity records, business and community organization information, and job and volunteer postings. The preliminary findings at Northwest Tower Apartments suggested the role that residents and the community can play in not only defining community space, but also providing input to a technology project that strengthens relationships within that domain. Toward that end, the accomplishments at Northwester Tower heavily informed and shaped the methodology of a subsequent project that was conducted at another housing development in Roxbury, MA.

Camfield Estates, Roxbury, MA

Camfield Estates, formerly Camfield Gardens, is a predominantly African American, low- to moderate-income housing development in the Roxbury/South End section of Boston, Massachusetts. Of the approximately 350 residents, 75 percent are African American, whereas the Hispanic and Non-Hispanic split across all races is 32 percent and 68 percent respectively. The average age at Camfield is 27 years as a result of a large youth population under 18 (45 percent), and an appreciable adult population 30 and above (39 percent). The majority of the residents at Camfield are female (55 percent), including the CTA board of directors, which consists of seven women and one man. All residents qualify as "low-income" or "very low-income" according to the guidelines set forth by HUD.

Camfield is a participant in HUD's Demonstration-Disposition or "Demo-Dispo" program (HUD/MHFA, 1998). HUD implemented Demo-Dispo in 1993, as a strategy to deal with its growing inventory of foreclosed multifamily housing, much of which was in poor physical and financial condition (MHFA, 2001). Through this national demonstration program, approved only in the City of Boston, the Massachusetts Housing Finance Agency (MHFA) was designated to oversee the renovation and sale of HUD properties to resident-owned organizations. As a result, the 136 low- to medium-rise apartments of Camfield Gardens were demolished in 1997 and residents were relocated throughout the greater Boston area. Reconstruction of the property was completed in 2000 as residents returned to Camfield Estates – 102 units of newly built town houses. The renovated property also includes the Camfield Community Center that houses meeting space, management offices, and the Neighborhood Technology Center (NTC) – a CTC and HUD Neighborhood Networks site, managed by Williams Consulting Services, and supported by MHFA. Finally, in 2002, HUD will dispose (transfer ownership) of the property to the non-profit Camfield Tenants Association, Inc. (CTA), making Camfield the first of several participants in the Demo-Dispo program to successfully complete the process.

The Camfield Estates–MIT Creating Community Connections Project (Pinkett, 2002; Pinkett and O'Bryant, 2002) was initiated in January 2000 by graduate students and faculty from the MIT Media Laboratory, MIT Department of Urban Studies and Planning, MIT Center for Reflective Community Practice, and MIT Laboratory for Computer Science. These researchers shared an interest in the role of technology for the purpose of building community, empowerment, and self-sufficiency in a low-income community. Camfield was identified as an excellent site to examine these issues and conduct a longitudinal study for numerous reasons, including the strong leadership exemplified by CTA, the cable-modem Internet capabilities in each unit, and the presence of NTC, along with its associated course offering and ongoing technical support. However, what made Camfield particularly attractive were the prospects to sustain the initiative as a result of their leading role in the Demo-Dispo program and impending ownership of the property.

The W. K. Kellogg Foundation provided primary support for the project in the form of a monetary grant, followed by in-kind donations from Hewlett-Packard Company (computers), RCN Telecom Services (cable-modem Internet service), Microsoft Corporation (software), and ArsDigita Corporation (software and technical support), with additional support from MHFA, Williams Consulting Services, Lucent Technologies, HUD, the Institute for African-American eCulture (iAAEC), YouthBuild of Boston, and the William Monroe Trotter Institute at the University of Massachusetts at Boston. Exploratory meetings between CTA, MIT, Kellogg, and Williams Consulting took place during the winter of 2000, culminating in final approval of the project by CTA. The project officially began in June 2000.

During the summer of 2000, the project team developed a pre-assessment survey instrument to collect data in the following areas: community interests and satisfaction, social networks (strong and weak ties), neighboring, awareness of community resources, community satisfaction, community involvement, empowerment, self-sufficiency, computer experience, hobbies, interests and information needs, assets and income, and demographics. The survey was designed for two purposes. First, to provide strategic direction for the initiative by identifying the interests and needs of residents – this information would shape the nature of online and offline activities to be planned in the future. Second, to provide baseline and formative data for the research study. This information would be used to perform a comparative analysis of a similar data set to be gathered approximately one year later.

During this same period, an awareness campaign was conducted to inform residents about the initiative. A series of mailings were distributed describing the project's goals and objectives, and offering a new computer, high-speed Internet connection, and comprehensive courses at NTC, for adults 18 years and older that completed the courses, completed the preliminary interview, and signed an informed consent form granting permission to track the web-traffic at Camfield through a proxy server (aggregate patterns of use only, and not individually attributable). An open forum was also held in the community center for questions and answers. While families were encouraged to attend the training, at least one adult from each household had to fulfill these requirements in order to receive the computer and Internet access. Given the fact that NTC was primarily used by youth at this time (O'Bryant, 2001), it was the decision of the committee to restrict participation to adults only, as we believed it would motivate parents to attend the training for the benefit of their children. August 2000 marked the deadline to sign-up for the project, and 32 of the 66 occupied units at Camfield elected to participate in Round I.

From September to October 2000, introductory courses were offered at NTC to Round I participants. The activity-based curriculum lasted eight weeks (two sessions per week, two hours per session) and covered various aspects of computer and Internet use. Meanwhile, a second instantiation of the C3 system was co-designed by residents and MIT researchers. This version of the system incorporated additional features to support community communication and expression, such as personal home pages, discussion forums, calendar of events, email lists (listservs), chat rooms, news and announcements, surveys and polls, and a geographic information system (GIS) module that represented community assets in the form of a map with hyperlinked symbols for various resources. In November 2000, specialized courses were offered on how to use the C3 System, which was made available through the Camfield Estates website (http://www. camfieldestates.net), as shown in Figure 12.2.

In November 2000, 26 families received computers, software, and subsequent high-speed Internet access, having fulfilled the aforementioned requirements. In January 2001, a second awareness campaign was conducted and aimed at the 47 families still eligible for the project (the number of occupied units had increased from 66 to 80). There were 27 families who participated in Round II, raising the total number of families participating in the project to 59 out of 80 eligible units. A more detailed discussion of Round II is beyond the scope of this chapter. A third awareness campaign and Round III are currently under consideration.

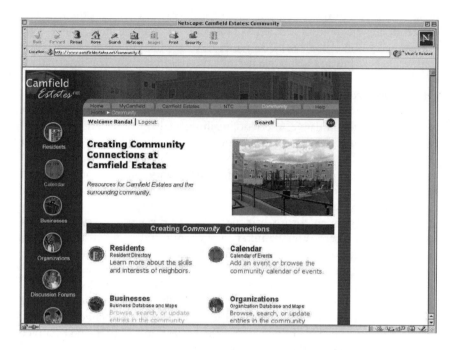

Figure 12.2 The Creating Community Connections (C3) System v2.0

Sociocultural constructions are physical, virtual, and cognitive artifacts that are resonant with a given social environment and its culture as mediated by technological fluency. Asset-mobilization involves the establishment of productive and meaningful connections between residents, organizations, institutions, and businesses, which previously did not exist, toward achieving specific outcomes, as facilitated by asset-mapping.

A resident-led asset-mapping took place during the summer 2000, with technical assistance from researchers at MIT. It consisted of mapping all the organizations, institutions (e.g. libraries, schools, etc.), and businesses within an approximately 1.5-mile radius of Camfield, as shown in Figure 12.3. This broad attempt to identify community resources was done to obtain local information of potential benefit to residents that would eventually be made available through C3, and as a preparatory step for individual capacity mapping to be conducted after analyzing the results of the pre-assessment. Not surprisingly, the mere process of gathering this information served to heighten residents' awareness of assets in their own neighborhood. For example, the first-pass general asset-map was conducted within a few square blocks of the property. Residents soon discovered there were very few organizations and institutions in this catchment area, and only a small cluster of businesses. The decision was then made to

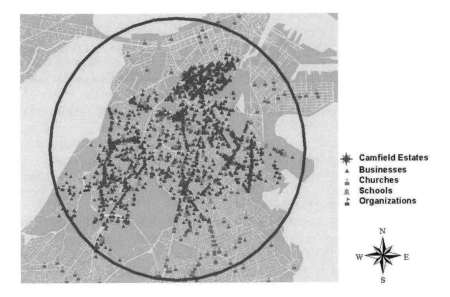

Figure 12.3 Camfield Estates catchment area

expand the radius of the asset-map to 1.5 miles, which captured approximately 757 businesses, 178 organizations, 67 churches, and 29 schools, as shown in Figure 12.3.

Asset-mapping of residents' individual capacities began in November 2000, and consisted of documenting the formal and informal skills of residents. This took place during the final two weeks of the introductory and specialized courses. Using C3, residents entered their formal and informal skills and interests, by selecting from an inventory of more than 150 items. Given this information, residents could now use C3 to identify neighbors who could perform plumbing, babysitting, web design, etc., or neighbors who were interested in learning these skills.

In April 2001, the results of the preliminary assessment were compiled. These results suggested the following strategies: (1) offer more activities for youth, (2) improve community communication and social interaction at the development, (3) augment current safety and security measures, and (4) expand employment opportunities for residents. Although seniors' concerns were not visibly represented in the results of the assessment, another recommended strategy was to offer more activities for seniors in addition to youth. With this information, a series of meetings took place among members of the project committee to discuss these findings and address the issues raised by residents. Because sociocultural constructions and asset-mobilization manifest themselves online and offline in the context of an integrated community technology and community building initiative, these discussions focused on ways to effect change in both physical and virtual settings.

A number of strategies were undertaken in response to these findings including: use of the C3 system to improve communication and information flow at the development; activities during Black Family Technology Week that paired youth with seniors to create PowerPoint presentations; the establishment of a newsletter in both paper-based and electronic formats; thematic workshops for adults on the topics of "Online Educational Services," "Online Banking Services," "Online Shopping Services," "Online Government Services," and "Online Housing Services"; and the establishment of a Cisco Networking Academy at NTC, a program that teaches students how to design, build, and maintain computer networks toward becoming certified as a Cisco Certified Network Associate (CCNA). Note that an in-depth discussion of these strategies is beyond the scope of this chapter.

In August 2001, a post-assessment and evaluation was conducted with the head-of-household from the 26 out of 32 families who completed the introductory course. The post-assessment and evaluation consisted of a comparative analysis against the pre-assessment as well as other sources of data (proxy server logs, C3 server logs, direct observation) to quantify and qualify the initiative's progress to-date. Some of the early results from the post-assessment are highlighted below (Pinkett, 2002; Pinkett and O'Bryant, 2002).

First, participants have strengthened their personal connections to family members and local friends. The number of residents that were recognizable by name increased from 30 to 40 out of a possible 137 adults; the number of residents contacted via telephone and email doubled; and 53 percent of participants reported that they were more connected to family and friends in the local area.

Second, participants are making better use of community resources as a result of increased awareness of these resources. The number of City of Boston services, programs, and/or departments that participants had heard of or used increased from an average of 34 to 43; there were statistically significant increases in residents' awareness and use of community resources in four out of a possible nine categories (a fifth category was nearly statistically significant), including the following: (1) residents' skills and abilities, (2) volunteer opportunities in the neighborhood, (3) social services and programs provided for the community, (4) community projects, activities, and events, and (5) employment opportunities in the community; the Camfield Estates website and the C3 system received high marks from participants when asked to rate its usefulness in this regard.

Third, participants are better informed about what is happening locally and there is an improved communication and information flow at the development. Almost half of participants (47 percent) reported that they are more aware of what is going on at Camfield when compared to before the project was started; the most popular C3 modules were the resident profiles (31 percent of traffic), calendar of events (18 percent of traffic), and discussion forums (13 percent of traffic) on the Camfield Estates website, and while these modules experienced moderate use, their traffic has steadily increased since the site went live.

Fourth, participants have been inspired through use of the Internet to stay informed locally, nationally, and internationally. Although the pre-survey revealed that a significant number of Camfield residents already possessed a strong personal commitment to their local community, in the post-survey the data suggest they have been using these tools to obtain information both within and beyond the local area. Respectively 84 percent and 90 percent of participants went on-line frequently and/or occasionally to obtain information local to the City of Boston and national information (news, sports, etc.). Furthermore, a strong majority of participants (95 percent) felt motivated to find out more about what is going on in the world.

Fifth, participants are using the Internet to gather information that can help address basic interests and needs. With nearly 90 percent of participants reporting that they are more aware of human and health services in their community, residents have begun to develop a cadre of options for themselves to support their essential needs. Eighty-nine percent of respondents felt that they could find housing through the Internet if they needed to, while 84 percent stated the same with respect to finding a job. Shopping online for retail goods such as clothes, books, music, movie tickets, etc. was also very popular with participants (74 percent). These results show an emergence of using the Internet to address basic interests and needs.

Finally, participants have cultivated the meta-competence of a renewed confidence in themselves and their ability to learn. Qualitative responses from the one-on-one interviews revealed a shift in participants' attitudes and perceptions of themselves as learners. Several participants described their personal transition of moving from a reticence toward technology to envisioning themselves as (or taking actual steps to becoming) web designers, network administrators, and programmers. In particular, their participation in the training has given them a greater appreciation of their strengths, and it has given the community a greater appreciation of its most basic assets, the skills and abilities of its residents.

Towards a new paradigm of community building and community technology

Many lessons can be learned from Northwest Tower Apartments and Camfield Estates projects as well as recommendations presented to community technology and community building practitioners, researchers, funders, government agencies, and public policy-makers. In this final section, we outline three policy suggestions and recommendations. First, the praxis of an asset-based approach to community building and community technology calls for community-driven strategies to be applied to resident-defined issues. The issues at Northwest Tower were related to individual capacity building and workforce development.

At Camfield Estates, the issues were identified as youth, seniors, community, safety/security, and employment. Accordingly, residents' efforts to address these issues have been focused on achieving positive outcomes in each area as opposed to merely obtaining access to technology. In *From Access to Outcomes: Raising the Aspirations for Technology Initiatives in Low-Income Communities*, the Morino Institute (2001) emphasized the importance of placing technology in the appropriate context. They write,

> focusing on outcomes is easiest when the application of technology represents just one component of a comprehensive solution to a need. It is much harder to focus on outcomes when launching a stand-along technology project, such as providing wiring for a school or community center.
>
> (Ibid.: 8)

Second, an asset-based approach to community building and community technology upholds the true power of building community online as enhancing, rather than supplanting face-to-face or offline community interaction. Therefore, perhaps the most effective strategy for building community online is building community offline. A good example of integrating online and offline was the Black Family Technology Week celebration at Camfield. Before the week, a Black History contest was conducted online. During the week, a day was designated for seniors and youth to work together face to face at NTC searching the web for additional Black History facts. At the end of the week, a dinner was organized to recognize participants. After the week, pictures were posted to the Camfield website to capture the event.

Our third recommendation is to encourage bottom–up, inside-out revitalization when addressing the introduction of community technology. Our work at both Northwest Tower and Camfield Estates has drawn upon the ideas of a capacity-oriented approach that focuses on assets, instead of a deficiency-oriented approach that focuses on needs. Consequently, we need to identify guidelines for capacity-oriented funding when designing and evaluating proposals. This includes soliciting proposals that clearly identify how the skills, abilities, capacities, and assets of local residents and citizens associations will be mobilized and enhanced before funding is initiated. The data and stories that have emerged at Northwest Tower and Camfield Estates hopefully demonstrate the value of such an approach to philanthropy. By funding community technology and community building initiatives in this manner, foundations and other grant-makers can take better steps to ensure that their dollars are being used effectively and in a way that is consistent with the voice and the pulse of the community.

Our contribution to the fields of community building and community technology add to the discussion of how to combine these movements, as well as the debate on how to build information and communication infrastructures that can address the digital divide and closely related content divide. Since many low- to moderate-income citizens have not been engaged in this debate, we believe the combination of community building principles through an asset-based framework and individual and community engagement with technology through a sociocultural constructionist paradigm can provide an approach towards their holistic integration.

Chapter 13

Community network development and user participation

Murali Venkatesh, Julia Nosovitch and Wayne Miner

Introduction

In 1995, as part of a settlement of a regulatory case before the New York State Public Service Commission, a major telephone company (hereafter provider) committed $50 million to deploy broadband services in the state's poor and underserved areas.[1] A program was set up to solicit proposals for broadband services from consortia of eligible organizations – which referred to public institutions (e.g. city and county government agencies, K–12 schools, healthcare agencies), small non-profits (hereafter community-based organizations, or CBOs), and small businesses. Organizations had to be located in or provide services to approved postal codes to be eligible for the subsidies sanctioned under the program. State and federal government agencies were not eligible to participate, neither were individual residents or households. Two rounds of grants were awarded before the program concluded in 2000. In all, 22 projects were funded – 14 urban/suburban, six rural, with two qualifying as urban/suburban/rural combination projects.

The program awarded competitive grants based on proposals from eligible consortia. The grant selection committee comprised representatives from state government and public interest groups. Eighty percent of the grant went back to the provider to cover costs associated with the development and deployment of network infrastructure[2] and approved broadband connectivity options (options that offer data transmission speeds of 200,000 bits per second or more). The remaining 20 percent could be used for customer premise equipment (CPE) and/or training for network subscribers (users). Grant funds could not be used toward technical support or consultants, or for software applications. Subscribers would pay subsidized monthly rates for broadband connectivity and were required to connect to the shared network infrastructure. The infrastructure (called backbone) linked all subscriber sites and thus served as an inter-organizational network (recall that only eligible *organizations,* not individuals or households, could subscribe) for the area as well as a high-speed Internet access ramp. That is, subscribers could use the shared infrastructure to connect to other subscribers and the Internet.

The program's stated objective was to bring broadband connectivity to "economically disadvantaged areas of New York State that would not be available in the near future on account of limitations in the advanced telecommunications infrastructure and related equipment marketplace" (Evaluation Report, 2001). Implicit were the social objectives. Grant selection committee members interviewed by the first author hoped that the grant, and the inter-organizational network infrastructure resulting from it, would help bring together public institutions, CBOs and small businesses to meet local needs and address local problems. To qualify for an award, proposals had to show sustainable, broad-based support for the project within the local community. Selection committee members spoke of a program-funded network serving as a *community network* in grantee *communities* (groupings of proximate postal code areas) – a mechanism to strengthen inter-organizational social ties across functional sectors so that a K-12 public school, for example, used the network infrastructure to connect not only to another area school but to CBOs and the local zoo as well to serve a cross-section of needs. Remarkably, their emphasis on strengthening inter-organizational linkages is consistent with assertions in the community development literature on the centrality of such linkages for community cohesion (Warren, 1978). Psychological benefits from using the network to strengthen inter-organizational linkages were variously described as "community networking," the forging of "coalitions and partnerships," and "finding common ground" in communities receiving a program grant. Many of the projects did not meet these self-set goals, but the intent of the projects and of the program was quite clear in its orientation.

We tracked the work of volunteer *planners* affiliated with five projects over several months. These project sites are located in different parts of the state. Each site, however, covers physically proximate postal code areas. These projects (one urban/suburban, four rural) received over $11,000,000 total under the program's second round. Grants ranged from around $1,000,000 to under $4,000,000. Planners were technical and non-technical volunteers representing eligible organizations; as such, they spoke for prospective users of the network. They had drafted the project proposal and constituted the project steering committee. At the time of this research, they were participants in network design with the provider's design personnel (hereafter designers) from sales, marketing, and engineering functions. Our focus here is on the design (technical specification) process as it pertains to these five projects. We do comment on some of the uses of these networks. Early indications are that these networks cater to the needs of resource-rich institutions and at present boast a negligible number of CBOs and small businesses as subscribers. Not surprisingly, available applications serve the needs of the resource-rich. However, it must be noted that these networks have only been operational for about 18 months on average at this writing, so they are still evolving.

Impediments to user participation

The designers were open to planner participation in design. But participation proved challenging for all involved. We identify six factors that impeded participation.

The knowledge barrier

Lack of access to necessary knowledge impeded participation and independent evaluation of design options by planners. Two types of knowledge are needed to participate in design: knowledge about design options and experience with those options (Kensing and Munk-Madsen, 1993). We discuss the first here; the second is discussed next. Prospective users cannot expect to possess technical knowledge at the level of technology professionals, but they need to be adequately informed to participate meaningfully in design. A respondent observed that the more creative designs in first- and second-round projects had resulted from well-informed planners pushing designers to explore contextually sensitive solutions. Another said: "We need information on technology. Why is this surprising? How can we make decisions if we don't know the technology?" Consequently, the most common questions from planners were: How does it work? What can I do with it? How does it compare with other available options? Will it work with what I have now? And, what are the costs?

The RFP's emphasis on applications helped planners focus proposals on how the network would be used. But as the design effort intensified, planners increasingly felt under-informed and struggled in their role as participants. As one frustrated planner noted: "Technology specifics emerged in importance much later." Planners needed objective information from sources independent of the provider in order to evaluate the designers' suggestions, and many did not know where to look for this information. One project rejected a design because they were unable independently to evaluate it. According to the county data processing chief who headed up the project, planners (including herself) were "clueless" on how to proceed on their own. They felt they had lost control of the design process.

Planners' knowledge shortfalls were pervasive and concerned the backbone, the access network (which connected the subscriber site to the backbone), CPE, and software applications. In addition, they had many unanswered questions on the ins and outs of the contracting process for technical support services (such as network management).

Both planners and program authorities concurred that lack of access to know-how was a critical barrier to participation. Note that program funding could not be used to hire consultants, and only one of the projects covered in this research had independent funds to hire technical help. Knowledge shortfalls were especially acute in CBOs and small businesses and explained their low level of participation. One respondent noted: "Smaller agencies may be more creative, and may be more aware of what the community needs are. They may not have the technical expertise, but may understand [community] needs better." "In-depth technical assistance" would have helped them benefit from the program subsidies and make those benefits available to the publics they served, she added.

Not surprisingly, knowledge shortfalls were relatively higher in rural communities. In the urban/suburban communities, shortfalls got steeper the farther one got from the city. Shortage of technical support staff in-house (i.e. on-site) significantly affected an organization's ability to participate in the design process.

Knowledge shortfalls had been a significant problem in the first round as well. The first round RFP had asked proposers to specify technologies as well as applications, but proposers were unable to provide this information. A program representative observed: "Either they asked for things the provider couldn't do, or they simply didn't know what to ask for. There was widespread lack of understanding and knowledge of technology specifics." This had delayed implementation.

Continuance of program subsidies to aid what we have termed CBOs ("community action agencies, day care centers, Head Start providers, community centers, community health care clinics, legal aid offices, and other service providers located within low income communities") was recently (and unsuc-cessfully) proposed before the state Public Service Commission (Public Utility Law Project, 2001). Importantly, in addition to subsidized monthly service charges and CPE support, the document seeks assistance to cover technical help at the subscriber site.

Lack of "show-how"

Lack of concrete illustrations of design options via functional prototypes was a barrier to participation, and it exacerbated knowledge shortfalls. Planners were frustrated that they could not visualize the network or its uses. The designers used computer-generated network diagrams and flow-charts at design meetings. These can be useful early in design to illustrate a technology's possibilities. But they are less useful later, when users have questions on implementation specifics in actual use settings. Planners felt that working prototypes may have helped answer many such questions. Prototyping, or "show-how," can be a powerful complement to and elucidator of know-how.

Functional prototypes can have symbolic value as well. At most project sites, the long gap (an average of 14 months) between proposal submission and the start of the design process had blunted public interest in the project and contributed to planner attrition. Prototypes can refresh interest in and impart momentum to a stalled project.

Project delays

The projects surveyed here experienced long delays for a number of reasons. The monthly service charges that users would have to pay and the CPE relief they could expect remained ambiguous well into the design process, delaying a decision by prospective users on whether or not to subscribe to the network. Questions from prospective users on issues they considered key to this decision were conveyed to the project steering committee en route to the program authorities. Clarifications obtained from the authorities often resulted in more questions, leading to further delays.

Planner participation was negatively affected by project delays. The result was lack of personnel continuity in varying degrees. Even among personnel that stayed on, enthusiasm diminished for a project that seemed to go on and on with no end in sight. Planner turnover contributed to project delays, and project delays led to planner turnover. As the design process unfolded, planners found it increasingly difficult to find time to attend meetings. Small businesses and CBOs were especially hard-pressed for time, and their participation dropped steeply as project delays lengthened.

Delays proved fatal for one project in the southern portion of the state. This project had started out with a high level of local involvement. Two planners interviewed for this research said they had been "impressed with the level of community involvement early on. But now it has evaporated. Government officials on the (steering) committee are now reluctant to attend meetings because their superiors do not see the need to waste more time on this." Delays affected this project in many ways. "The public safety group . . . was interested in a high-speed link between county court house and public safety building for video arraignment. Now they are going with three ISDN (a broadband option not approved for use in the program) lines because they couldn't wait," noted one member of the steering committee. ISDN service is not a program-eligible service, "which means the video arraignment link will be outside the community network in terms of access and interoperability," she said. This project has since dropped out of the program and returned the grant. Project delays contributed to the decision.

In a positive light, delays can help by giving planners an opportunity to step back and consider the design options and propose modifications. But this did not happen in the project surveyed. The delays were often unanticipated, which meant that the time between design steps did not lend itself to productive or creative use by planners. For these and other reasons (knowledge shortfalls), the wait periods were not conducive to creative reworking of design options.

Project scope change

Project scope ambiguity and change can impede participation. The project scope changed significantly in four out of the five projects surveyed. Project scope change can alter network priorities and objectives. A planner affiliated with the project that returned the grant said: "The network's priorities have changed . . . what started as a regional proposal linking several agencies in three communities . . . now has been pared down . . . to link a few agencies in one county." Planners who had been affiliated with this particular project moved when the project was broken up, and new players had to be brought in and brought up to speed. Planner "churn" from this and other sources (attrition) did not help continuity.

Formulaic approaches to design

In the present research, design flexibility appeared to depend on the designers assigned to the project and on how informed the planners were.

Some designers were creative and resourceful, and were very successful in working with planners. One respondent said: "Bottom line, it depended on the individual characteristics of the engineer." Another said: "It (the design) depended on the engineer assigned to the project. Some had a broader understanding than others. If an engineer had worked with a particular technology, then there was a greater probability that he would back that technology." He continued: "The provider has tried to keep it simple . . . The only time we have gone beyond cookie cutter (formulaic) solutions is when we have had informed participants at the community level."

An engineer who led the design in many second round projects described the "backwards" nature of the design challenge he faced: "Typically, the customer asks sales for a product, sales talks to engineering, and passes along customer needs. With these projects, we didn't have a [well-defined] customer . . . I'm designing a circuit for someone who didn't know what he wanted."

Divergent design objectives

Eligible organizations often had divergent views on the primary function of the network. For example, in one of the projects surveyed, CBOs and small business entities saw the network as a high-speed Internet access ramp. Many did not have Internet access, and those that did wished to upgrade from dial-up access. Public institutions were more interested in using the subsidized services to meet their intra-organizational networking needs. Many already had high-speed Internet access, and meeting internal networking needs cost-effectively was very attractive to them. The smaller agencies were equally clear on what they wanted. "I see no need for agencies to be linked to other agencies. It is more important to be linked to the Internet," a CBO representative argued at a design meeting. It must be emphasized that it was not an either/or issue: the network could support both types of connectivity and indeed, design proposals in the projects surveyed covered both types.

However, the network's basic character would be different depending on its primary function. If the design had emphasized the network-as-Internet access ramp function, the subscription costs would likely have been low to facilitate access by resource-poor agencies. As it turned out, the network-as-intra-organizational connectivity solution gained momentum as the design process unfolded. This meant relatively higher subscription costs, which restricted subscription to resource-rich entities like the public institutions. Divergence in objectives confronted the steering committees involved with a moral dilemma: What should the defining character of the network be? They, like administrative bodies in general, were far more competent to tackle project management and budgetary matters than moral choices. Consequently, such matters were either avoided entirely or not addressed adequately in the design process. The steering committees surveyed appeared unprepared to deal with such questions.

The view favored by the CBOs and small business entities did not prevail. As a group, they lacked financial clout in design deliberations. They constituted a relatively small market for telecommunications services. The public institutions, on the other hand, constituted a much larger market and were more influential. At least in one of the projects surveyed, their willingness and capacity to pay for the higher-end broadband services was interpreted by the steering committee as "insurance" that the project would go forward as planned. Just ensuring that the project stayed on time and on budget was a daunting enough job for these committees, and they performed competently under the circumstances. However, had they been sensitive to the relationship between power and participation (participation as an expression of and as limited by power) their construal of their own role as planners, and as participants in design, might have expanded to include advocacy. Both participation and planning are political in that they are about the exercise of power.

The politics of participation (and the politics of planning)

> Indeed, it might be argued that an exclusion of power in the consideration of participation . . . is something akin to describing free enterprise capitalism without talking about the profit motive.
>
> (Spiegel, 1973: 372)

Participation by prospective users of a system is generally a good thing. As one analyst remarked of citizen participation in social change programs: "The idea of citizen participation is a little like eating spinach; no one is against it in principle because it is good for you" (Arnstein, 1969: 216). In practice, however, user participation may not be as effective as proponents would like, or it may not occur at all for any number of reasons. When participation is examined within the context of public projects, as was the case in the present research, the analyst cannot ignore the broader, embedding social setting. In the present case, we argue that user participation in community network development cannot be analyzed without reference to the social systems and social relations characterizing the host communities. This is the realm of social structure. A community's social structure may be described as patterned relations among its constituents – individuals, groups, and organizations (Laumann *et al.*, 1978). Constituents are related through the *positions* they occupy in the social network, and these positions represent vested interests (Archer, 1995) and differential access to resources (Wellman, 1997). It would be naïve indeed to assume that constituents are all equally powerful. Some (such as the public institutions in the projects surveyed here) enjoy considerable power in communities by virtue of the resources they command: this is an example of structural power (Brint and Karabel, 1991). A structural view problematizes the notion of participation by examining it in terms of the social relations, interests, and relative power that characterize a social order. Structural power imbalances can fundamentally affect who participates and how effectively, and what social groups and interests fail to find a voice.

We identified a number of constraints that combined to render participation by CBOs and small businesses less effective. Lack of access to necessary knowledge and resources was a barrier to participation by these entities. The resource-rich entities could participate far more effectively to shape the outcomes of design. In the face of such inequalities, what should the goal of participation be? What is the proper role of representative bodies such as the project steering committee?

Participation can occur at different levels and with different goals. Typologies of citizen participation have been proposed to characterize the aims of involvement. Arnstein (1969), for example, developed a ladder of participation ranging from non-participation to citizen control, where "have-not citizens obtain the majority of decision-making seats, or full managerial power" (ibid.: 217). The rhetoric in these formulations is shaped by concern for the politically powerless ("have-not citizens"), and by the recognition that redistribution of power through effective participation is a valid goal. Social programs like community action furnished the context for Arnstein, but we would argue that the same political goal is relevant to community networking projects. This in turn argues for an explicitly political view of planning – planning viewed as an enterprise designed to give voice to the voiceless and secure equitable outcomes. This rests on a characterization of politics as the negotiation of power relations (Gregory, 1998) and entailing the articulation of positions, active advocacy, and working through the resulting conflict. When the planning context involves public projects with stated social aims, it would be hard to argue for a purely technical-rational view of planning, which was largely how the planners surveyed here viewed their job.

The planners' apolitical construal of their job betrayed their naïveté about the distribution of power in the social order. Explicitly or implicitly, they appeared to subscribe to the outlook summarized by a political analyst. Social planning, he notes, is "rooted in a pluralistic assumption about the distribution of power . . . Communities are said to be governed by interest groups . . . which can still be brought together in a rational manner to act in the "public interest" which overrides their specific concerns . . ." (Rose, 1973: 317). Rose's conclusion was prompted by failed social planning strategies of the 1970s, but it sheds light on what we discerned in the present research. Contrary to pluralist-rational assumptions the "public interest," which was quite explicitly stated in the project proposals in line with program expectations, was not persuasive in the later design stages. Instead of the public interest overriding the "specific concerns" of powerful entities, the latter often prevailed, often at the expense of broad-based benefits. A politically aware and activist set of planners would have actively advocated the needs of the resource-poor organizations to better approximate the "public interest."

For a number of reasons, the CBOs and small businesses failed to unite and speak with one voice to secure their interests. Most simply did not have the flexibility in their schedules and the necessary "warm bodies" to be present at the planning and design meetings to press their interests. This was particularly the case in the later (and crucial) stages of the projects when attrition rates spiked sharply. Resource-rich entities were much better off in terms of time and bodies and were less affected by the long drawn-out process. Current theorizing on collective action views social capital as a resource and as a necessary condition for initiating such action (Gualini, 2002). As atomized entities, the CBOs and small business units lacked "presence" in the deliberations. Although equally atomized, the resource-rich entities were a compelling presence because of their individual buying power – the telephone company or the project steering committee could not ignore them.

What can politically aware technology planners do to change the state of affairs in a progressive direction? First, the resource-poor must be empowered (provided technical assistance and training) so that they may participate meaning-fully. Second, they must be helped to organize around preferred outcomes. Last but not least, how should participation be institutionalized? What enabling structures should be developed so that participation is substantive, broad-based, and ongoing? In the projects surveyed above, steering committees have evolved into standing bodies with formal authority and fiduciary powers. They manage the network and set and enforce policy. The other half of the picture – partici-patory structures for community residents to register their voice in community network governance – is far less developed and formal in nature.

Conclusion

Descriptive and non-evaluative characterizations of the term "community" start with locality: in its most basic sense, a community is physically definable and tied to a particular geographical location. Such an entity is also a social entity to the extent that it supports human residents and their day-to-day needs. A sociological view of community encompasses these dual meanings of the term: a community is a physical location with the necessary support structures

– physical, social – to sustain "ordinary social life" (Selznick, 1996). Warren (1978) expands on this view: ". . . by *community* we mean the organization of social activities to afford people daily local access to those broad areas of activity that are necessary in day-to-day living" (ibid.: 9, italics in original). In the present research, we embrace such a view: community as a geographically defined social entity. The program that funded the projects under scrutiny here defined *community* similarly but more specifically, to refer to selected, proximate postal code locations in urban and rural settlements that qualified as *economically poor* and *underserved* areas under the program. Recall that only such areas were eligible for program funding.

Insofar as community refers to a proximate physical-social space, the availability of amenities and services in support of "ordinary social life" would be an integral part of such a space. A community, at a minimum, would be expected to offer safe housing, paved roads and public transportation, a water and sewer system, a law enforcement system, schools, and healthcare services. In strictly administrative terms, such amenities may not all be available in the same locality. A municipality may or may not provide all of them within the confines of a proximate, administratively defined area, but to a prospective resident, convenient access to basic amenities would arguably be important as a quality-of-life criterion. A locality-based understanding of *community*, in other words, would also recommend an instrumental (or utilitarian) appreciation of it. While program authorities were sensitive to the psychological benefits from linking organizations (recall the "forging common ground" sentiment) to a shared backbone, they tended to view a program-funded network primarily as facilitating coordinated delivery of public and social services, including affordable broadband access to the Internet, in grantee communities.

A community, however, is more than a geographical area. A community is socially constructed. It is a complex amalgam of place, identity, cultural signification, and politics, and implicates social groups and their (often divergent and competing) interests. It is a product of such interests, in pursuit of which or in resisting which social groups in a proximate physical area may build coalitions with groups and institutions within and outside that area. Some analysts have defined (locality-based) community exclusively in social constructivist terms: ". . . community is a power-laden field of social relations whose meanings, structures and frontiers are continually produced, contested and reworked in relation to a complex range of socio-political attachments and antagonisms" (Gregory, 1998: 11). Such a view, of course, stems from a social structural understanding of community organization (outlined earlier) in terms of the interests and relations of power that characterize the constituents of a physical-social space.

If a community is socially constructed, a community network, as a technological artifact, is also socially constructed. Drawing on arguments in Bijker (1995) among others, we would argue that a community network must be understood as the product of social power and influence. As we argued earlier, it would be naïve to assume that all relevant interests in a given social order have equal power or resources to participate in the community network development process. A social structural view would argue against such an assumption. If a community's prevailing institutions and value systems are shaped by the interests of its dominant groups and bear the imprint of its distribution of power, a community network, as located in and developed within this social context, cannot be immune from such influences. A community network is a social and political artifact as much as it is a technological artifact and competing interests will therefore view them as sites of contestation. In fact, as we noted, the projects referenced above tended to reproduce the host community's dominant interests. Advanced technology may *systematically* inhibit participation by the resource-poor and less powerful interests. A social constructivist view (versus a technology determinist view) of community network development would vigorously resist the implication that the biases evident in the above projects stemmed from the advanced nature of the technology. It would, instead, recommend corrective action as a matter of policy. Our discussion of radical technology planning praxis is inspired by a social constructivist view of technology development, which rests on the belief that alternative developmental trajectories are always possible.

Technologically advanced community networks can offer significant benefits to communities interested in innovative service delivery. They can disembed service delivery from the physical infrastructure of roads and transportation. For example, healthcare delivered over video-conferencing can dramatically enrich the remote consulting experience for the doctor and the patient without compromising convenience. Video can be used to bypass literacy barriers and to deliver sign language services to hearing impaired patients from remote locations. From a utilitarian viewpoint, advanced technology networks can augment and extend a community's social support structures for meeting residents' day-to-day needs.

Such a function can increase convenience while also empowering the resident who avails of network-delivered services. The Medicaid program in the US helps the needy with medical expenses. The applicant for Medicaid benefits is certified as eligible after a complex process, a key step of which is a face-to-face interview with a Medicaid "specialist" at the administrative offices. We developed a video-conferencing-based application prototype for possible use with one of the networks surveyed here. The prototype was successfully used with 25 actual applicants. The prototype permitted the specialist to interview the applicant at the nursing home (where applicants tended to be at the time they applied for benefits) and not at the Medicaid offices, making it more convenient for the applicant. The applicant's family members could be co-present during the interview, providing moral support through this difficult process while also helping fill in the gaps of the applicant's financial information for the Medicaid specialist. Furthermore, the technology allowed the nursing home caseworker, the applicant, and the Medicaid specialist to work together in real time on the application, which resulted in fewer errors and miscommunication and improved the quality of the information gathered through the interview. Because the technology allowed co-work in real time by all involved, only one out of the 25 applicants used an attorney as an intermediary during the interview. Normally, one in two applicants relied on an attorney to shepherd them through the interview process because they were so afraid of it. The prototype was empowering in the most fundamental sense by giving control over the benefits certification process to the applicant and their family, not to the attorney or to the county Medicaid specialist. Despite its success, video-based benefits certification is currently stalled in this community for a number of "bureaucratic" reasons and may never be an option for applicants.

Service delivery would be a legitimate and valuable function of a community network. However the economics of service delivery and the politics of needs often (invariably) intersect to determine which needs are recognized and which are not, and one can be certain that political-economic criteria will be critical to decisions on using advanced technology networks for service delivery given their high costs. So where does that leave such artifacts? Are they doomed to be elitist toys? A social constructivist view would argue against such fatalism.

A social constructivist view would argue that the community network should provide the means for residents to form into groups to press for new services as new needs arise. In other words, it is not enough if the network provides services; it should serve progressive ends as well. So for example, applicants for Medicaid benefits should be able to use the network, among other means, to mobilize other applicants and lobbyists and concerned others to press for video-based interviewing as a standard option. A social constructivist view understands community as a product of politics. Proponents attempt to realize and sustain preferred interpretations through conflict and negotiation. In a normative sense, we see a tension between the utilitarian and the progressive political in uses of a community network. This tension is dialectical to the extent it implicates (a) the community's prevailing hierarchy of needs, which is reflective of its social organization and distribution of power, and (b) the constitution of new needs as a community's demographics change. In the first case, local government agencies may use the network to meet certain needs, including their own internal ones. In the latter case, social groups may use the same network to organize around unmet needs and challenge the community's entrenched needs hierarchy. The establishment, definition, and fulfillment of needs are fundamentally political concerns (Fraser, 1989). By facilitating formation of online and offline coalitions and interest groups, a community network can aid political mobilization and help expand the space of politics and participation. It can be a means to collective power.

The networks surveyed are currently used to deliver a range of services – some of which are open only to network subscribers (paying customers). At least in one case, subscribers use the network for linking branch campuses to their organizational headquarters. By offering subscribers plenty of bandwidth, advanced technology may recommend such use, which in this case is not easily defensible considering the broad social aims of the funding program. But such use may not be avoidable. As noted earlier, in this case, resource-rich entities stepped forward with commitments to subscribe when a broadband option they preferred was approved for program subsidies. Resource-poor entities were not yet ready to commit as they could not afford any of the available broadband options. By their willingness to subscribe, the resource-rich effectively became guarantors of the project going forward. As such, their interest in using the project to meet their internal connectivity needs assumed legitimacy in the planners' eyes. But the planners failed to use this interest by the resource-rich entities to negotiate concessions from them that would have helped the social aims of the project. A planner argued that the resource-rich entities were obligated to the community in whose name the grant (and the subsidies) had been obtained in the first place, and that they should see themselves as resource providers and help the less resource-poor entities to get connected. However, the project leadership never pursued this line of reasoning. A plausible explanation for this failure was that the planners did not see themselves as political actors pursuing the project's (and the program's) stated social goals; rather, they saw themselves as working with the telephone company design professionals on specifying the network so that it could be built.

The political economy of broadband telecommunications may confront the radical planner with just such a scenario. Happily, two projects (not among those referenced here) came up with creative ways to provide some protection for the interests of the resource-poor while also satisfying the needs of the resource-rich. In one case, the project steering committee saved a portion of the CPE funds in an escrow account for the resource-poor entities to draw on when they were ready to sign up. In the second case, resource-rich entities could negotiate better terms (e.g. lower rates) with the steering committee in exchange for assisting resource-poor entities to get connected (e.g. by sharing technical know-how). A social constructivist construal of community network development would argue vigorously against the stance that the technology *determined* biased outcomes. While the nature of the technology certainly played a role, enlightened, socially responsive choices were available to planners if they were sufficiently concerned about equity and solidarity. Social action is key to ensuring that network governors recognize the value of progressive political use of the community network and that (a) utilitarian use is not narrow or purely private but is in fact broad-based in its reach, and (b) the network is open to broad-based participation and is responsive to changing needs in the broader community. The latter, relying on "bottom-up" collective action, would help ensure that the community network stays responsive to the community it is designed to serve.

Notes

1 "Economically disadvantaged areas means zipcodes within Standard Metropolitan Statistical Areas (SMSA's) and cities, towns and villages outside SMSA's that are within the operating territory for (the telephone company) in New York State . . . Median household incomes for the listed zipcodes, cities, towns and villages are below 75 per cent of the statewide median household income" (New York State Diffusion Fund Committee, 1996). Underserved zipcodes were defined as these "where the percentage of households without telephone service is at least 50 per cent above the statewide average . . ." (New York State Diffusion Program, 1996).

2 "Network infrastructure means electronics, equipment, hardware and software associated therewith, and materials of (telephone company) required to establish connections, either dedicated or switched, necessary to support an advanced telecommunications application within (telephone company's) operating territory in New York State" (New York State Diffusion Program, 1996).

Chapter 14

Community Informatics Systems

A meeting place for useful research

Wal Taylor and Stewart Marshall

Introduction

Information Communication Technologies (ICT) are posing fundamental questions for society, government, and commerce in economic, social, educational, cultural, and democratic processes within and across nation states in terms of access, equity, and security. Electronic networks, which can operate outside nation states with hitherto unknown volume and velocity, are changing the architecture of power and culture (Bollier, 2003).

Many governments and global agencies have recognized the growing issues associated with inequitable ICT access and have provided funded programs aimed at addressing specific needs within nation states. However, there is growing evidence that many of these programs have failed to deliver on their desired aims and that the societal and community-based disadvantages resulting from uneven societal adoption of ICT are growing (Castells, 2000). There is now increased understanding that the provision of ICT access, either high or low capacity, through government and private sector efforts by itself is insufficient to address the substantial concerns that face the world as a direct result of ICT.

In direct recognition of this, the United Nations (UN) through the International Telecommunications Union (ITU) committed to sponsor two World Summits on the Information Society[1] (WSIS) in Geneva in December 2003 and Tunis in 2005. By adopting General Assembly Resolution 56/183, the UN explicitly recognized three sectors, namely government, civil society, and private sector, to play meaningful roles in these summits. This was the first time that the UN had formally recognized civil society and its concerns as an equal participant in UN deliberations. This, in itself, raised issues of participation and representation and resulted in proposals for the establishment of a Civil Society Bureau, which were ratified by the Geneva PrepCom held in February 2003. This initiative provided challenges for global civil society in general and specifically for the agencies which purport to represent the interests of the civil society.

Universities, because of their key roles in independent teaching and research, have been identified as one of the ten key family groups that comprise civil society as defined by the WSIS process. In addition, there have been responses at national and international levels to encourage collaborations of university-based research on the impact of ICT on society. An example of this is the EU 6th Framework program,[2] which is allocating significant funds for research on a "User Friendly Information Society." However, many developed and developing countries have not yet come to fully recognize the potential of this area of research, and this goes to the heart of the challenge facing higher education and research in benefiting the network society. There appears to be little academic discussion on how the needs of civil society in the information age can best be met and little development of any theoretical frameworks to meet these needs. This lack of leadership by universities in what is one of the major "ages" in human development, and one in which universities have the inherent intellectual base, is reflected by the general lack of civil society recognition of the potential and fundamental rationale for universities to deliver on the challenge.

The chapter discusses the use of ICT within a societal construct, particularly how the technology and the information it accesses can be delivered through knowledge into beneficial action and how these issues may be framed for examination and discussion in both research and praxis. It begins by charting the development of Information Systems (IS) as a discipline, provides a context for the emerging discipline of Community Informatics Systems (CIS), discusses the concept of community practice as a delivery mechanism for local engagement and provides a proposed framework for the categorization of CIS practice and research.

Information systems

The traditional discipline of Information Systems (IS) is currently undergoing a major evolutionary step into societal applications (as opposed to organizational applications in business, education, and service delivery). Harris (2002) has proposed a discussion framework for the emergence of Information Systems as a discipline (see Table 14.1). Whilst the time frames in this proposition may be considered arbitrary, depending upon location, and the descriptors used unnecessarily prescriptive, the proposition does, none the less, chart a development base for Information Systems as a discipline. It also makes the powerful point that the Information Systems discipline is now increasingly moving outside of organizational boundaries and into society. This domain is much more difficult to adequately define in terms of both form and function at the operational level.

In making this step, the discipline of Information Systems is mixing with hitherto unfamiliar disciplines that have community engagement as an operating premise. The term Community Informatics has recently emerged to describe the use of ICT for local community benefit and more recently, international researchers and funding agencies have moved towards the term Community

Table 14.1 Information Systems as an emerging discipline

Dominant technology	Information systems locus	Work group focus	Dominant referent discipline	Scope
1960–70 Main frame computers	Electronic data processing	Clerical staff	Computer science	The organization
1970–80 Mini-computers	Management information systems	Managers	Management	
1980–90 Personal computers	End user computing	Knowledge workers	Organizational behaviour	
1990–2000 Networks	Strategic information systems	Shareholders	Economics and marketing	
2000 The Internet	**Community Informatics**	Citizens	Social science	**Society**

Source: Harris, 2002.

Informatics Systems (CIS) as a parallel for Management Information Systems (MIS) (Gurstein, 2003).

At the beginning of the twenty-first century, the emerging field of CIS, which is attracting researchers, policy-makers, funders, and practitioners across the globe, is drawing from a range of academic disciplines and social practices. For example, Schmidt provides a quote from the now unavailable call for papers for the Informing Science Conference held in Krakow June 19–22, 2001, which described Community Informatics in the following manner:

> The term Community Informatics (CI) refers to an emerging area of research and practice, focusing on the use of Information Technology (IT) by human communities. It links economic and social development at the community level with emerging opportunities in such areas as electronic commerce, community and civic networks, electronic democracy, self help, advocacy and cultural enhancement. CI brings together concepts of IT and information systems with the concept of community development. As an area of research, CI is a growing body of theory underlying one of the most exciting phenomena of the last decade, namely the diffusion and use of Internet technologies within communities.
>
> (Schmidt, 2000)

As such, the emerging development of CIS is leading the reframing of concepts of "Digital Divide" from access and the marketing of computers/Internet (which in the longer term serve the economic interests of developed countries), into qualitative issues affecting the use of ICT as an enabler of all aspects of community life including economic, cultural, and social development as well as democratic empowerment.

As briefly outlined above, this emerging field has substantial international interest and support. However, in many countries in both the developed and the developing world, there have been few attempts to develop delivery systems around a CIS agenda. Where these have occurred, they have been mostly fragmented in a range of traditional service delivery disciplines in government agencies and in community development approaches.

The contextual framework for a Community Informatics Systems (CIS) research approach

As proposed above, CIS research can fit within an Information Society framework which may be depicted as outlined in Figure 14.1. To date, much of the energy in the application of ICT for the Information Age has been in the technology, business, and organizational domains. Thus, ICT has been treated more like a technology good in the sense of technology development, organizational efficiency, commerce, and a service-delivery enhancer within an embedded culture of the *homo economicus*[3] approach. These legitimate domains are displayed in the three middle boxes in Figure 14.1 (Business/organization, Government services and Technology).

The outside boxes of Civil society and Contemporary communication recognize that ICTs in their emerging role radically expand on notions that limit their application, usefulness, and evaluation into *homo economicus* or technological deterministic frame.

Technological determinism views ICT development as being independent of society and its needs, and holds that ICT development shapes society but is not reciprocally influenced by society. Researchers such as Day (2001) contend that ICT development is often shaped by economic factors such as cost reduction, rationalization, and increasing revenues or efficiency measures in order to sustain capitalist patterns of power authority and ownership.

Further, authors such as Castells (1989, 1996, 2000) and Schiller (1985) point to the diffusion of Internet technologies and the commodification of information as reinforcing the hierarchical power of capitalism. Under these scenarios Internet technologies have been seen to centralize power and work against the interests of community through calculative rationality (Falconer *et al.*, 2000).

However, whilst there is abundant evidence for this position which is continually reinforced in the mass media, the social shaping of Internet technology is an emerging interest which has its basis in the concepts of CIS as

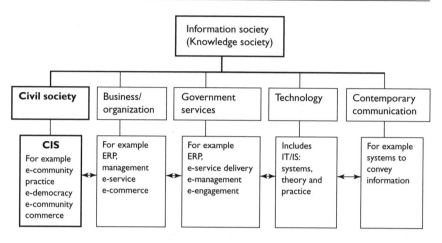

Figure 14.1 Contextual framework for Community Informatics Systems

espoused by Schuler (1996), Gurstein (2000), Day (2001), Harris (2002) and others, as well as being the foundation for national and international collectives such as AFCN,[4] EACN,[5] GCNP,[6] CIRN.[7] This approach is in direct contrast to the concepts of technological determinism, techno-economic capitalism, social exclusion, and cultural capitalism, which not only reinforces and centralizes power structures within communities but disadvantages sections of society in developed and developing countries. The concept of social shaping of ICT provides the philosophical underpinning for a CI approach, which in turn is recursive in strengthening both the applications and the communities.

The interaction of these two largely opposing philosophies forms the basis of simultaneous and sequential interacting effects of Internet technologies shaping society and society affecting the structural use of ICT. A process described by Giddens (1984), Orlikowski and Robey (1991) and others as structuration.

Structuration theory appears to offer a means to address the dialectical nature of diffusion/adoption of ICT within a system that can include a community/societal construct. Taylor (2002) identified the interaction between structures and people in shaping each other as an important construct in examining adoption of ICT for community development in a regional setting. At the same time structuration appears to be able to accommodate a case study approach and meet some of the inadequacies identified in other adoption/diffusion approaches and theories. However, as Towers (1996) concluded, his attempts at developing a structuration model of innovation could at best be seen as "only a component contributing to the understanding the interactions between communication and information technologies, social settings and human agents" (Towers, 1996: 357).

Community practice as the delivery of knowledge

The delivery of the benefits of ICT in equitable and tangible ways to society is being recognized as a more complex issue than the mere provision of access or the creation of knowledge *per se*. Experience in developed countries is showing many of the high-cost IT infrastructure programs are failing to meet their stated aims in equity of end use and that there is a glass ceiling in the adoption of ICT for either local community benefit or society at large (Gurstein, 2003; Taylor *et al.*, 2003). Further, it is increasingly obvious that, without proactive approaches, the application of ICT in social constructs that favour a *homo economicus* approach has a natural tendency to centralize power and decision-making. The lessons clearly point to the need for *a mechanism of doing* if the technology is to be harnessed in ways that benefit local communities and society as a whole. The concept of community practice provides such a basis for the harnessing of ICT in these ways and for taking acquired knowledge in to tangible social benefit. Community practice is used in this chapter to describe both the process of community capacity building and the outcomes in terms of social, economic and cultural capital derived from the process.

Glen (1993) identifies three approaches to community practice:

- Community development – this is concerned with the empowerment of communities to define and meet their own needs.
- Community action – this consists of organizing and campaigning to achieve community goals.
- Community services – this involves altruistic and compulsory (statutory) forms of assistance.

Community practice has multi-disciplinary characteristics. For instance, it is simultaneously economic, political, and social and can be viewed as a science, a social movement, as social engineering, as a program, and as a product (Voth, 1989). It can be viewed as a black box into which proponents of various disciplines apply their own particular theories.

The concept of community practice within a CIS approach has an embedded notion of people using ICT to apply knowledge in a "doing sense." As such it also has parallels with development theory. "Development research is informed by development theory as increasing human capability to make decisions to control the way they live" (Benjamin, 2001: 8). In this development research construct, the role of the development professional or researcher is to support the empowerment of the people who are part of the project, rather than to extract knowledge purely for the edification of other "experts"; it is a process of collaborative learning that impacts on and is impacted by the process (Chambers, 2002). The power of a strategic compact amongst key organizations in setting of a development dynamic has been found to be a key issue in the success of CIS projects in an international review of Community Networks approaches held in Zurich in October 2001.[8] This concept of a strategic compact points to the need for partnerships in delivering CI approaches which turn knowledge (obtained locally and through ICT) into action which addresses the fundamental issues of the digital divide.

Experience clearly points to the need for patron agencies to at least initiate and in most cases sustain CIS initiatives. Dependency upon short-term public agency, foundation funds, or community subscription has problems of sustainability. For instance, in an examination of Community Network projects in Western Europe, Day (2001) illustrates that bureaucratic demands of government agency funding not only inhibit but also often cause CI approaches to fail. In examining the underlying causes of failure of CIS projects, Romm and Taylor (2000) proposed the Harmony/Autonomy model, which identifies local autonomy in establishing, managing, and delivering CIS projects as a critical factor.

An approach to addressing problems of autonomy and sustainability has been the basis for suggestions of local partnerships. Traditionally, local partnerships have been developed between public and private sectors within the confines of an economic development framework. This type of partnership concentrates on economic and infrastructural capital overlooking the potential contribution of social capital as described by Cox (1997), Loury (1977), and Putnam (2000). This approach concentrates power in the economic, regulatory, and administrative domains in respect to local development, excluding the third sector, the civil society, from effective participation (Day and Schuler, 2000).

A development of this is a cross-sectoral approach involving local government, universities, and private and voluntary sectors (Harris, 1996). However, experience with these arrangements suggests that the agenda is invariably narrowly focused on economic development and disempowers or totally excludes the community through referent and expert power; see for example Garlick (1998). In such partnership models, the private and government agency sectors need to have legitimate roles to make profits and to administer policy. They need to have form and function to enable them to maximize efficiency in a calculative rationalist manner and operate in a unitary organizational mode. In these systems operatives are socialized in these modes by training and promotion (Falconer et al., 2000).

What is missing in the development of new partnerships is the opportunity for a pluralist approach that not only addresses issues of politics and power but also provides a mechanism for delivery of community benefit to be legitimized. This can be achieved by using a CIS approach which is based in community and provides legitimacy for community development, community action as well as service provision through established agencies.

In addressing the call for new forms of partnerships to initiate and deliver CIS activities, Day (2001) outlines a tripartite approach which involves the private, public, and community sectors in a participative manner that requires a directional shift from the dominant techno-economic model that presently exists

(Shearman, 1999). Success in tripartite partnerships requires fundamental changes to the way that bureaucracies function and the practices relating to the power of administrators (Day, 2001: 72). This approach recognizes that the development of local communities cannot be shaped by economics alone as this is only one element of the human condition, which requires communication and participation with others as part of the social fabric. It also recognizes that rich creativity exists in local communities and that this creativity can be harnessed to benefit the delivery of a CIS approach which is just a means to an end for empowering community. The social inclusion agenda, which is fundamental to a CIS approach, is based on principles of participation, self-actualization and individual responsibilities to the rest of the community. As such these principles inculcate a participative form of democracy being advocated by many involved with CI approaches including Schuler (1997) and Shearman (1999).

The issue of new forms of partnership and community engagement go to the very heart of educational responsibility and local governance. It puts the potential of CIS at the centre of not only new forms of community representation but also community participation. It is not the availability of, nor necessarily access to, ICT that is the limitation to the adoption of a CIS approach. But the limitations are to be found within existing structures that were designed to serve community's best interests and also in community's understanding, willingness, and capacity to respond to pressures of modern living, which reduce participation (Putnam, 2000). As Schuler points out, these are fundamental issues that are worsening because of the increased efficiencies that ICT has brought to traditional structures at the expense of community's interests (Schuler, 1997, 2001). In order to address this imbalance of power between governance, the private sector, and the community Schuler (1997, 2001) and others including Day (2001) and Gurstein (2000) propose new forms of partnerships, a focus on creating civic intelligence, and acceptance by universities and local governance of their responsibilities in this regard (Harkavy, 1998; and Campus Compact[9]).

In the next section a new framework for research and practice is proposed. This framework allows both research into the societal needs and community practices of the information age to be described and linked.

CIS: a meeting place for innovative research

From what has been discussed so far, it is apparent that CIS is a meeting place in an exciting and emerging area for many research disciplines. It builds on previous research within organizational frameworks and extends into a new paradigm which to date has been not widely understood. Hence, it provides the opportunity to examine new approaches and new combinations to theory building, evaluation, and praxis, which allow researchers, practitioners, service-providers and policy-makers from many disciplines to interact. Further, it stretches the bounds of some traditional methodologies. For example, the power of story-telling in establishing decision-making, cultural understanding, and analysis is becoming more widely recognized in community practice research. Extensions to this can be many and varied and include approaches such as ethnodrama in which expression and participation interact in real time.

By way of contextualizing a starting place for CIS research and praxis, it is useful to consider the community concept from "familial" to the broader construct of "society" and then to apply this to the current paradigms of segmented benefit which are used by many in resource allocation evaluations and policy development.

Table 14.2 provides a conceptual framework that may be useful in categorizing some possible descriptors for research, evaluation, and policy development. This framework can promote discussion on the interaction between the use of CIS processes in a community practice construct and their impact on some of the more traditional evaluative constructs. How these constructs can be effectively measured is still open for interpretation depending upon the various worldviews that researchers, funders, communities, governance structures, and policy-makers hold. However, what is certain is that the impacts of CIS can vary across the community subsets categorized in Table 14.2 and that these subsets may have desires, needs, and wants. Segmenting CIS through such a matrix provides a means to commence discussion on the complexities of society ("the third sector") as an equal to business and government and to consider this sector as potentially proactive rather than just as a client or a customer. As such it provides a basis to supplement representative processes with participative processes and

Table 14.2 Conceptual framework for the categorization of analysis of CIS research

	Assessable				Impact	
	Social	Economic	Cultural	Health	Governance	Service delivery
Community subset						
Familial						
Social networks						
Special interest networks						
Spatial communities						
Government						
Society						

Source: Taylor et al., 2003.

give more substance to current interests in "community engagement" being sought by many government agency service delivery arms.

A new framework for CIS practice and research

Given the categorization of CIS analysis suggested above, there still remains the issue of how this may be adequately described within a community practice construct which of its very essence implies continuing activity. A framework which may assist in the process of mapping CIS practice and research as an ongoing interactive development is proposed in Figure 14.2. This framework borrows heavily from a number of texts and writings of CI practitioners, particularly Shearman (1999).

The framework suggests that the adoption and use of Internet technologies and ICT for community practice should be seen within a community practice paradigm and ICT applied to this paradigm.

Processes for achieving this can be described in terms of a cyclical process of community building, leading to social inclusion, resulting in social mobilization, which delivers community renewal. Figure 14.2 presupposes community building is a prerequisite for social inclusion, which is a prerequisite for social mobilization, which in turn is a prerequisite for community renewal. However, whilst these issues may be depicted as sequential, it is important to note that they can, and often do, operate in parallel both within and between particular applications occurring in the community. Alternatively this mechanism can be viewed as developing competence (community building), leading to connectedness (social inclusion), resulting in the development of community practice concepts (mobilization and renewal). The framework demonstrates that each of the main components have their own inputs which produce outputs to allow either a strengthening within each of the components or the capacity to move to the next component. Figure 14.2 provides some examples of the sorts of issues and practices which can form either inputs or outputs for each of the community practice descriptors or phases. For example, an output of a CIS approach in the Community Building component maybe an increased interest in learning and increased confidence in using CIS approaches. Further an output of the Social Inclusion component may be a growth of pluralism within and between secular community groups in the pursuit of increased local participation and self-reliance. The ICT and Internet technology products and services used in the pursuit and development of CIS approaches can either emanate from the generic ICT arena (for example, email etc.) or from specially developed applications as a result of community actions within the various components. For example, a community group interest in a medical condition may lead to specific ICT-enabled developments which meet the demand created by the group.

The use of this framework would enable a wider range of aspects of CIS from basic training to community activism and social entrepreneurship to be

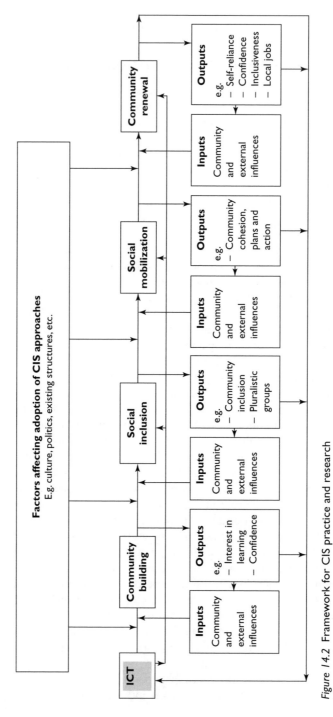

Figure 14.2 Framework for CIS practice and research

considered in a way that provides a relationship with other components of the diverse and complex subject of CIS. The presentation of this alternative CIS framework is presented here with a view to initiating discussion on the desirability of having such a descriptive framework. An advantage of this framework is that it enables practitioners and researchers to interact in a more meaningful manner as suggested by Gurstein (2000). As such it responds to the calls for this interaction between the stakeholders in a CIS approach (AFCN; Benjamin, 2001; Bowles and Gintis, 1986, 1997; Day, 2001; EACN; GCNP; Gronski and Pigg, 2000; Schuler, 1997, 2001; Sellar, 2001; Shearman, 1999).

The foregoing call is a challenge to the diversity of priorities and competing outcomes sought by participants in the process. For example these include:

1   The community which has interest in immediately visible deliverables;
2   The policy-makers who are essentially public agency employees with mixed loyalties to concepts of community emancipation;
3   Researchers whose interests are largely in determining reportable findings and hence have a bias towards segmentation, reductionism, and the short term, whereas the problems in community are largely an antithesis of this position;
4   Governance with issues related to visibility, the short term, and allocatable credit when compared to community practice which is about shared long-term benefits;
5   Business which is interested in rational decision-making based on profit; and
6   Service provider agencies, whose interests, as this research has shown, are vertically aligned around an expert-based, service delivery approach.

However, the framework is advanced for discussion by CI researchers and practitioners in order to begin the process of harnessing the available resources in a collective and collaborative manner in order to benefit spatial communities through the use of CIS.

Conclusion

There is a significant multi-focused international movement examining the impact of ICT in and on society as a construct that is separate from government and business. This area of effort goes to the very heart of some of the promises of an electronically enabled age in delivering on the worthy aims underpinning the broad titles of the "Information Society" and the "Knowledge Society." This chapter has outlined a gap in academic research and practice in providing for the emerging needs of the Information Society to address the issues not only of equity of access but of utilization of ICT for local community benefit, i.e. Community Informatics Systems.

It has proposed both a positional framework and a research and practice operational framework for Community Informatics Systems. These frameworks implicitly recognize the importance of contextualization, the conflict between existing unitary structures, and the reality of plurality in harnessing CIS and the need to treat the concept of civil society in a more adequate fashion. Clearly context counts and policy or analysis which relies upon a homogeneous view within a *homo economicus* paradigm has not yet delivered on the altruistic social capital agendas which many believe is an area of "community commons."

Further, it stands to basic reason that any new view which fundamentally challenges structures which have been built over hundreds of years and which have incrementally "built-in" societal dependence will be heavily scrutinized. The unitary focus of many structures in business and government service delivery has served succession and service delivery well, but in many cases failed to valorize internal power and politics in a way that allows for the reality of plurality or flexibility in dealing with changing societal knowledge or acceptability. Environmental issues and corporate responsibility are but two cases in point. Structuration has been proposed to describe the conflict between plurality and unitarianism. ICT products and services are now providing new opportunities for engagement, increased self-reliance, and emerging forms of community living which are challenging existing systems. They are doing this in the same way that other major technological advances such as printing, internal combustion engines, industrialization, etc. have done in the past.

In this particular instance, universities hold both a privileged position and a responsibility in providing leadership that allows an Information Civil Society to flourish alongside Information Government and Information Business. To meet this responsibility, it is essential that an independent process for inquiry and analysis be developed. This chapter has attempted to contribute to this agenda. The UN-led process for the World Summits on the Information Society (WSIS) has created a global dynamic. It provides new opportunities for teaching and research to benefit local communities. It is now up to individuals in positions of influence and those with capacity and knowledge to grow the necessary practice.

Notes

1 http://wsis.itu.int
2 http://europa.eu.int/comm/research/fp6/index_en.html
3 The *homo economicus* approach, which underpins the free market doctrine, assumes all individuals permanently display and make decisions on high levels of rationality, self-interest, and knowledge. For a discussion on this matter refer to http://www.korpios.org/resurgent/L-homoeconomicus.htm
4 http://www.afcn.org/afcnorg.html
5 http://www.communities.org.uk/eacn/main.htm
6 http://www.globalcnpartnership.org
7 http://www.ciresearch.net
8 http://www.hsw.fhso.ch/ruddy/chrono.htm
9 http://www.compact.org

Conclusion

Chapter 15

Integrating practice, policy, and research

Peter Day and Douglas Schuler

Introduction

In Chapter 1 we considered what we meant by community practice and illustrated the existence of an inextricable link to community policy. We argued that changes in the culture and mind-sets of policy and practice were necessary, especially in the integrated cyclical activities of policy development and implementation, for both to successfully achieve their goals. However, such changes will not occur without a deepening and enrichment of knowledge about how communities work and what they need. The processes of data/information collection, classification, and analysis that will enable such an augmentation of understanding of community practice and policy in the network society is the responsibility of research. More specifically, it is the responsibility of those researchers, both academics and practitioners, who form the emerging field of community communication technology research – commonly known as community informatics (Schuler, 1996; Gurstein, 2000; Keeble and Loader, 2001; and Marshall *et al.*, 2004).

Traditionally, research is viewed as an academic process in which knowledge is developed through the exploitation of scientific methods and analysis. In this way scientific knowledge is acquired and expanded. For community research to be successful, however, the cultivation of scientific knowledge is only part of the equation. Because the behaviour of people is often unpredictable and does not respond as uniformly as inert substances such as rocks, or with the calculable precision of mechanical systems, social knowledge, often tacit in nature and embedded in community culture, must also be advanced. Scientific method and analysis must find a way of working alongside, and in partnership with, social method (practice) and analysis. It was with this in mind that we invoked Howard Rosenbrock's metaphor of the Lushai Hills,[1] to support our contention that the understanding, knowledge, and technological directions accepted as scientific fact in today's network society are not necessarily the only "truths" in terms of socio-technological development. We believe that other pathways exist to network society knowledge, pathways that have yet to be traveled. With this in mind we considered the relationship between community practice and community policy as being significant to the creation of a more accessible route to network society knowledge and understanding.

We do not suggest that the arguments raised here are by any means exhaustive. Nor that the integrated practice, policy, and research framework we are about to present is *the* one best way of using community technologies for building and sustaining healthy communities. Our purpose, with this book, has been to provide a frame of reference for those practitioners, researchers, and policy-makers wishing to engage in a dialogue about community communication technologies, in the hope that this will ultimately result in socially productive action. To this end we have brought together a collection of chapters that provide critical evaluation of a normally neglected area of the information age discourse – community practice. The next section of this chapter examines how the emerging field of community informatics might make such a contribution to scientific and social knowledge.

Community informatics: consideration of an emerging research and development agenda

Although the last two decades have borne witness to a spate of development programs directed at community-based ICT projects internationally, most are predicated on underlying assumptions of technological determinism and economic rationalism – illustrations of this can be found in the chapters by Marshall, Robinson, Courtright and Alkalimat in Part 2, "Snapshots of community practice" (Chapters 6–9) of this book. Traditionally, the normal practice of such programs has been to offer up short-term funding for the purpose of providing a degree of public access to ICT – often with inadequate training and little contextualized relevance to the social environment in which they are placed.

No matter how well-intentioned, top-down development programs such as these often parachute projects into geographic communities (Day, 2001) with little knowledge of local needs or wants, much less an understanding of how such projects might assist in achieving community goals (Day and Harris, 1997). All too often their strategic, if not operational, rationale appears to be driven by the need to achieve information society policy performance targets and indicators rather than any constructively considered plan that might improve the quality of community life. A case in point is the UK Online Centres program, proclaimed by the government to be an indicator of their determination to "bridge" the digital divide in the UK. However, since initial short-term funding ran out, the Audit Commission has expressed concerns that significant numbers of UK Online Centres, especially in the most socially excluded areas, are in danger of closing (NAO, 2003).

Governments across the world and at all levels should take note. If communication systems are to be serious components of their plans to contribute toward building healthy and sustainable communities in the network society, then the planning, design, implementation, and ongoing development of such systems must be grounded in the social networks and social capital of local community life. They must be considered as integral elements of the community infrastructure, in much the same ways as public libraries are.

> The kind of communication that creates community must be that of active interpersonal communication, leading to a common sense of purpose and solidarity. It seems sufficient for our purposes to view the art of community-building as that of creating effective communication linkages. These enable people to define their own problems, set their own goals, come up with their own solutions, and optimise individual and group abilities to learn, resolve their differences, and to act on their own behalf.
>
> (White, 1999: 29)

White's quote – from an edited collection of participatory approaches to grassroots communication – draws attention to the centrality of communication to the processes of community practice. Communication is pivotal, not only to the activities and mechanisms of everyday community life, but also in creating or building community in the first instance. If we accept White's proposition that communication gives rise to community, it takes no great leap of imagination to understand that ICT can be used as tools for underpinning community practice in the network society. Of course, ICT is a generic term covering a wide range of media technologies and applications. Communication technologies offer communities a range of media to exploit information and communicate in a variety of different ways. Community newsletters, radio, TV, video, and resource centers are among applications contributing to the growing strength of the community technology movement.[2]

The key to the social significance of the use of such technological applications is to be found in the appropriateness of any given media to their social environments. In other words, to the material conditions experienced by people in the community in question. Increasingly, the Internet is heralded as a community technology, often with all the hype that accompanies use of this communications medium. However, the Internet is not a cure-all or miracle panacea for every development ill. It is not *the* solution to every community problem that exists. In fact, it is important to remember that solutions to social problems can only be found through social interaction and communication between people. Technology might assist us in implementing solutions but it does not and cannot create the solutions itself. This is just as true with the Internet. It can, and very often does, facilitate access to important new information resources that enable communities to find solutions to their problems. Similarly, it can be utilized to provide a range of new communication channels and opportunities for communities. It does not, however, select the solution or implement it – people do that!

Within a community practice context, the appeal of the Internet – as with community technologies in general – lies not in the technology or even the information it provides access to, but with the interactions and exchanges between *people* that it facilitates. In other words, it is the potential for supporting communication in and between communities that makes community Internet initiatives socially significant. However, as a number of contributors to this book have suggested (e.g. Boyd-Barrett and Sclove), the Internet can also be used in ways that are or can be damaging to healthy communities. The potential danger of the Internet to community life should not be underestimated, just as the potential benefit should not be overstated. Within a community context, the Internet is a paradox. As with all ICT and technology in general, the paradox lies in its potential for duality. Technology, any technology, is designed, developed, and utilized to suit specific social purposes, and as such, is socially shaped. However, this social shaping does not always follow the same direction or pathway. The design, development, and intended use of technology is dependant on the social agenda of those responsible for shaping these processes. To date, as was seen in Chapter 1, the technologies that underpin the network society, ICT, are primarily shaped by the economic influences of the capitalist system within which we live. However, and this is a significant point, not all ICT development is economically driven, e.g. community networks, the open source movement, Indymedia, and antiwar campaigning are examples of technological developments driven by agenda of co-operation, collaboration, and social conscience rather than competition and financial gain.

Rejecting the techno-economic agenda of recent, grand information-age policy visions (Gore, 1993; Commission of the EC, 1993, 1994a and 1994b; Blair, 2002), we assert that community communication systems should be shaped by community visions of how technology might be utilized to underpin community practices and support the plans and activities of community groups, organizations, networks, and institutions to build and sustain community life. Not because it is technologically feasible, nor because it is socially fashionable, and not because research and development funding might exist and a convincing proposal can be crafted, but because the community has a vision of how ICTs might support communities achieve the "good life" (Chapman, 2004).

To date, most community informatics research has focused on the study of community technology systems – as a number of the chapters in this book illustrate. Whilst such an approach provides useful operational insights into community technology practice, it often lacks strategic understanding. In order to develop a more rounded and richer picture of the interactions and tensions between community practice and community policy, a more grounded approach is required. An approach in which research contributes not only to the development of academic knowledge and understanding but also, through active collaboration, to the development of knowledge and understanding for the purposes of community practice and policy.

The need for practitioner/researcher collaboration

However, such an approach is not without its detractors. Traditionally social scientists have often avoided activist, advocacy, or participatory approaches to research, believing that only totally "neutral" or non-partisan research is acceptable. However, such a view is becoming increasingly untenable. "With perhaps some rare and only imaginable exceptions, all participants in social interaction are partisans" and although researchers should not "bias results to suit an audience," they cannot but help take an orientation "from one of various explicitly recognized partisan interests each playing its role in the resolution of policy conflict" (Lindblom and Cohen, 1979: 62).

While researchers are often prone to voice both their objectivity and independence, the reality tends to be more complex. Educational and scientific research, as an enterprise, is embedded in a constellation of social, economic, and political relationships. Agencies and organizations that fund higher educational research have obvious influences on the research agenda. The increasing dependence on the corporate sector for much of this funding consequently puts increased emphasis on projects with financial payoffs.

In this respect, researchers are part of the world in which they live. Observing critical and, possibly, irreversible changes in communication technology as passive and dispassionate spectators is not defensible from an academic or ethical perspective. Researchers, especially those concerned with the effects of technology on society, have a number of significant roles to play in both the understanding and the development of communication technology in the network society. If the social science community turns its back on community problems it is likely to become ever more insular and out of touch. By the same token, if the public perception of higher education, particularly the social sciences, is that it is not relevant to their daily lives then they will be less inclined to support higher education through taxation.

Grounds for collaboration between practice and research

It would be unwise to underestimate the potential difficulties of collaborative partnerships between practice and research, especially as the cultures of the two worlds are often so very different. However, across the world there are glowing examples of where collaboration can and does work. It should be noted that such collaboration demands a lasting interest in and commitment to the community and its needs, from researchers. Similarly, collaborative community research requires an a priori commitment to the development of knowledge, not just as an academic construct – although this is obviously of importance to the researchers – but as a means of finding solutions to community problems and, equally as important, as a communal resource to be accessed, drawn upon, and updated as and when necessary.

Collaboration that is grounded in mutuality and reciprocity not only provides researchers with insights and data that more traditional methodological approaches could never hope to elicit but also reacquaints community members with the many facets of their lived community experience and in so doing makes it possible for them to develop an understanding of their experience. The processes of community articulation, collection, classification, critical evaluation, and examination that emerge from collaborative research provide a potential for the discovery of solutions to community problems. They can also be enormously empowering, stimulating new community activity and breathing renewed life into shared community experiences.

Sharing expertise and knowledge can be of mutual benefit to both researcher and practitioner alike. The know-how and skills of community practitioners together with the historical "lived experience," local knowledge (often tacit), and understanding of the social environment possessed by local community citizens combine to make an impressive and, most importantly, indispensable research resource. Often untapped, such a knowledge base, based as it is in the social capital of a community, can be of enormous significance to community researchers. In fact, we would goes as far as to say that without access to such data, community research has little real social relevance or meaning.

By the same token, community (technology) practitioners need to learn how to learn more effectively. They need to learn how to adjust their future activities based on their learning. Here, researchers, who after all do this for a living, have knowledge and expertise that can be of practical use to practitioners. Learning through research comprises a conscious, cyclical process of question formulation and/or hypothesizing about social phenomena, designing methods of data collection that effectively lead to an understanding of social phenomena, data collection, classification, analysis, reporting, and evaluation. Ideally, the steps are repeated based on what was learned through previous traversals of the cycle. Researchers are familiar with these processes and can help guide communities and community practitioners in collaborative research initiatives.

Collaboration, however, does not mean a lack of criticism. In fact, a healthy two-directional critical dialogue is an important aspect of meaningful collaboration. Researchers and practitioners must learn to listen to one another and integrate their concerns into an action research program that both groups can understand, participate in, and learn from.

Community informatics – the need for a participatory approach

It is worth noting that collaborative research partnerships do not materialize out of thin air. They are built on trust and mutual respect. Collaborative community research must be conducted sensitively. It should be completely open, beyond reproach, and sanctioned by the community itself. Community research should empower the community, not be isolated from it. Both research process and product should address community need. It is for these reasons that we advocate participatory action research (PAR) as an appropriate methodological approach for community informatics research and development in the network society. For the purposes of this discussion, we adopt the definition of PAR provided by Deshler and Ewert:

> [A] process of systematic inquiry, in which those who are experiencing a problematic situation in a community or workplace participate collaboratively with trained researchers as subjects, in deciding the focus of knowledge generation, in collecting and analyzing information, and in taking action to manage, improve, or solve their problem situation.
>
> (1995)

At this point it is important to make an important distinction between what we are and are not advocating. We do not suggest that all investigations of community technology initiatives or projects using traditional research instruments such as questionnaires, surveys, and case studies have no place in community informatics. Indeed, such tools have provided a wealth of useful insights that contribute to the development of community technology knowledge. We do, however, assert that community informatics research, whatever the specifics of the data collection methods being used, should be grounded in an ethos of participatory action research. PAR is a methodological approach (not a specific method) that can both inform and sustain community practice through its emphasis on participatory collaboration. Where community research is intertwined with community development – as is often the case with community technology activities – the PAR methodology is useful for facilitating the requisite relationship conditions of mutual trust, respect, and reciprocity between community and researchers.

PAR encourages the development of equitable partnerships that draw from and share the knowledge, skills, and expertise of all participating partners. Relationships are founded on equability of knowledge rather than hierarchies of knowledge. Community solutions are not dependent solely on the knowledge of external "expertise" (the researchers). By embedding research collaboration in community need, community members will identify with and feel a sense of ownership of the research being conducted, viewing it as something to benefit the community rather than rather than resenting it as an intrusion.

This is especially important, as a major problem in the past has been that researchers will often abandon community projects the moment funding stops, sufficient data is acquired, school term ends, or project personnel changes. Such behaviour is often resented in the community who feel that the time and energy they invested was more or less stolen so a privileged researcher could advance his or her career

Integrating community and university

The efforts of community researchers to ground community research in the needs of local communities and develop the requisite trust within collaborative community research partnerships are often undermined by the intransigence and lack of flexibility of university organizational cultures. Unfortunately academic community partnerships are prone to a variety of structural problems that need to be addressed if sustained relationships are to be formed. Universities can often appear distanced from the communities in which they are situated. Like hermetic bastions of academic endeavor, they are located in, but not of, the local community. Clearly the university impacts on the local community. It creates jobs; stimulates the local economy, and every year an influx of students swells the local population. However, generally speaking, universities have a poor record when it comes to contributing to the social fabric and quality of life of the community, in ways that are tangible to local people.

In order to address this situation, it is important to design and implement ways to integrate the community into university affairs (as active members, learners, researchers, etc.) and vice versa, creating a more permeable university in which, for example, citizens could more easily use university facilities, attend classes, etc. As Richard Sclove (1995) and others have written, the government, the military, and the corporate sector have long dictated the role of the university. There is a growing desire, among many in academia and elsewhere, to change this situation.[3] With this in mind the creation of an ongoing public dialogue on the role of the university in the community would be a healthy antidote to the hitherto rather exclusive tradition of many universities.

A practical example of this growing desire among some universities to forge stronger links with communities can be found in the UK city of Brighton and Hove. In March 2003, the University of Brighton (Peter Day's home university) launched a venture to build partnerships between local community and university – in the form of its Community University Partnership Project (CUPP).[4] CUPP's aim is to build stronger connections between the university and local communities that bring together the university's values, expertise, and assets with community skills, aspirations, and needs. Particular emphasis is placed on achieving systematic and systemic benefit for both community development and university practice.

Although the University of Brighton has a long tradition of community engagement and extensive experience of working with local community groups this has tended to be centered around the efforts of specific research interests or academic activity, rather than any concerted strategic effort on the part of the university. CUPP will enable the institution to build stronger connections with communities, providing coherence for much of the important work that has been done for some years. The intention is to extend the nature, range, and quality of the university's teaching, learning, and research while delivering real gains for local people through the development of partnerships working together on community projects.

Currently in the first stage of its development cycle, CUPP has just completed an initial information-gathering exercise designed to map both the needs and priorities of local communities and existing community–university activities and links. A number of pilot projects have been established, including a project intended to encourage refugees into higher education and an access to arts project for people with learning disabilities. By the time this book is published, the second stage of the partnership, which is expected to start in January 2004, will have started and will be the focus of the main component of CUPP's work. This main programme of activity will run until February 2007 and is likely to concentrate on four strategic themes: (1) community research, project development and evaluation; (2) access to education for excluded groups; (3) releasing student capacity for community benefit; and (4) Higher Education learning opportunities for people working in and with communities. Action teams will be established for each theme – comprising experts and stakeholders from the university and community – to take responsibility for furthering the work in each area.

The University of Brighton is not alone in its activities, nor is it the first academic institution to consider the social importance of developing partnerships with the community. The home school of Douglas Schuler, the Evergreen State College in Olympia, Washington, recently established the new Center for Community Based Learning and Action (CCBLA) to help promote effective community–academia partnerships. Evergreen's pedagogy and structure, which focuses on interdisciplinary, collaborative teaching and learning, provides fertile ground for effective community-based learning. In fact, Evergreen has been doing this type of work for years. The primary work of the center is supporting and enhancing work that Evergreen faculty and students already do. For that reason, one of the first efforts will be to interview faculty, students, and community members to capture some of the knowledge that may have ordinarily been lost and to publish it on the CCBLA web site as part of a community (in the broadest sense) resource.

The CCBLA (1999) will, according to their founding documents,

> serve as a point of contact between academic programs and community organizations, serve as a clearinghouse and archive of opportunities and past work, stimulate curricular innovation involving community-based learning, consider strategies and approaches for evaluating community-based learning, and negotiate, broker and coach community-academic partnership projects.

The center will run institutes for faculty development and curricular revitalization that involve community-based learning. It will promote the college's commitment to diversity by actively seeking partners from diverse communities; and promote and nurture – in close co-operation with faculty – long-term, collaborative relationships with community organizations and academic programs.

Emerging strategies linking community informatics to community practice

The contributions to this book are an indication of the diversity of connections that exist between academics and communities at a range of levels. Some links are forged through the development of curricular activities that contribute to, and find a resonance in, community life. Examples of our own personal experience of such curricular community/academic partnerships include information and library students at the University of Brighton who, in conjunction with the Sussex Community Internet Project and as part of their final year dissertation projects, worked with local communities to identify their information and communication needs, as part of an ongoing city-wide community network development program. Similarly, students at Evergreen, working in small teams, develop web applications for communities all over the world in a one-year Community Information Systems program which is offered every other year. Students in the recently commenced "Community Practice and Digital Social Change" program will develop media or software projects that help link community members in Olympia to community members elsewhere in the world.

Other forms of community/academic association have emerged in recent years which run parallel to global network society developments. As the hegemony of private and public sectors continues to grow in what Castells calls the "space of flows," a form of alternative "space of flows" is beginning to emerge. A space in which an alliance of geographic communities, communities of interest, social movements, academics, and other parties from civil society around the world are making use of ICT to form globally networked public spheres in which issues of concern are considered and social action organized.

An example of such network alliance-building – of interest to the subject matter of this book – is the recent formation of the community informatics Research Network (CIRN). An international network of practitioners and researchers, CIRN was established in October 2003 and is the outcome of several years of informal discussions and action by a global network of active academics and practitioners. In practice, community informatics is often seen as bringing together people involved with electronically enabling communities: local, virtual, and communities of practice. However, this is only part of what actually happens because community technology does not occur in a social vacuum, as if not connected to everyday community life. Community informatics is concerned with structuring collaborations between researchers and practitioners in these three community domains. The complexities involved in achieving such structural collaborations highlighted the need for the development of a more permanent network of international research-based community technology advocates and activists. Such a network would articulate issues of concern to community practice in the network society through evidence-based research and social networking. Clearly CIRN is still in its infancy but already the network has been successful in winning two significant nationally funded research projects in Canada and the UK, which it is hoped will provide evidence to support the kind of approach being advocated in the pages of this text.

Computer Professionals for Social Responsibility (CPSR), in particularly its biannual Directions and Implications of Advanced Computing (DIAC) symposium, which helped give rise to this volume, are also actively engaged in global community networking. The DIAC symposium is now one of the oldest conferences dedicated to the implications of computer technology and how it should be directed for human needs. The goals of the conference include fostering community and promoting human needs in computing as a legitimate scholarly pursuit. As part of these CPSR activities, the Public Sphere Project (PSP) was launched to help promote more effective and equitable public spheres all over the world. An outgrowth of the "Shaping the Network Society" DIAC symposium held in Seattle in May, 2000, the Public Sphere Project is intended to provide a broad framework for a variety of interrelated activities and goals including event organizing and maintains a number of online resources (with others under development) including public sphere bibliography, calendar of events, and educational and technological links.

The Pattern Language for Participation, Action, and Change is one of the PSP's most prominent projects. The pattern language project is intended to help integrate hitherto disconnected efforts in public sphere activities. Too often, people are unaware of work that is happening in other locations, or of work that may have profound implications for their future work. The premise that increased, strengthened relationships – both intellectual and action-oriented – could empower the movement for democratic media gives rise to many questions. How can "traditional" forms such as public libraries or physical meeting venues inform technological development? What observations from rural environments are relevant in urban ones – and vice versa? What policies open up opportunities, which ones can restrict them? What services can be provided for people who are illiterate? How best to support multiple languages, different cultures? In general: what works, what doesn't and why?

To help answer these questions and, more generally, demonstrate and explore the deep relationships between the important aspects of this work an open worldwide participatory pattern language project was launched in 2001, which adopts the "pattern language" concepts of architect Christopher Alexander (Alexander et al., 1977). Patterns, when taken as a group and ordered from most general to most specific, can present a comprehensive vision of a built environment that is beautiful, is on a human scale, and, most importantly, promotes human values. Each pattern contains a problem, discussion, and a solution followed by the solution portrayed diagrammatically.

There are now over 240 pattern submissions in the system. In order to set the "pattern" ball rolling, we used patterns as the sole submission method for the 2002 DIAC "Shaping the Network Society" symposium. We gathered over 100 submissions in just a few months. The authors of these submissions represented over 20 countries. Some of the pattern proposals submitted thus far include, "Targeted Entertainment," "Value Sensitive Design," "Meeting Space," "Civic and Community Indicators," "Online Museum," "International Networks of Alternative Media," "Mobile ICT Learning Facilities for 3rd World Communities," "Online Deliberation Using Roberts Rules of Order," "World Summit," and "Universal Voice Mail."

Finally, a brief mention of the first United Nations World Summit on the Information Society (WSIS), which will have taken place by the time this book is printed, is in order. In Geneva in December 2003 (with a follow-up in Tunis in 2005) activists from civil society will have an opportunity to meet with their counterparts around the world. Civil society players have historically been denied substantial standing in proceedings likes this. While it seems likely that the civil society actors will not succeed in pushing an agenda that does not meet the approval of the resource-richer representatives from governments and the private sector, the prospect of tens of thousands of people from all over the world talking about the work they are doing and their visions is compelling. This process of civil society interaction, together with the activist networks that they will undoubtedly establish, should become an extremely powerful social resource as time goes by.

Framework for the future of community practice in the network society

Although the core theme of this book is community practice in the network society, we have shown how community practice is connected to both community policy and community research. To understand community practice it is first necessary to understand its relationship with the other two elements of what is a synergistic trilogy of community in the network society. Although each field has its own parameters, goals, actors, and audience, the purpose, population, and performance of each are inescapably interwoven with that of the others. Each draws from, contributes to, and sustains the others in a network of community services, actions, relationships, communication, and outcomes. It has been our intention that the contents of this book will contribute to the development of such an understanding.

In concluding our contribution to the community practice discourse, we present a framework of democratic principles relating to community practice, policy, and research in the network society.

Democratic principles for community technology practice

Whatever the composition and balance of the three interrelated elements of community practice, i.e. community services, community development, and community action, a shared value base that prioritizes the identification and realization of community need as the motivating force of community technology initiatives (CTIs) is required if they are to be socially sustainable. Subordinating community technology systems and artifacts to the needs of community members is fundamental to this process.

1   For CTIs to become integral and contributing components of community life they must first be grounded in local community values (solidarity, participation, and coherence). Their planning, design, implementation, and ongoing development should therefore be undertaken through processes of community engagement.
2   The goals, activities, services, and outcomes of CTIs should meet the needs of the community, identified through sustained and meaningful dialogue. The needs and interests of the marginalized and socially excluded should form an important element here.
3   In addition to providing a wide range of community services, CTIs should stimulate and promote both community development and community action with a view to empowering communities to identify and, where possible, address their own needs.
4   Contribute to a public space for shared communication that facilitates inter and intra community conviviality.
5   Recognize and celebrate diversity of opinions, beliefs, values, cultures, and norms, whilst avoiding actions and behavior that promote intolerance and disrespect.
6   Promote self-actualization through CTI activities and services that stimulate life-long learning and active citizenship in the community.
7   Develop a sense of community identity with, and ownership of, CTIs.

Democratic principles for community technology policy

Healthy communities are predicated on the active participation of community members, groups, and organizations in shaping community life. However, a shared value base[5] with community policy-makers is crucial to the formulation of policies that support the building and sustaining of healthy communities. By developing an understanding of what *community* means at the local level, it is possible to develop policies that are meaningful and relevant to communities in the network society.

1   Avoid policies that establish authoritarian or elitist social relations.
2   Encourage participatory community action in pursuit of community goals and promote CTI autonomy.
3   Invest in social capital by harnessing the indigenous knowledge and creativity that exists in communities, focusing on common community interests and concerns and promoting open dialogue and reciprocal knowledge sharing.

4 Stimulate the social fabric, or core values, of the local community as well the local economy. Schuler's six core values of community (conviviality and culture, education, strong democracy, health and human services, economic equity, opportunity and sustainability, and information and communication) (1996) can provide some useful structure in this dialogue.

5 Promote cross-sectoral or tripartite partnerships that facilitate meaningful engagement with community groups and organizations based on equality of power and mutual respect.

6 Facilitate collaborative interaction and exchange within and between communities. Communities are dynamic and active social structures that are both the progenitor and recipient of a range of services, products, and activities.

Democratic principles for community (informatics) technology research

To date much of the research in the realm of community informatics has been undertaken using more traditional social science research methods. It is our belief that, in order to develop the quality of knowledge and enriched understanding of community practice necessary to facilitate socially sustainable CTIs, research processes must fully engage with communities, not only as research subjects but also as research partners.

1 Communities should be involved in all stages of research design, implementation, and analysis from the earliest possible point.

2 The processes and outcomes of community research should be of benefit to community life and address community need.

3 Partnerships developed between researchers and community members should be extended beyond the life of the project. The broadening of community/university partnerships to include community service learning approaches and the opening of a public dialogue to consider the role of universities as accessible community assets is essential. Although it may not be obvious to all academics, nearly all university departments could adopt at least some CTI research without losing sight of their principal orientation. A variety of possibilities are suggested in Schuler (1997).

4 Academic researchers can assist community members, by teaching a range of research and learning skills and techniques, to become empowered enough to undertake their own research projects that address community needs that they themselves have identified.

5 Communities see a lot of traditional social science research as being abstract and irrelevant. Community research can, through community engagement, be shaped and targeted to ensure relevance and appropriateness to the issues of the community environment.

Looking forward and back

The "network society" can be construed in two basic ways. It can be seen in purely technological terms as the existence of a densely meshed system of computers (and other digital devices) and the media and protocols that link them. With that perspective, knowledge is "content," comprised of bits. People of course become "information processors." In economic terms they are more often consumers, sometimes producers, of information.

Another version is possible, although time for such an alternative may be running out. This competing version places human values at the center and people are the designers and developers of the communication systems that they use. This view asserts that values and human actualization are at least as important as the economic imperative, much beloved of large corporations and "free-market" rhetoricians.

We believe that it is critical right now to look at our communities and think about what is worth protecting – and enhancing – in this "traditional" (and usually "non-virtual") venue. At the same time we must look forward to new emerging realities and consciously incorporate our findings into our actions. How do new forms of communications affect our communities, enhance our communities, threaten our communities? And what must be done?

The authors in this book are concerned with the need to understand as well as the need to act. The offerings in this book necessarily provide only a small glimpse into the vast universe of community and civic undertakings that are now underway. We are proud to be working, directly and indirectly, with all of these visionary and principled people. If they are successful, the information and communication systems of the future will be more responsive to human – both individual and collective – needs. If they are not, we are likely to see a mindless replication of broadcast television that is distracting at best, deceptive and destructive at worst. It is our hope that this volume can in some small measure contribute to their success.

Notes

1 See Chapter 1.
2 http://www.comtechreview.org
3 The Campus Compact based on the civic purposes of higher education is a coalition of over 900 colleges and universities. Founded on the notion of campus/community partnerships the compact promotes community service with a view to developing students' citizenship skills and values. http://www.compact.org
4 http://www.brighton.ac.uk/hubs/about/cupp.html
5 See Chapter 1.

Bibliography

Accenture, Markle Foundation, and UNDP (2001) "Creating a development dynamic: Final report of the Digital Opportunity Initiative." Online. Available: http://www. opt-init.org/framework/onepage/onepage.html (accessed 13 September 2002).

Acheson, D. (1998) *Independent Inquiry into Inequalities in Health,* London: Stationery Office.

Aguilar, R. (1996, October 29) "Net realty for sale," *C | Net NEWS.COM,* The Net. Online. Available http://www.news.com/News/Item/0,4,4896,00.html (accessed 9 April 2003).

Alexander, C., Ishikawa, S., and Silverstein, M. (1977) *A Pattern Language: Towns, Building, Construction,* New York: Oxford University Press.

Alkalimat, A. (2000) "Africana Studies 4900, cyberspace and the black experience, at U. of Toledo," *Chronicle of Higher Education,* 19 May 2000, p. A18. Online. Available http://www.academics.calpoly.edu/diversity/digitaldivide/Cyberspace .htm (accessed 17 March 2003).

Alkalimat, A. and Williams, K. (2001) "Social capital and cyberpower in the African American community: a case study of a community technology center in the dual city," in L. Keeble and B. Loader (eds.) *Community Informatics: Shaping Computer Mediated Social Relations,* London: Routledge, 2001. Online. Available http://www. communitytechnology.org/cyberpower/ (accessed 17 March 2003).

Allen, R. and Miller, N. (2002) "Panaceas and promises of democratic participation: reactions to new channels, from the wireless to the World Wide Web," in S.Wyatt *et al.* (eds.) *Technology and In/equality,* London: Routledge.

Alperovitz, G. (1996) "The reconstruction of community meaning," *Tikkun,* 11, 3: 13–16, 19.

Analysys Consulting (2000) *The Network Revolution and the Developing World* (Analysys Report No. 00–216), Washington, DC: The World Bank. Online. Available: http: //www.infodev.org/library/WorkingPapers/400.doc (accessed 13 October 2002).

Andersen, I.-E. (ed.) (1995) "Feasibility study on new awareness initiatives: studying the possibilities to implement consensus conferences and scenario workshops." Online. Available http://www.cordis.lu/interfaces/src/feasibil.htm (accessed 10 November 2002).

Anderson, R. H. *et al.* (1995) *Universal Access to E-Mail: Feasibility and Societal Implications,* Santa Monica, CA: RAND.

Archer, M. (1995) *Realist Social Theory: The Morphogenetic Approach,* Cambridge, UK: Cambridge University Press.

Arnstein, S. R. (1969) "Ladder of citizen participation," *Journal of the American Institute of Planners*, 35, 4: 216–224.

Article 19 Global Campaign for Free Expression (2003) "Statement on the right to communicate." London, 13 February. Online. Available http://www.article19.org (accessed 9 April 2003).

Asociación Infocentros (2002) "Web site of Asociación Infocentros de El Salvador." Online. Available: http://www.infocentros.org.sv (accessed 13 October 2002).

Aspen Institute (1997). *Voices from the Field: Learning from the Early Work of Comprehensive Community Initiatives,* Washington, DC: The Aspen Institute. Online. Available http://www.aspenroundtable.org/voices/index.htm (accessed 1 November 2002).

Associated Press (2000) "Governors say congress shouldn't bar state internet sales tax," *New York Times*, 29 Feb. Online. Available http://query.nytimes.com/search/advanced/ (accessed 4 April 2003).

Associated Press (2000) "Loans.com domain sells for $3 million," *New York Times*, 31 Jan. Cybertimes.

Attewell, P. (1992) "Technology diffusion and organizational learning: The case of business computing," *Organization Science*, 3, 1: 1–19.

Bagdikian, B. H. (1997) *The Media Monopoly (5th edition)*, Boston: Beacon Press.

Balas, J. (1998) "Debating public access to the Internet," *Computers in Libraries*, 18, 3: 42+. Online. Available HTTP: http://www.ebsco.com (27 January 1999).

Balka, E. and Peterson, B. J. (1999) *Jacques and Jill at VPL: Citizenship and the Use of the Internet at Vancouver Public Library: Preliminary Report (Assessment of Technology in Context Design Lab (ATIC-DL) Report 9903)*, Burnaby: Authors.

Balka, E. and Peterson, B. J. (2002) "Jacques and Jill at VPL: citizenship and the use of the Internet at Vancouver Public Library', in M. Pandakur and R. Harris (eds.) *Citizenship and Participation in the Information Age,* Toronto: Garamond.

Banco Central de Reserva (2001) "Informe Económico 2000," San Salvador: BCR. Online. Available: http://www.bcr.gob.sv/inform01.htm (accessed 29 June 2001).

Barabasi, A.-L. (2002) *Linked: The New Science of Networks,* Cambridge, MA: Perseus.

Barber, B. (1984) *Strong Democracy: Participatory Politics for a New Age*, Berkeley: University of California Press.

Barlow, J. P. (1990) "Crime and puzzlement, Electronic Freedom Foundation," June 8. Online. Available http://www.eff.org/Publications/John_Perry_Barlow/crime_and_puzzlement.1 (accessed 9 April 2003).

Barlow, J. P. (1997) "The best of all possible worlds," *Communications of the ACM* 40, 2: 68–74.

Barnouw, E. (1966) *A Tower in Babel: A History of Broadcasting in the United States, Volume I,* New York: Oxford University Press.

Barnouw, E. (1968) *A Tower in Babel: A History of Broadcasting in the United States, Volume II,* New York: Oxford University Press.

Beamish, A. (1999) "Approaches to community computing: bringing technology to low-income groups," in D. Schön, B. Sanyal, and W. J. Mitchell (eds.) *High Technology in Low-Income Communities: Prospects for the Positive Use of Information Technology* (pp. 349–368), Cambridge, MA: MIT Press. Online. Available http://web.mit.edu/sap/www/colloquium96/papers/index.html (accessed 1 November 2002).

Bell, D. (1973) *The Coming of Post-Industrial Society: A Venture in Social Forecasting.* Harmondsworth: Penguin, Peregrine Books.

Bell, D. (1979) "The information society: the social framework of the information society," in T. Forester (ed.) *The Microelectronics Revolution*, Oxford: Blackwell, pp. 500–549.

Bell, D. (1980) *Sociological Journeys, 1960–1980*, London: Heinemann.

Bell, D. (1987) "The post-industrial society: a conceptual schema," in A. E. Cawkell (ed.) *Evolution of an Information Society*, London: ASLIB.

Benjamin, P. (2001) "Telecentres and universal capability." Unpublished thesis, University of Aalborg.

Benton Foundation (1997) "The Benton Foundation's Telecommunication Act of 1996 Homepage." Online. Available http://www.benton.org/Policy/96act/ (accessed 4 April 2003).

Bergmann, M. K. (2002) "The deep web: surfacing hidden value," BrightPlanet Corporation. White Paper. Online. Available http://www.brightplanet.com/deepcontent/tutorials/DeepWeb/index.asp (accessed 3 April 2003).

Bijker, W. E. (1995) *Of Bicycles, Bakelites, and Bulbs: Toward a Theory of Sociotechnical Change*, Cambridge, MA: MIT Press.

Bijker, W. E. *et al.* (eds.) (1987) *The Social Construction of Technological Systems: New Directions in the Sociology and History of Technology*, Cambridge, MA: MIT Press.

Bimber, B. and Guston, D. H. (eds.) (1997) "Technology assessment: the end of OTA," special issue of *Technological Forecasting and Social Change*, 54, 2 and 3: 125–286.

Birdsall, W. F. (1998) "A Canadian right to communicate?' *Government Information in Canada/Information gouvernementale au Canada*, Number/Numéro 15 (September).

Birdsall, W. F. and Rasmussen, M. (2000) "Citizens at the crossroads: the right to communicate," *Government Information in Canada/Information gouvernementale au Canada*, Number/Numéro 20 (February).

Bix, B. (1996) "Natural law theory," in Dennis Patterson (ed.) *A Companion To Philosophy of Law and Legal Theory,* Cambridge, MA: Blackwell.

Blair, T. "Prime Minister's Key Note Speech to e-Summit 19 November, 2002." Online. Available http://www.number-10.gov.uk/output/Page1734.asp (accessed 25 April 2003).

Bollier, D. (2003) "The rise of netpolitik: how the Internet is changing international politics and diplomacy," a report to the 11th annual Aspen Institute roundtable on Information Technology, Washington, DC: Aspen Institute. Online. Available http://www.aspeninstitute.org/AspenInstitute/files/CCLIBRARYFILES/FILENAME/0000000077/netpolitik.pdf (accessed 20 April 2003).

Bouguettaya, A. *et al.* (2001) "Helping citizens of Indiana: ontological approach to managing state and local government databases," *IEEE Computer*, February.

Bouguettaya, A. *et al.* (2002) "Supporting data and services access in digital government environments," in W. McIver and A. K. Elmagarmid (eds.) *Advances in Digital Government: Technology, Human Factors, and Policy*, Boston: Kluwer.

Bourgon, J. (1997) "Connecting Canadians: public service in the information age." Ottawa, ON: Government of Canada. Online. Available HTTP: http://www.pco-bcp.gc.ca/ClerkSP-JB/Gtech_e.htm (accessed 10 April 1999).

Bourgon, J. (1998) "Fifth Annual Report to the Prime Minister on the public service of Canada," Ottawa, ON: Government of Canada. Online. Available HTTP: http://www.pco-bcp.gc.ca/default.asp?Page=Publications&Language=E&doc=5rept97/cover_e.htm (accessed 30 October 2002).

Bowers, C. A. (2000) *Let Them Eat Data: How Computers Affect Education, Cultural*

Diversity, and the Prospects of Ecological Sustainability, Athens, GA and London: University of Georgia Press.

Bowles, S. and Gintis, H. (1998) "The moral economy of community: structured populations and evolution of prosocial norms," *Evolution and Human Behavior*, 19, 1: 3–25.

Bowles, S. and Gintis, H. (1986) *Democracy and Capitalism: Property, Community, and the Contradictions of Modern Social Thought*, New York: Basic Books.

Boyd-Barrett, O. (1980) *The International News Agencies*, London: Constable.

Boyd-Barrett, O. (2003a) "The 'New Model' News Agency," in APA – Austria Presse Agentur (ed.) *The Various Faces of Reality. Values in News (Agency) Journalism*, Vienna: Innsbrucker Studienverlag, pp. 91–96.

Boyd-Barrett, O. (2003b) "US global cyberspace," in D. Schuler and P. Day (eds.) *Shaping the Network Society*, Cambridge, MA: MIT Press.

Boyd-Barrett, O. (2003c). "Doubt foreclosed: US mainstream media and the attacks of 9–11," in N. Chitty *et al.* (eds.) *Studies in Terrorism*, Penang: Journal of International Communication/Southbound Press.

Boyd-Barrett, O. and Rantanen, T. (2003) "State news agencies: time for a re-evaluation," in APA – Austria Presse Agentur (ed.) *The Various Faces of Reality. Values in News (Agency) Journalism*, Vienna: Innsbrucker Studienverlag, pp. 79–90.

Brin, S. and Page, L. (1998) "The anatomy of a large-scale hypertextual web search engine," paper presented at the Seventh International World Wide Web Conference. Brisbane, Australia. 14–18 April, 1998.

Brint, S. and Karabel, J. (1991) "Institutional origins and transformations: the case of American community colleges," in W. W. Powell and P. J. DiMaggio (eds.) *The New Institutionalism in Organizational Analysis,* Chicago: University of Chicago Press.

Broersma, M. (1998) "Analysts: MSN will give portals a fight," *ZDNet News*, July 24.

Brzezinski, Z. (1998) *The Grand Chessboard: American Primacy and Its Geostrategic Imperatives*, New York: Harper Collins.

Bullen, D. (2001) "Right to communicate," in *New Code Words for Censorship*. World Press Freedom Committee.

Burdsey, T. (2002) "Nottingham CityNet: tackling social exclusion through participatory approaches to ICT," paper presented at Health Development Agency Conference on Social Action for Health and Wellbeing, London, June 2002. Online. Available http://www.social-action.org.uk/conference/conference.html (accessed 10 November 2002).

Burk, D. L. (1995) "Trademarks along the Infobahn: a first look at the emerging law of cybermarks," *Richmond Journal of Law and Technology* 1. Online. Available http://law.richmond.edu/jolt/v1i1/burk.html (accessed 9 April 2003).

Butcher, H. (1993) "Introduction: Some examples and definitions," in H. Butcher, A. Glen, P. Henderson, and J. Smith (eds.) *Community and Public Policy*, London: Pluto Press, pp. 3–21.

Calhoun, C. (1997) "Nationalism and the public sphere," in J. Weintraub and K. Kumar (eds.) *Public and Private in Thought and Practice*, Chicago: University of Chicago Press, pp. 75–102.

Calhoun, C. (ed.) (1992) *Habermas and the Public Sphere*, Cambridge, MA: MIT Press. Cambridge, MA: Harvard Law School.

Campbell, C. *et al.* (1999) *Social Capital and Health,* London: Health Education Authority.

Canada's SchoolNet (1999) "Canada's SchoolNet: Programs," Ottawa, ON: Government of Canada. Online. Available HTTP: http://www.schoolnet.ca/home/e/programs/ (10 April 1999).

Canadian Heritage (1999) "PRI data development. Survey on citizens' access to, and use of, information communication technologies," Ottawa, ON: Government of Canada. Online. Available HTTP: http://policyresearch.schoolnet.ca/keydocs/prdg/prdg-se1-e.htm (accessed 10 April 1999).

Carey, J. (1988) *Communication as Culture*, New York: Routledge.

Castells, M. (1989) *The Informational City: Information Technology, Economic Restructuring and the Urban-Regional Process*, London: Blackwell.

Castells, M. (1996) *The Rise of the Network Society. The Information Age: Economy, Society and Culture*, Volume I, Oxford: Blackwells.

Castells, M. (1997) *The Power of Identity. The Information Age: Economy, Society and Culture*, Volume II, Oxford: Blackwells.

Castells, M. (1998) *End of Millennium. The Information Age: Economy, Society and Culture*, Volume III, Oxford: Blackwells.

Castells, M. (2000) "Information technology and global capitalism," in W. Hutton and A. Giddens (eds.) *On the Edge: Living with Global Capitalism*, London: Jonathan Cape.

CCBLA – Community Service Learning DTF (1999) *The Engaged Campus Report and Recommendations Community-Based Learning DTF*. Online. Available http://www.evergreen.edu/dtf/communitylearning/report.html

Central Intelligence Agency (2000) *The World Factbook 2000: El Salvador*, Washington, DC: CIA. Online. Available: http://www.odci.gov/cia/publications/factbook/geos/es.html (accessed 24 June 2001).

Chambers, R. (2002) "Relaxed and participatory appraisal: notes on practical approaches and methods for participants in PRA/PLA-related familiarisation workshops," Brighton: Institute of Development Studies. Online. Available http://www.ids.ac.uk/ids/particip/research/pra/pranotes02.pdf (accessed 11 March 2003).

Chanan, G. et al. (2000) *The New Community Strategies: How to Involve Local People*, London: Community Development Foundation.

Chapman, G. (2004) "Shaping technology for the 'Good Life': the technological imperative versus the social imperative," in D. Schuler and P. Day (eds.) *Shaping the Network Society*, Cambridge, MA: MIT Press.

Children's Partnership (2000) *On-line Content for Low-Income and Underserved Americans: The Digital Divide's New Frontier*, Santa Monica, CA: The Children's Partnership. Online. Available http://www.childrenspartnership.org (accessed 1 November 2002).

Chomsky, N. and Herman, E. S. (1988) *Manufacturing Consent*, New York: Pantheon.

CIRCLE/CCRN Round Table. (2000) "Conference Report: making connections: Culture and social cohesion in the new millennium (26 & 27 May, 2000)," Edmonton, AB: University of Alberta. Online. Available http://www.boekman.nl/circle/canada3.htm (accessed 5 January 2003).

Clausing, J. (1997) "Ad hoc group takes up technical issues of domain expansion," *New York Times*, 6 Sept. Cybertimes.

Clausing, J. (1997) "The public jumps into the domain-name dispute," *New York Times*, 15 Aug. Cybertimes.

Clausing, J. (1997) "US public provides comment, but little consensus, on domain names," *New York Times*, 23 Aug. Cybertimes.

Clausing, J. (1998) "Internet registrar plots its post-monopoly future," *New York Times*, 20 Jan. Cybertimes.

Clausing, J. (1998) "Private group warns of US Internet Registry Plans," *New York Times*, 23 Jan. Cybertimes.

Clausing, J. (1998) "US releases report on governing internet," *New York Times*, 30 Jan. Cybertimes.

Clement, A. and Shade, L. R. (1996) "What do we mean by 'Universal Access'?: Social perspectives in a Canadian context," paper presented at *INET96: The Internet – Transforming Our Society Now*, Montreal. Online. Available http://www.isoc.org/inet96/proceedings/f2/f2_1.htm (accessed 19 April 2003).

CNet ".com stands for competition" (1996, August 22) *C|Net NEWS.COM*. Online. Available http://news.com.com/2100–1023–222281.html?legacy=cnet (accessed 9 April 2003).

CNET (1996) "Top ten stupidest domain names," *Digital Dispatch*, 2, 6. San Francisco: C/Net. Online. Available HYPERLINK http://web.archive.org/web/20010219024137/http:/coverage.cnet.com/Community/Welcome/Dispatch/dd44.html 1 "6" http://web.archive.org/web/20010219024137/http:/coverage.cnet.com/Community/Welcome/Dispatch/dd44.html#6 (accessed 12 February 2004).

Commission of the European Communities (1993) *Growth, Competitiveness, Employment: The Challenges and Ways Forward into the 21st Century – White Paper*, COM (93) 700 Final, Luxembourg: Office for Official Publications of the European Communities, 1994, 107–115. Online. Available http://europa.eu.int/en/record/white/c93700/contents.html (accessed 15 April 2003).

Commission of the European Communities (1994a) *Europe and the Global Information Society: Recommendations to the European Council* [The Bangemann Report] CD-84–94–290-EN. Online. Available http://europa.eu.int/ISPO/infosoc/backg/bangeman (accessed 15 April 2003).

Commission of the European Communities (1994b) *Europe's Way to the Information Society: An Action Plan*, Brussels: CEC COM(94) 347 final, 19/7/94. Online. Available http://europa.eu.int/ISPO/infosoc/backg/bangeman.html#chap6 (accessed 15 April 2003).

Community Services, City of Vancouver (1999) *Vancouver Local Areas, 1996: Data from the Canadian Census*, Vancouver: Community Services.

Computer Professionals for Social Responsibility (1999) "One planet, one net: principles for the Internet era." Online. Available http://www.cpsr.org/onenet/onenet.html (accessed 9 April 2003).

Computer Professionals for Social Responsibility (2001) "Telecommunication policy." Online. Available http://www.cpsr.org/cpsr/nii/cyber-rights/web/current-telecom.html (accessed 4 April 2003).

Conectándonos al Futuro de El Salvador (1999) *TechNet Think Tank: Building a Learning Society in El Salvador*, Washington, DC: TechNet. Online. Available: http://www.vita.org/technet/esls/ (accessed 20 October 2002).

Connecting Canadians (1999) *Connecting Canadians. The Initiative: Introduction*, Ottawa, ON: Government of Canada. Online. Available http://www.connect.gc.ca/English/Initiative/IntroductionENG /index.htm (accessed 1 October 1999).

Connecting Canadians (2002) *Connecting Canadians*, Ottawa, ON: Government of Canada. Online. Available http://connect.gc.ca/en/100-e.htm (accessed 11 December 2002).

Contractor, N. and Bishop, A. P. (1999) *Reconfiguring Community Networks: The Case of PrairieKNOW,* Urbana-Champaign, IL: Department of Speech Communication, University of Illinois at Urbana-Champaign.

Cordes, C. and Miller, E. (2000) *Fool's Gold: A Critical Look at Computers in Childhood,* College Park, MD: Alliance for Childhood. Online. Available: http://allianceforchildhood.net/projects/computers/computers_reports_fools_gold_contents.htm (accessed 4 April 2003).

Courtright, C. (1997) *Information and Development in El Salvador: Preliminary Notes (translation),* San Salvador: Fundación Nacional para el Desarrollo. Online. Available: http://php.indiana.edu/~ccourtri/ElSalvadorInfoDev.pdf (accessed 20 October 2002).

Courtright, C. *et al.* (1999) *Estrategia para la creación de una sociedad de aprendizaje en El Salvador/Strategy for Building a Learning Society in El Salvador,* San Salvador: Conectándonos al Futuro de El Salvador. Online. Available: http://www.conectando.org.sv (accessed 20 October 2002).

Cox, E. (1997) "Building Social Capital", *Health Promotion Matters* 4: 1–9.

Cragg Ross Dawson (1998) "Qualitative evaluation of D-Code," unpublished report, Health Education Authority.

Cronin, B. and Davenport, E. (1991) "The compound eye/I: an introduction to social intelligence," *Social Intelligence* 1, 1: 1–6.

Curran, J. (1992) "Mass media and democracy," in J. Curran and M. Gurevitch (1992) *Mass Media and Society,* London: Edward Arnold, pp. 82–117.

Dag Hammarskjöld Foundation (1981) *Development Dialogue,* 1981: 2, A journal of international development cooperation published by the Dag Hammarskjöld Foundation, Uppsala. Published in cooperation with the Latin American Institute for Transnational Studies (ILET).

Dag Hammarskjöld Foundation (1989) "The right to inform and be informed: another development and the media," *Development Dialogue,* February, 2: 1–115.

Dane, P. (1996) "Conflict of laws," in Dennis Patterson (ed.) *A Companion To Philosophy of Law and Legal Theory,* Cambridge, MA: Blackwell.

d'Arcy, J. (1969) "Direct broadcast satellites and the right to communicate," in L. S. Harms, Jim Richstad, and Kathleen A. Kie (eds) *Right to Communicate: Collected Papers,* Honolulu: University of Hawaii Press, 1977, pp. 1–9. Originally published in *EBU Review* 118 (1969): 14–18.

Day, P. (2001) "The networked community: policies for a participative information society," unpublished PhD thesis: University of Brighton.

Day, P. (2002) "Community informatics – policy, partnership and practice," in S. Marshall *et al.* (eds.) *IT in Regional Areas (ITiRA) 2002 Conference Proceedings,* Rockhampton, Australia: Central Queensland University Press.

Day, P. and Harris, K. (1997) *Down-to-Earth Vision: Community Based IT Initiatives and Social Inclusion* [The Commit Report], London: IBM/CDF.

Day, P. and Schuler, D. (2000) "Shaping the Network Society: the future of the public sphere in cyberspace," paper presented at the DIAC 2000 International Symposium, Seattle, Washington, May 2000.

De la Paz Sylva, M. and Robinson, S. S. (2000) *Telecentros: Ciudadanía Y Gestión Municipal (México): Una Cronología,* Ottawa, Canada: IDRC. Online. Available http://www.idrc.ca/pan/panlacscodoc1.doc (accessed 2 April 2003).

de Saint-Exupéry, A. (1943) *The Little Prince,* trans. Katherine Woods, New York: Harcourt, Brace and World.

Department of Health (1999) *Saving Lives: Our Healthier Nation*, London: Department of Health.

Department of Health and Social Security. Working Group on Inequalities in Health (1980) *Inequalities in Health: Report of a Research Working Group*, London: DHSS.

Deshler, D. and Ewert, M. (1995) "Participatory action research: traditions and major assumptions," personal communication, paper sent by Gary Chapman of the University of Texas 7/7/95 ~ gary.chapman@mail.utexas.edu

Dewey, J. (1954) *The Public and Its Problems*, Chicago: Swallow Press.

DiMaggio, P. *et al.* (2001) "Social implications of the Internet," *Annual Review of Sociology* 27: 307–336.

Douglas, S. J. (1987) *Inventing American Broadcasting: 1899–1922*, Baltimore: Johns Hopkins University Press.

Duff, A. S., David, C. and McNeill, D. A. (1996) "A note on the origins of the 'information society'," *Journal of Information Science*, 22, 2: 117–122.

Dunn, A. (1996) "A corporate land grab in cyberspace," *New York Times*, 7 Jan. Cybertimes.

Dutton, W. H. (1997) "Multimedia Visions and Realities," in H. Kubicek, W. H. Dutton, and R. Williams (eds.) *The Social Shaping of Information Superhighways: European and American Roads to the Information Society*, Frankfurt: Campus Verlag, pp. 133–155.

Dyson, E. *et al.* (1994) "Cyberspace and the American dream: a magna carta for the knowledge age" (Release 1.2, August 22), *The Information Society* 12, 3 (Jul–Sept. 1996): 295–308.

East Sussex, Brighton and Hove Health Authority (1999) *First Health*, Spring 1999: 13.

Electronic Freedom Foundation (EFF) (1990) "New foundation established to encourage computer-based communications policies," Press Release, July 10. Online. Available http://www.eff.org (accessed 9 April 2003).

Etzioni, A. and Etzioni, O. (1999) "Face-to-face and computer-mediated communities, a comparative analysis," *The Information Society*, 15, 4: 241–248.

Evaluation Report (2001) *New York State Advanced Telecommunications Project: Diffusion Fund Program*, White Plains, NY: Magi Educational Services (mimeo).

Falconer, D. *et al.* (2000) "Critical approaches to Information Systems planning: refining the research agenda," paper presented at the Americas Conference on Information Systems, Long Beach, CA.

Federal Trust, (1995) *Network Europe and the Information Society*, London: Federal Trust.

Felix, D. (1995) "The Tobin tax proposal: background, issues and prospects," in H. Cleveland *et al.* (eds.) *The United Nations: Policy and Financing Alternatives*, Washington, DC: Global Commission to Fund the United Nations, pp. 195–208.

Flink, J. J. (1988) *The Automobile Age*, Cambridge, MA: MIT Press.

Fraser, N. (1989) *Unruly Practices: Power, Discourse, and Gender in Contemporary Social Theory*, Minneapolis, MN: University of Minnesota Press.

Frederick, H. (1994) "People's Communication Charter," e-mail list INTCAR-L. Online posting. Available http://muhu.www.ee/mailing_lists/pointers/msg00017.html (accessed 9 April 2003).

Freeman, C. (1994) "The diffusion of information and communication technology in the world economy in the 1990s," in R. Mansell (ed.) *The Management of Information and Communication Technologies – Emerging Patterns of Control*, London: Aslib, pp. 8–41.

Froomkin, A. M. (1999, May 19) "A Commentary on WIPO's *The Management of*

Internet Names and Addresses: Intellectual Property Issues." Online. Available http://www.law.miami.edu/~amf/commentary.htm (accessed 9 April 2003).

Gallagher, D. F. (2002) "New economy: a copyright dispute with the Church of Scientology is forcing Google to do some creative linking," *The New York Times.* 22 April, p. C4.

Garfinkel, S. (2000) *Database Nation: The Death of Privacy in the 21st Century*, Sebastopol, CA: O'Reilly.

Garlick, S. (1998) "Creative associations in special places: enhancing the partnership role of universities in building competitive regional economies," Dept Education Employment Training and Youth Affairs. Online. Available http://www.dest.gov.au/archive/highered/eippubs/eip98-4/execsum.htm (accessed 20 April 2003).

Garnham, N. (1990) *Capitalism and Communication,* Newbury Park, CA: Sage Publications.

Garnham, N. (1994) "Whatever happened to the information society?" in R. Mansell (ed.) *The Management of Information and Communication Technologies*, London: Aslib, pp. 42–51.

Garrett, L. (2000) *Betrayal of Trust: The Collapse of Global Public Health*, New York: Hyperion.

Gates, B. (1995) *The Road Ahead*, New York: Penguin.

Gates, B. (1999) *Business @ the Speed of Thought: Using a Digital Nervous System*, New York: Warner Books.

Gehl, J. and Gemzøe, L. (1996) *Public Spaces – Public Life, Copenhagen 1996*, trans. Karen Steenhard, Copenhagen: The Danish Architectural Press and the School of Architecture, Royal Danish Academy of Fine Arts.

Giddens, A. (1984) *The Constitution of Society*, Berkeley, CA: University of California Press.

Gigante, A. (1997) "'Domain-ia': the growing tension between the domain name system and trademark law," in B. Kahin and J. H. Keller (eds.) *Coordinating the Internet*, Cambridge: MIT Press, pp. 136–153.

Glen, A. (1993) "Methods and themes in community practice," in H. Butcher *et al.* (eds.), *Community and Public Policy*, London: Pluto Press, pp. 22–40.

Goldhaber, M. H. (1997) "The attention economy and the Net," *First Monday* 2, 4.

Goldstein, J. (1976) *The Experience of Insight*, Boulder, CO: Shambhala Press.

Gómez, R. and Ospina, A. (2001) "The lamp without a genie: using telecenters for development without expecting miracles," *Journal of Development Communication*, 12, 2: 16–25.

Gore, A. (1991) "Infrastructure for the Global Village," *Scientific American*, 265 (September): 108–111.

Gore, A. (1993) Speech to the Press Club. Online. Available.

Gorgeç, A. *et al.* (1999) *An Analysis of Internet Use in the Public Library*, Vancouver: School of Library, Archival and Information Studies, University of British Columbia. Online. Available HTTP: http://www.schoolnet.ca/ln- rb/e/about/ubc/index.html (accessed 3 June 1999).

Governor-General of Canada (2002) "The Canada we want: speech from the Throne to open the second session of the thirty-seventh Parliament of Canada," Ottawa: Government of Canada. Online. Available HTTP: http://www.sft-ddt.gc.ca/hnav/hnav07_e.htm (accessed 30 October 2002).

Greenbaum, J. and Halskov Madsen, K. (1993) "Small changes: starting a participatory design process by giving participants a voice," in D. Schuler and A. Namioka (eds.) *Participatory Design: Principles and Practices,* Hillsdale, NJ: Lawrence Erlbaum Associates.

Gregory, S. (1998) *Black Corona: Race and the Politics of Place in an Urban Community,* Princeton, NJ: Princeton University Press.

Gronski, R. and Pigg, K. (2000) "University and community collaboration," *The American Behavioral Scientist,* 43, 5: 781–792.

Grube, G. M. A. (ed.) (1974) "Plato circa 380 B.C.E." *The Republic in Plato's Republic,* Indianapolis, IN: Hackett.

Gualini, E. (2002) "Institutional capacity building as an issue of collective action and institutionalization: some theoretical remarks," in G. Cars *et al.* (eds.) *Urban Governance, Institutional Capacity and Social Milieux,* Aldershot, UK: Ashgate.

Guernsey, L. (1999) "The Web: new ticket to a pink slip," *New York Times,* 16 Dec. pp. E1, E8.

Guglielmo, C. (1998) "Microsoft cries foul over Netscape Communicator 4.5," *Inter@ctive Week.*

Guice, J. (1998) 'Looking Backward and Forward at the Internet," *The Information Society,* 14, 3: 201–211.

Gurstein, M. (2000) *Community Informatics: Enabling Communities with Communications Technologies,* Hershey, PA: Idea Group Publishing.

Gurstein, M. (2003) "Perspectives on urban and rural community informatics: theory and performance, community informatics and strategies for flexible networking," in S. Marshall *et al.* (eds.) *Closing the Digital Divide: Transforming Regional Economies and Communities with Information Technology,* Westport, CT: Greenwood Publishing Group.

Gurstein, M. (2003) "Communities: the hidden dimensions of ICTs," The Cris Campaign: Issue Paper No. 7. Online. Available http://www.nervesane.net/projects/cris/issues/7_community_ICTs.doc (accessed 2 April 2003).

Gutstien, D. (1999) *e.con: How the Internet Undermines Democracy,* Toronto: Stoddart.

Hakala, D. and Rickard, J. (1996) "A domain by any other name," *Boardwatch,* October.

Hamelink, C. J. (1994) *The Politics of World Communication: A Human Rights Perspective,* London: Sage.

Hamelink, C. J. (n.d.) "The People's Communication Charter (PCC)." Online. Available http://www.pccharter.net/charteren.html (accessed 9 April 2003).

Hamilton, D. (2002) "Sustainability of a community technology center: action research at the Murchison Community Center, Toledo, Ohio," MA Thesis, University of Toledo.

Hammond, A. S. (1997) "The Telecommunications Act of 1996: codifying the digital divide," *Federal Communications Law Journal,* 50, 1 December.

Hardesty, D. (2001a) "2001 SSTP Wrap-Up." Online. Available http://ecommercetax.com/doc/123001.htm (accessed 4 April 2003).

Hardesty, D. (2001b) "Internet Tax Freedom Act Extended." Online. Available http://ecommercetax.com/doc/120201.htm (accessed 4 April 2003).

Hardin, R. (1982) *Collective Action,* Baltimore: Johns Hopkins University Press.

Hargittai, E. (1998) "Reinventing universal broadcasting: parallels between radio's early years and the Internet's emergence," in *INET 1998 Proceedings of the Internet Summit,* Geneva, Switzerland: The Internet Society. Online. Available http://www.isoc.org/inet98/proceedings/2f/2f_1.htm (accessed 9 April 2003).

Hargittai, E. (2000) "Open portals or closed gates? Channeling content on the world wide web," *Poetics,* 27, 4: 233–253.

Hargittai, E. (2000) "Radio's lessons for the Internet," *Communications of the ACM* 43, 1: 50–57.

Hargittai, E. (2002) "Second-level digital divide: differences in people's online skills," *First Monday* 7, 4.

Harkavy, I. (1998) "School-community-university partnerships: effectively integrating community building and education reform," paper presented at the Connecting Community Building and Education Reform: Effective School, Community, University Partnerships – A Joint Forum of the US Department of Education, US Department of Housing and Urban Development, Washington, DC.

Harmon, A. (1998a) "Internet group challenges US over Web addresses," *New York Times*, 26 Jan. Cybertimes.

Harmon, A. (1998) "US Plan on Internet Names Lacks Support From Users," *New York Times*, 2 Feb. Cybertimes.

Harms, L.S. (n.d.) "Some essentials of the right to communicate." Online. Available http://www.righttocommunicate.org (accessed 9 April 2003).

Harris, K. (1996) "Social inclusion in the information society," in D. Wilcox (ed.) *Inventing the Future: Communities in the Information Society*, Brighton: Partnership Books.

Harris, R. (2002) "Research partnerships to support rural communities in Malaysia with information and communication technologies," in J. Lazar (ed.) *Managing IT/ Community Partnerships in the 21st Century*, Hershey, PA: Idea Group Publishing.

Hart, J. A. *et al.* (1992) "The Building of the Internet: implications for the future of broadband networks," *Telecommunications Policy*, 16, 8: 666–690.

Haywood, T. (1995) *Info-rich Info-poor: Access and Exchange in the Global Information Society*, London: Bowker-Saur.

Health Development Agency (2002) *Assessing People's Perceptions of their Neighbourhood and Community Involvement*, London: Health Development Agency. Online. Available http://www.social-action.org.uk/hdaresearch/hdaresearch.html (accessed 22 January 2003).

Health Education Authority (1998) *D-code*, London: Health Education Authority.

Heath, S. B. (1980) "The functions and uses of literacy," *Journal of Communication*, 30, 1: 123–133.

Heeks, R. (1999) "Information and communication technologies, poverty and development" (Development Informatics Working Paper Series 5), Manchester, UK: Institute for Development Policy and Management. Online. Available: http://idpm. man.ac.uk/wp/di/di_wp05abs.htm (accessed 20 October 2002).

Heiskanen, V. (1999, May) *Commercial Concern vs. Public Interest: Reconciling the Internet Domain Name System and the Protection of Intellectual Property Rights*, Helsinki, Finland: Institute of International Economic Law, University of Helsinki. Manuscript in preparation.

Henwood, F. *et al.* (2003) "'Ignorance is bliss sometimes': constraints on the emergence of the 'informed patient' in the changing landscapes of health information," *Sociology of Health and Illness*, special issue: *Media and Health*, 25, 6: 589–607.

Hess, D. R. (1999) "Community organizing, building and developing: their relationship to comprehensive community initiatives," Working paper series for COMM-ORG: The On-Line Conference on Community Organizing and Development, June. Online. Available http://comm-org.utoledo.edu/papers99/hess.html (accessed 1 November 2002).

Hiler, J. (2002) "Google loves Blogs," in *Microcontent News*. Online. Available http://www.microcontentnews.com/articles/googleblogs.html (accessed 6 April 2003).

Hirsch, P. M. (1972) "Processing fads and fashions: an organization-set analysis of cultural industry systems," *American Journal of Sociology*, 77, 4: 639–659.

Hoffman, D. L. and Novak. T. P. (1999) "The growing digital divide: implications for an open research agenda. eLab," Owen Graduate School of Management, Vanderbilt University (Nov. 29), Online. Available http://elab.vanderbilt.edu/research/papers/pdf/manuscripts/DigitalDivideNov1999-pdf.pdf (accessed 9 April 2003).

Holstein, W. J. *et al.* (1990) "The stateless corporation," *Business Week*, 14 May, pp. 98–106.

Hooper, P. K. (1998) "They have their own thoughts: children's learning of computational ideas from a cultural constructionist perspective," unpublished PhD Dissertation, Cambridge, MA: MIT Media Laboratory.

Howard, P. E. N. *et al.* (2001) "Days and nights on the Internet: the impact of a diffusing technology," *American Behavioral Scientist*, 45, 3: 383–404. http://www.eff.org/Infra/Govt_docs/gore_nii.speech (accessed 15 April 2003). http://www.ntia.doc.gov/ntiahome/domainname/dnsdrft.htm (accessed 9 April 2003).

HUD/MHFA (1998) *Demonstration Disposition Program Information Packet,* Boston, MA: MHFA.

Hughes, T. P. (1983) *Networks of Power: Electrification in Western Society, 1880–1930*, Baltimore: Johns Hopkins University Press.

Ibarra, R. (2000) *La red en El Salvador,* Eugene, OR: Network Startup Resource Center. Online. Available: http://www.nsrc.org/db/lookup/ISO=SV (accessed 20 October 2002).

Illich, I. (1973) *Tools for Conviviality*, New York: Harper and Row.

Information Highway Advisory Committee (IHAC) (1995) *Access and Social Impacts: The Human Dimension,* Ottawa, ON: Government of Canada. Online. Available HTTP: http://strategis.ic.gc.ca/SSG/ih01027e.html (accessed 10 April 1999).

Information Infrastructure Task Force (1993) *National Information Infrastructure [NII]: Agenda for Action.* Washington, DC: National Telecommunications & Information Administration (NTIA) Online. Available http://www.eff.org/Infra/Govt_docs/nii_agenda_govt.paper (accessed 15 April 2003).

Information Infrastructure Task Force (1994a) Information Infrastructure Task Force, *National Information Infrastructure. Progress Report September 1993–1994*, Washington, DC: Office of the Vice President, The Secretary of Commerce. Online. Available http://www.eff.org/Infra/Govt_docs/nii_prinicples_progress.report (accessed 15 April 2003).

Information Infrastructure Task Force (1994b) Information Infrastructure Task Force, Committee on Applications and Technology, *Putting the Information Infrastructure to Work*, Washington, DC: National Institute of Technology. Online. Available http://www.eff.org/Infra/Govt_docs/nii_task_force.report (accessed 15 April 2003).

Information Infrastructure Task Force (1994c) Information Infrastructure Task Force, Committee on Applications and Technology, *The Information Infrastructure: Reaching Society's Goals*, Washington, DC: National Institute of Technology. Online. Available http://www.eff.org/Infra/Govt_docs/iitf_goals_nii.paper (accessed 15 April 2003).

International Telecommunication Union (1999) *Country Data for El Salvador,* Geneva:

ITU. Online. Available: http://www7.itu.int/bdt_cds/CDS/Country_Data.asp? Country=ELS (accessed 24 June 2001).

Internet Assigned Numbers Authority, The, and Internet Society, The (1997, February 28) "Establishment of a Memorandum of Understanding on the generic top level domain name space of the internet domain name system." Online. Available http://www.gtld-mou.org/gTLD-MoU.html (accessed 9 April 2003).

Introna, L. and Nissenbaum, H. (2000) "Shaping the Web: why the politics of search engines matters," *The Information Society*, 16, 3: 1–17.

James, J. A. (1996) *Resisting State Violence: Radicalism, Gender, & Race in US Culture*, Minneapolis: University of Minnesota Press.

Jansen, B. J. and Pooch, U. (2001) "A review of Web searching studies and a framework for future research," *Journal of the American Society for Information Science and Technology*, 52, 3: 235–246.

Jewkes, R. and Murcott, A. (1996) "Meanings of community," *Soc. Sci. Med.* 43, 4: 555–563.

Johnson, V. and Webster, J. (2000) *Reaching the Parts . . . Community Mapping: Working Together to Tackle Social Exclusion and Food Poverty*, London: Sustain.

Kagan, A. (2000) "The growing gap between the information rich and the information poor both within countries and between countries: a composite policy paper," *IFLA Journal*, 26, 1: 28–33.

Kalil, T.A. (1997) "The Clinton–Gore National Information Infrastructure Initiative," in H. Kubicek, W. H. Dutton, and R. Williams (eds.) *The Social Shaping of Information Superhighways: European and American Roads to the Information Society*, Frankfurt: Campus Verlag, pp. 45–59.

Karr, T. (2002) "Who sets the world news agenda," paper presented to the Global Community Journalism Conference at the Journalism Resources Institute, Rutgers University, 31 May.

Keeble, L. and Loader, B. D. (eds.) (2001) *Community Informatics: Shaping Computer-Mediated Social Relations*, London: Routledge.

Kensing, F. and Munk-Madsen, A. (1993) "PD: Structure in the toolbox," *Communications of the ACM*, 36, 4: 78–85.

Kesan, J. P. and Shah, R. C. (2001) "Fool us once shame on you – fool us twice shame on us: what we can learn from the privatizations of the Internet backbone network and the domain name system," *Washington University Law Quarterly*, 79: 89–220.

Kilgour, D. (1998) *Preparing Canada for a Knowledge-based Economy: Expanding Access to the Information Highway*, Ottawa, ON: Government of Canada. Online. Available HTTP: http://www.e- view.com/davidkilgour/new/infohwy.htm (accessed 10 April 1999).

Klein, H. (2002) "ICANN and Internet governance: leveraging technical coordination to realize public policy," *The Information Society*, 18, 2: 193–207.

Kling, R. (1998) "Technological and social access to computing, information and communication technologies," White Paper for Presidential Advisory Committee on High-Performance Computing and Communications, Information Technology, and the Next Generation Internet. Online. Available http://www.slis.indiana.edu/kling/pubs/NGI.htm (accessed 10 November 2002).

Korten, D. C. (2001) *When Corporations Rule the World*, 2nd edn, Bloomfield, CT: Kumarian Press.

Kretzmann, J. P. and McKnight, J. L. (1993) *Building Communities from the Inside Out: A Path Toward Finding and Mobilizing a Community's Assets,* Chicago, IL: ACTA Publications.

Kubicek, H. and Dutton, W.H. (1997) "The social shaping of information super-highways: an introduction," in H. Kubicek, W. H. Dutton, and R. Williams, (eds.) *The Social Shaping of Information Superhighways: European and American Roads to the Information Society,* Frankfurt: Campus Verlag, pp. 9–44.

Labonte, R. and Laverack, G. (2001) "Capacity building in health promotion: Part 1: for whom? And for what purpose?' *Critical Public Health,* 11, 2: 111–127.

Lacey, M. (2000) "Clinton to seek US subsidies to help the poor get online," *New York Times,* 22 Jan, p. A7.

Lagerfeld, S. (1998) "Who knows where the time goes?" *Wilson Quarterly,* 22, 3 (Summer): 58–70.

Lake, D. (2000) "The Web: growing by 2 million pages a day," *Computerworld,* June, Vol. 5.

Landolt, P. *et al.* (1999) "From hermano lejano to hermano mayor: the dialectics of Salvadoran transnationalism," *Ethnic and Racial Studies,* 22, 2: 290–315.

Laumann, E. O., Galaskiewicz, J. and Marsden, P. V. (1978) "Community structure as interorganizational linkages," *Annual Review of Sociology,* 4: 455–484.

Lawrence, S. and Giles, C. L. (1999) "Accessibility of information on the Web," *Nature,* 400: 107–109.

Lazarus, W. and Mora, F. (2000) *Online Content for Low-income and Underserved Americans: The Digital Divide's New Frontier,* Santa Monica, CA: The Children's Partnership. Online. Available: http://www.childrenspartnership.org/pub/low_income/index.html (accessed 20 October 2002).

Le Duc, D. R. (1977) "The right to receive communications: a thought worth entertaining," in L. S. Harms, and J. Richstad (eds.) *Evolving Perspectives on the Right to Communicate,* Honolulu: University Press of Hawaii.

Lee, J. (1999) "For at least some domains, there's money in the names," *New York Times,* July 15. Cybertimes.

Leiner, B. M. *et al.* (1998, February 20) "A brief history of the Internet," version 3.1. Online. Available http://www.isoc.org/internet/history/brief.shtml (accessed 9 April 2003).

Lessig, L. (2002) *The Future of Ideas: The Fate of the Commons in a Connected World,* New York: Vintage Press.

Lindblom, C. and Cohen, D. (1979) *Usable Knowledge: Social Science and Social Problem Solving,* New Haven, CT and London: Yale University Press.

Loader, B. D. (1998) *Cyberspace Divide: Equality, Agency and Policy in the Information Society,* London: Routledge.

Lopes, P. D. (1992) "Innovation and diversity in popular music industry, 1969 to 1999," *American Sociological Review,* 57, 1: 56–71.

Loury, G. (1977) "A dynamic theory of racial income differences," in P. A. Wallace and A. Le Mund (eds.) *Women, Minorities and Employment Discrimination,* Lexington, MD: Lexington Books, pp.153–186.

Lycos, Inc. (1998) "Annual Report pursuant to Section 13 or 15(D) of the Securities and Exchange Act of 1934. Commission File Number 0–27830."

Macintyre, S. (1997) "The Black Report and beyond: what are the issues?" *Social Science and Medicine,* 44, 6: 723–745.

Mackay, H. (2001) "Theories of the information society," in H. Mackay *et al.* (eds.) *Investigating the Information Society*, London: Open University/Routledge.

Malanczuk, P. (1991) "Freedom of information and communication – recent developments in the Helsinki Process (Conference on Security and Cooperation in Europe)," in A.-Ch. Kiss/ J. G. Lammers (eds.) The Association of Attenders and Alumni of the Hague Academy of International Law, *The Hague Yearbook of International Law/ Annuaire de la Haye de droit international*. Dordrecht: Martinus Nijhoff Publishers, Vol. 3, pp. 89–104.

Mander, J. and Goldsmith, E. (eds.) (1996) *The Case Against the Global Economy and For a Turn Towards the Local*, San Francisco: Sierra Club Books.

Mansell, R. and Wehn, U. (1998) *Knowledge Societies: Information Technology for Sustainable Development*, Oxford: Oxford University Press.

Marks, S. P. (1981) "Emerging human rights: a new generation for the 1980s?" *Rutgers Law Review*, 33 (Winter): 435–452.

Marshall, A. (2000) "ICTs for health promotion in the community: a participative approach," unpublished thesis, University of Brighton.

Marshall, S., Taylor, W. and Yu, X. (2004) *Using Community Informatics to Transform Regions*, London: Idea Group Publishing.

Marvin, C. (1988) *When Old Technologies Were New: Thinking About Electric Communication in the Late Nineteenth Century*, New York: Oxford University Press.

Massachusetts Housing Finance Agency (2001) "MHFA's Demonstration Disposition (DemoDispo) Program History." Online. Available http://www.mhfa.com/dev/dp_ddhistory.htm (accessed 1 November 2002).

McChesney, R. W. (1993) *Telecommunications, Mass Media, and Democracy: The Battle for the Control of US Broadcasting, 1928–1935*, New York: Oxford University Press.

McChesney, R. W. (1999) *Rich Media, Poor Democracy: Communication Politics in Dubious Times*, Urbana and Chicago: University of Illinois Press.

McConnell, S. (2000) "A champion in our midst: lessons learned from the impacts of NGO's use of the Internet," *Electronic Journal on Information Systems in Developing Countries* 2. Online. Available: http://www.is.cityu.edu.hk/research/ejisdc/vol2.htm (accessed 20 October 2002).

McGreevy, M. (2002) "First Saturday: mobilizing a community for achievement and empowerment," unpublished thesis (MA), University of Toledo.

McIver, W. J., Jr. and Birdsall, W. F. (2002) "Technological evolution and the right to communicate: the implications for electronic democracy," The European Institute for Communication and Culture (EURICOM 2002) Project: Electronic Networks and Democratic Life. Electronic Networks & Democratic Engagement Colloquium, Nijmegen, The Netherlands, October 9–12, 2002.

Menou, M. J. (1995a) "The impact of information – I. Toward a research agenda for its definition and measurement," *Information Processing & Management* 31, 4: 455–477.

Menou, M. J. (1995b) "The impact of information – II. Concepts of information and its value," *Information Processing & Management*, 31, 4: 479–490.

Menou, M. J. (1999) "Impact of the Internet: some conceptual and methodological issues, or how to hit a moving target behind the smoke screen," in R. Gómez and P. Hunt (eds.) *Telecentre Evaluation: A Global Perspective*, Ottawa: International Development Research Centre. Online. Available: http://www.idrc.ca/telecentre/evaluation/nn/24_Imp.html (accessed 20 October 2002).

Menou, M. J. (2001) "Digital and social equity? Opportunities and threats on the road to empowerment," paper presented at the LIDA 2001 Annual Course and Conference, "Libraries in the Digital Age," Dubrovnik, Croatia. Online. Available: http://www.ffzg.hr/infoz/lida/present.htm (accessed 23 June 2001).

Menou, M. J. (ed.) (1993) *Measuring the Impact of Information on Development*, Ottawa: International Development Research Centre.

Menou, M. J. (1991) "National information policy in the less developed countries: an educational perspective," *International Library Review*, 23: 49–64.

Menou, M. J. and Potvin, J. (2000) *Toward a Conceptual Framework for Learning about ICTs and Knowledge in the Process of Development*, Ottawa: The Global Knowledge Learning and Evaluation Action Program (GKLEAP). Online. Available: http://www.bellanet.org/gkaims/documents/docs/LEAP_Concept_2May2000.HTM (accessed 20 October 2002).

Mills, D. L. (1981, September) *RFC 799: Internet Name Domains*, Internet Engineering Task Force, Network Working Group. Online. Available http://www.ietf.org/rfc/rfc0799.txt?number=799 (accessed 9 April 2003).

Mitchell, D. *et al.* (1997) "In whose domain? Name service in adolescence," in B. Kahin and J. H. Keller (eds.) *Coordinating the Internet*, Cambridge MA: MIT Press, pp. 258–270.

Mitchell, W. J. (1999) *E-topia: "Urban Life, Jim – But Not as We Know It,"* Cambridge, MA: MIT Press.

Mockapetris, P. (1983, November) *RFC 882: Domain Names – Concepts and Facilities*, Internet Engineering Task Force, Network Working Group. Online. Available http://www.ietf.org/rfc/rfc0882.txt?number=882 (accessed 9 April 2003).

Mockapetris, P. (1987, November) *RFC 1034: Domain Names – Concepts and Facilities*, Internet Engineering Task Force, Network Working Group. Online. Available http://www.ietf.org/rfc/rfc1034.txt?number=1034 (accessed 9 April 2003).

Moore, G. (1983) *Lifeline Bill: Basic Minimum Telephone Service*, California Legislature – 1983–84 Regular Session, Assembly Bill 1348 (March 2).

Moore, N. (2000) "The international framework of information policies," in D. Law and J. Elkin *Managing Information*, London: The Open University Press, pp.1–19.

Morino Institute (2001) *From Access to Outcomes: Raising the Aspirations for Technology Initiatives in Low-Income Communities*, Reston, VA: Morino Institute, July. Online. Available http://www.morino.org/divides/report.htm (accessed 1 November 2002).

Morino, M. (1994) "Assessment and evolution of community networking," paper presented at Ties That Bind, at Apple Computer, Cupertino, CA.

Morris, D. (2004) "Globalization and media democracy: the case of Indymedia," in D. Schuler and P. Day (eds.) (forthcoming) *Shaping the Network Society: The New Role of Civic Society in Cyberspace*, Cambridge, MA: MIT Press.

Mueller, Jr., M. L. (1997) *Universal Service: Competition, Interconnection, and Monopoly in the Making of the American Telephone System*, Cambridge, MA: MIT and Washington, DC: AEI Press.

Nathenson, I. S. (1997) "Showdown at the domain name corral: property rights and personal jurisdiction over squatters, poachers, and other parasites," *University of Pittsburgh Law Review*, 58, 4.

National Audit Office (2003) "Progress in making e-services accessible to all – encouraging use by older people" [Report by the Controller and Auditor General

HC428 Session 2002–2003: 20 February 2003]. Online. Available http://www.nao. gov.uk/publications/nao_reports/02–03/0203428.pdf (accessed 3 November 2003).

National Telecommunications and Information Administration (NTIA) (1995) "Falling through the Net: a survey of the 'Have Nots' in rural and urban America," Washington, DC: US Commerce Department (July). Online. Available http://www. ntia.doc.gov/ntiahome/fallingthru.html (accessed 9 April 2003).

National Telecommunication and Information Administration (NTIA) (1998) "Falling through the Net II: new data on the digital divide," Washington, DC: US Commerce Department. Online. Available http://www.ntia.doc.gov/ntiahome/net2/falling.html (accessed 9 April 2003).

National Telecommunication and Information Administration (NTIA) (1999) "Falling through the Net III: defining the digital divide," Washington, DC: US Commerce Department. Online. Available http://www.ntia.doc.gov/ntiahome/fttn99/contents. html (accessed 9 April 2003).

National Telecommunication and Information Administration (NTIA) (2000) "Falling through the Net IV: toward digital inclusion," Washington, DC: US Commerce Department. Online. Available http://www.ntia.doc.gov/ntiahome/fttn00/contents 00.html (accessed 9 April 2003).

Netcraft (2003) "Netcraft web server survey." Netcraft. Online. Available http://news. netcraft.com/ (accessed 3 April 2003).

Network Solutions (1993, January) "Network Information Services Manager(s) for NSFNET and the NREN: INTERNIC registration services. NSF Cooperative Agreement No. NCR-9218742." Network Solutions. Online. Available http:// www.cavebear.com/nsf-dns/nsf_nsi_agreement.html (accessed 9 April 2003).

Network Solutions (1995, September) "Cooperative Agreement No. NCR-9218742, Amendment 4." Network Solutions. Online. Available http://www.cavebear.com/ nsf-dns/amendment4.html (accessed 9 April 2003).

Network Solutions (2000) "Network Solutions at a glance." Online. Available http:// web.archive.org/web/20000815070941/http://www.nsol.com/corporate/glance.ht ml (accessed 9 April 2003).

New York State Diffusion Fund Committee (1996) Diffusion Program Request for Proposals, First Round. Albany, NY.

Nhat Hanh, T. (1987) Being Peace, Berkeley, CA: Parallax Press.

Nie, N. H. (2001) "Sociability, interpersonal relations, and the Internet: reconciling conflicting findings." American Behavioral Scientist, 45, 3: 420–435.

Nie, N. H. and Erbring, L. (2000) "Internet and society: a preliminary report," Stanford, CA: Stanford Institute for the Quantitative Study of Society.

Nye, J. S. and Owens, W. A. (1996) "America's information edge," Foreign Affairs, March/April, pp. 20–36.

O'Bryant, R. (2001) "Establishing neighborhood technology centers in low-income communities: a crossroads for social science and computer information technology," in A. Townsend (ed.) Projections: The MIT Student Journal of Planning – Making Places through Information Technology, 2, 2: 112–127.

Ordidge, I. (1998) "Multimedia in health promotion and the individual," in Health Education Authority, Multimedia – Interacting for Health? An Expert Seminar to Consider the Impact and Potential of Multimedia for Health Promotion, London: Health Education Authority.

Organization for Economic Co-Operation and Development (OECD) (1998) *Public Management Developments in 1998. 1998 Country Report: Canada*, Ottawa, ON: OECD. Online. Available HTTP: http://www.oecd.org/puma/gvrnance/surveys/ pubs/ report98/surv98ca.htm (accessed 10 April 1999).

Organization of American States (OAS) (1969) American Convention on Human Rights. Adopted at San José, Costa Rica, November 22, 1969, In force 18 July 1978.

Orlikowski, W. and Robey, D. (1991) "Information technology and the structuring of organizations," *Information Systems Research*, 2, 2: 143–167.

People's Communication Charter (PCC) (2000) "About the people's communication Charter." Online. Available http://www.pccharter.net (accessed 9 April 2003).

Peterson, Christopher (2002) "The Independent Media Center," paper presented to the Global Community Journalism Conference at the Journalism Resources Institute, Rutgers University, 31 May.

Peterson, R.A. and Berger, D.G. (1975) "Cycles in symbol production: the case of popular music," *American Sociological Review*, 40, 2: 158–173.

Pew Internet and American Life Project (2002) "Search engines: A Pew Internet project data memo." Online. Available http://www.pewinternet.org/reports/toc.asp? Report=64 (accessed 3 April 2003).

Piirto, R. (1994) "Why radio thrives," *American Demographics*, 16, 5: 40–46.

Pinkett, R. D. and O'Bryant, R. L. (2002) "Building community, empowerment and self-sufficiency: early results from the Camfield Estates – MIT Creating Community Connections Project," proceedings of Digital Communities 2001 Conference, Evanston, IL: Northwestern University, November 4–6. Online. Available http:// web.media.mit.edu/~rpinkett/papers/dc2002.pdf (accessed 1 November 2002).

Pinkett, R. D. (2000). "Bridging the digital divide: sociocultural constructionism and an asset-based approach to community technology and community building," paper presented at the 81st Annual Meeting of the American Educational Research Association (AERA), New Orleans, LA, April 24–28. Online. Available http://www. media.mit.edu/~rpinkett/papers/aera2000.pdf (accessed 1 November 2002).

Pinkett, R. D. (2002). "Creating community connections: sociocultural constructionism and an asset-based approach to community technology and community building," unpublished PhD dissertation, Cambridge, MA: MIT Media Laboratory, January 11. Online. Available http://llk.media.mit.edu/papers/2002/pinkett-PHD.pdf (accessed 1 November 2002).

Polanyi, K. (1957) *The Great Transformation: The Political and Economic Origins of Our Time*, Boston: Beacon Press.

Policy Research Initiative (1997) *Canada 2005: Global Challenges and Opportunities,* Ottawa, ON: Government of Canada.

Policy Research Initiative (1999) *Knowledge-Based Economy and Society (KBES) Pilot Project*, Ottawa, ON: Government of Canada. Online. Available http://policyresearch. schoolnet.ca/networks/kbes/kbes-e.htm (accessed 11 April 1999).

Pollack, A. (1999) "What's in a cyber-name? $7.5 million for the right address," *New York Times*, 1 Dec, Cybertimes.

Pool, I.d.S. (1983) *Forecasting the Telephone: A Retrospective Technology Assessment of the Telephone*, Norwood, NJ: Ablex.

Postel, J. (1983) *RFC 881: The Domain Names'Plan and Schedule*, Internet Engineering

Task Force, Network Working Group. Online. Available http://www.ietf.org/rfc/rfc0881.txt?number=881 (accessed 9 April 2003).

Postel, J. (1994) *RFC 1591: Domain Name System Structure and Delegation*, Internet Engineering Task Force, Network Working Group. Online. Available http://www.ietf.org/rfc/rfc1591.txt?number=1591 (accessed 9 April 2003).

Postel, J., and Reynolds, J. (1984, October) *RFC 920: Domain Requirements*, Internet Engineering Task Force, Network Working Group. Online. Available http://www.ietf.org/rfc/rfc0920.txt?number=920 (accessed 9 April 2003).

Powell, W. W. (1985) *Getting into Print*, Chicago: University of Chicago Press.

Power, R. and Hunter, G. (2001) "Developing a strategy for community-based health promotion targeting homeless populations," *Health Education Research*, 16, 5: 593–602.

Power, R. *et al.* (1999) "Health, health promotion, and homelessness," *British Medical Journal*, 318: 590–592.

Prettejohn, M. (1996) "The first year: August 1995–August 1996." Netcraft. Online. Available http://www.netcraft.com/survey/year1.html (accessed 3 April 2003).

Public Utility Law Project (2001) *Comments Filed before the New York State Public Service Commission*, Albany, New York (mimeo).

Putnam, R. C. (1998) Foreword. *Housing Policy Debate,* Vol. 9, Issue 1. Washington, DC: Fannie Mae Foundation. Online. Available http://www.fanniemaefoundation.org/research/policy/pdf/Putnam.pdf (accessed 1 November 2002).

Putnam, R. D. (2000) *Bowling Alone: The Collapse and Revival of American Community*, New York: Simon & Schuster.

Rheingold, H. (2002) *Smart Mobs: The Next Social Revolution*, New York: Perseus.

Rifkin, S. *et al.* (2000) *Participatory Approaches in Health Promotion and Health Planning: A Literature Review*, London: Health Development Agency.

Robinson, D. (2000) Paper presented at Eastern Touring Agency Conference on Surfin' and the 3 Rs, Birmingham, UK, March 2000. Online. Available http://www.getwired.org.uk/surf.pdf (accessed 10 November 2002).

Robinson, J. P. and Godbey, G. (1997) *Time for Life: The Surprising Ways Americans Use Their Time*, University Park, PA: Pennsylvania State Press.

Robinson, S. S. (2002) "Encuesta de cibercafes en cuatro estados de México." Online. Available ftp://ftp.chasquinet.org/pub/docs/politicas/ciber_mexico.doc (accessed 2 April 2003).

Robinson, S. S. (2004) "Rethinking telecentres: microbanks and remittance flows – reflections from Mexico," in D. Schuler and P. Day (eds.) *Shaping the Network Society: The New Role of Civic Society in Cyberspace*, Cambridge, MA: MIT Press.

Rochlin, G. (1998) *Trapped In The Net: The Unanticipated Consequences of Computerization*, Princeton, NJ: Princeton University Press.

Roman, R. and Colle, R. D. (2002) *Themes and Issues in Telecentre Sustainability* (Development Informatics Working Paper Series 10), Manchester, UK: Institute for Development Policy and Management.

Romm, C. and Taylor, W. (2000) "Explaining community informatics success prospects: the Autonomy Harmony Model," in F. Sudweeks and C. Ess (eds.) *Cultural Attitudes Towards Technology and Communication 2000*, Perth: School of Information Technology, Murdoch University, pp. 275–289.

Rose, S. M. (1973) "The transformation of community action," in R. L. Warren (ed.) *Perspectives on the American Community*, Chicago, IL: Rand McNally.

Rosenbaum, D. E. (15 August 1999) "Phone fee for school internet service seems to be too popular to overturn," *New York Times*, 15 Aug. Online. Available http://www.nytimes.com (accessed 9 April 2003).

Rosenbrock, H. (1990) *Machines with a Purpose*. Oxford: Oxford University Press.

Sanderson, I. (1999) "Participation and democratic renewal: from 'instrumental' to 'communicative rationality'?" *Policy & Politics*, 27, 3: 325–341.

Sanoff, H. (ed.) (1990) *Participatory Design: Theory and Techniques*, Raleigh, NC: North Carolina State University.

Schiller, A. and Schiller, H. (1988) "Libraries, public access to information, and commerce," in D. Gutstien (ed.) *e.con: How the Internet Undermines Democracy,* Toronto: Stoddart.

Schiller, H. (1983) "The world in crisis and the new information technologies," *Columbia Journal of World Business*, Spring 1983, pp. 86–90.

Schiller, H.I. (1996) *Information Inequality*, New York: Routledge.

Schmidt, S.W. (2000) "Community networks and community informatics: fast growth and deepening controversy on the application of information technology to citizen participation," DoctorPolitics.com. Online. Available http://www.doctorpolitics.com/communityinformatics.htm (accessed 20 April 2003).

Schor, J. B. (1997) "Civic engagement and working hours: do americans really have more free time than ever before?" paper prepared presented at Conference on Civic Engagement in American Democracy, 26–28 Sept. Portland, Maine. Online. Available http://www.swt.org/putok.htm (accessed 4 April 2003).

Schudson, M. (1995) *The Power of News*, Boston, MA: Harvard University Press.

Schuler, D. (1996) *New Community Networks: Wired for Change*, Reading, MA: Addison-Wesley.

Schuler, D. (1997) "Community computer networks: an opportunity for collaboration among democratic technology practitioners and researchers," paper presented at the Technology and Democracy Workshop, Oslo, Norway.

Schuler, D. (2001) "Cultivating society's civic intelligence: patterns for a new 'world brain'," *Information, Communication and Society*, 4, 2: 157–181.

Schuler, D. (2001) "What kind of platform for change? Democracy, community work and the Internet," in C. Werry and M. Mowbray (eds.) *Online Communities: Commerce, Community Action, and the Virtual University*, Upper Saddle River, NJ: Prentice Hall pp. 281–297.

Schuler, D. (2002) "Digital cities and digital citizens: new responses for new circumstances," in M. Tanabe, Pl. van den Besselaar and T. Ishida (eds.) *Digtal Cities II: Computational and Sociological Approaches*. Tokyo, Japan: Springer, pp. 71–85.

Schuler, D. and Day, P. (eds.) (2004) *Shaping the Network Society: The New Role of Civic Society in Cyberspace*, Cambridge, MA: MIT Press.

Schuler, D. and Namioka, A. (eds.) (1993) *Participatory Design: Principles and Practices*, Hillsdale, NJ: Lawrence Erlbaum Associates.

Sclove, R. and Scheuer, J. (1996) "On the road again?: If information highways are anything like interstate highways – watch out!" in R. Kling (ed.) *Computerization and Controversy: Value Conflicts and Social Choices*, 2nd ed., San Diego: Academic Press, pp. 606–612. Online in slight abridgment. Available http://www.loka.org/alerts/loka.1.6.txt (accessed 4 April 2003).

Sclove, R. E. (1995) *Democracy and Technology*, New York: Guilford Press.

Sclove, R. E. (1997a) "Historic, first-time US citizens' panel," *Loka Alerts* 4.2. Online. Available http://www.loka.org/alerts/loka.4.2 (accessed 10 November 2002).

Sclove, R. E. (1997b) "Telecommunications and the future of democracy," *Loka Alerts* 4.3. Online. Available http://www.loka.org/alerts/loka.4.3.htm (accessed 10 November 2002).

Sclove, R. E. (1996) "Town meetings on technology," *Technology Review*, 99, 5: 24–31. Online. Available http:www.loka.org/pubs/techrev.htm (accessed 4 April 2003), with supplementary information athttp://www.loka.org/pages/worldpanels.htm (accessed 4 April 2003).

Sclove, R. E. (1998) "For US science policy, it's time for a reality check," *Chronicle of Higher Education*, 23 Oct. pp. B1, B4-B5. Online. Available http://www.loka.org/pubs/chronicle102398.htm (accessed 4 April 2003).

Sclove, R. E. (1999) "Democratic politics of technology – the missing half: using democratic criteria in participatory technology decisions." Online. Available http://www.loka.org/idt/intro.htm (accessed 4 April 2003).

Sclove, R. E. (2000) "Counter the cybernetic Wal-Mart effect," *Loka Alert*, 7, 1 (29 March), sect. II. Online. Available http://loka.org/alerts/loka_alert_7.1.htm (accessed 4 April 2003).

Sclove, R. E. *et al.* (1998) *Community-Based Research in the United States: An Introductory Reconnaissance, Including Twelve Organizational Case Studies and Comparison with the Dutch Science Shops and with the Mainstream American Research System.* Amherst, MA: The Loka Institute and Washington, DC: Aspen Institute Nonprofit Sector Research Fund. Online. Available http://www.loka.org/CRN/case_study.htm (accessed 4 April 2003).

Sellar, G. (2001) "Can Regional Community Web Portals Become Sustainable? The Albany GateWAy: A Case Study," PhD thesis, Edith Cowan University, Perth.

Selznick, P. (1996) "In search of community," in W. Vitek and W. Jackson (eds.) *Rooted in the Land: Essays on Community and Place*, New Haven, CT: Yale University Press.

Shaw, A. C. (1995) *Social Constructionism and the Inner City: Designing Environments for Social Development and Urban Renewal*, unpublished PhD Dissertation, Cambridge, MA: MIT Media Laboratory.

Shaw, R. (1997) "Internet domain names: whose domain is this?" in B. Kahin and J. H. Keller (eds.) *Coordinating the Internet*, Cambridge: MIT Press, pp. 107–134.

Shearman, C. (1999) *Local Connections: Making the Net Work for Neighbourhood Renewal*, London: Communities Online.

Shenk, D. (1997) *Data Smog: Surviving the Information Glut*, San Francisco, CA: Haper Edge.

SHM Productions Ltd (1999a) "CityNet: building social capital for health." Online. Available http://www.phel.gov.uk/sarpdocs/CityNet building social capital for health Nottingham.pdf (accessed 10 November 2002).

SHM Productions Ltd (1999b) "Preliminary report into UK projects which aim to develop community involvement through Information and Communication Technology (ICT)," unpublished report, Health Education Authority.

Shuman, M. H. (1998) *Going Local: Creating Self-Reliant Communities in a Global Age*, New York: Free Press.

Silberman, S. (1997) "Would you buy Brooklynbridge.com from this man?" *Wired*, March 5: 50.

Silverstein, C. *et al.* (1999) "Analysis of a very large Web search engine query log," *SIGIR Forum* 33, 1: 6–12.

Simpson, H. M. (1981) *Makers of History*, Evansville, IN: Warren Publishers.

Skocpol, T. and Fiorina, M. P. (eds.) (1999) *Civic Engagement in American Democracy*, Washington, DC: The Brookings Institution and New York: Russell Sage Foundation.

Smulyan, S. (1994) *Selling Radio: The Commercialization of American Broadcasting, 1920–1934*, Washington: Smithsonian Institution Press.

Spiegel, H. B. C (1973) "Citizen participation in federal programs: a review," in R. L. Warren (ed.) *Perspectives on the American Community*, Chicago, IL: Rand McNally.

Spink, A. *et al.* (2002) "From e-sex to e-commerce: web search changes," *IEEE Computer*, 35, 3: 107–109.

Stagner, M. and Richman, H. (1996) *Hardship and Support Systems in Chicago, Volume 3: Help-Seeking and the Use of Social Service Providers by Welfare Families in Chicago*, Chicago, IL: Chapin Hall Center for Children, University of Chicago.

Sterling, C. H. and Kittross, J. M. (1990) *Stay Tuned: A Concise History of American Broadcasting*, 2nd ed., Belmont, CA: Wadsworth.

Stocking, B. *et al.* (1991) *Criteria for Change: The History and Impact of Consensus Development Conferences in the UK*, London: Kings Fund Centre.

Stoecker, R. and Stuber, A. (1997) "Building an information superhighway of one's own: a comparison of two approaches." Online. Available http://comm-org.utoledo.edu/drafts/uunn/UAApaper.htm (accessed 17 March 2003).

Stone, B. (2002) *Blogging: Genius Strategies for Instant Web Content*, Berkeley, CA: New Riders Publishing.

Street, P. (1997) "Scenario workshops: a participatory approach to sustainable urban living?' *Futures*, 2, 2: 139–158.

Streeter, T. (1996) *Selling the Air: A Critique of the Policy of Commercial Broadcasting in the United States*, Chicago: University of Chicago Press.

Su, Z. and Postel, J. (1982 August) "RFC 819: The domain naming convention for Internet user applications," Internet Engineering Task Force, Network Working Group. Online. Available http://www.ietf.org/rfc/rfc0819.txt?number=819 (accessed 9 April 2003).

Sullivan, D. (2003) "Nielsen//NetRatings search engine ratings." *Searchenginewatch.com*. Online. Available http://www.searchenginewatch.com/reports/article.php/2156451 (accessed 10 April 2003).

Sunstein, C. R. (2001) "The daily we: is the internet really a blessing for democracy?' *Boston Review*. Online. Available http://bostonreview.mit.edu/BR26.3/sunstein.html (accessed 4 April 2003).

Tarman, G. (2002) "Covering and participating in communications for social change," paper presented to the Global Community Journalism Conference at the Journalism Resources Institute, Rutgers University, May 31.

Taylor, W. (2002) "Factors affecting the adoption of internet technologies for community practice in a regional area," unpublished thesis, Central Queensland University.

Taylor, W. *et al.* (2003) "Factors affecting home internet use in Central Queensland," paper presented at Informing Science and IT Education Conference, Pori, Finland, 24–27 June 2003.

Tedeschi, B. (1999) "Local merchants going online rely on faith," *New York Times*, 26 July. Online. Available http://www.nytimes.com/library/tech/99/07/cyber/commerce/26commerce.html (accessed 4 April 2003).

Tedeschi, B. (2000a) "Real force in e-commerce is business-to-business sales," *New York Times*, 5 Jan.

Tedeschi, B. (2000b) "Critics press legal assault on tracking of web users," *New York Times*, 7 Feb. Online. Available http://nytimes.com/library.tech/00/02/cyber/commerce/07commerce.html http://query.nytimes.com/search/advanced (accessed 4 April 2003).

Temkin, K. and Rohe, W. M. (1998) "Social capital and neighborhood stability: an empirical investigation," *Housing Policy Debate,* 9, 1, Washington, DC: Fannie Mae Foundation. Online. Available http://www.fanniemaefoundation.org/research/policy/pdf/Temkin.pdf (accessed 1 November 2002).

Towers, S. (1996) "Diffusing videoconferencing in government organisations: a structualist analysis," unpublished thesis, Queensland University of Technology.

Turner, N. (1999). "Creating a neighborhood learning and employment network in West Town," unpublished report to Northwest Tower Resident Association (NRTA), DSSA & Associates, and Bank One.

Turner, R. (2000) *Unions and Technology*, Washington, DC: OMB Watch. Online. Available http://www.ombwatch.org/article/articleprint/324/-1/96/ (accessed 4 April 2003).

UN Development Program (2000) *Human Development Report 2000. Human Rights and Human Development*, New York: Oxford University Press.

UN Development Program (2001) *Human Development Report 2001. Making New Technologies Work for Human Development*, New York: Oxford University Press. Online. Available: http://www.undp.org/hdr2001/ (accessed 20 October 2002).

UN Development Program (2002) *Human Development Report 2002. Deepening Democracy in a Fragmented World*, New York: Oxford University Press.

UN Development Program (1999) *Human Development Report 1999. Globalization with a Human Face*, New York: Oxford University Press.

UNESCO (1980) *Many Voices One World: Towards a New More Just and Efficient World Information and Communication Order,* Paris: UNESCO.

United Nations (1993) *Human Rights: The International Bill of Human Rights: Universal Declaration of Human Rights; International Covenant on Economic, Social and Cultural Rights; and International Covenant on Civil and Political Rights and Optional Protocols,* New York: United Nations.

United Nations (1997) *Human Rights: A Compilation of International Instruments (Volume II Regional Instruments),* New York: United Nations.

United Nations (2000, March) "We the peoples: the role of the United Nations in the 21st Century. The Millenium Report of the Secretary-General." Online. Available http://www.un.org/millennium/sg/report/ (accessed 9 April 2003).

United Nations (September 2000) United Nations Millenium Declaration. Draft Resolution referred by the General Assembly at its fifty-fourth session, Item 61(b) of the provisional agenda. Online. Available http://www.un.org/millennium/declaration/ares552e.htm (accessed 9 April 2003).

United Nations Economic and Social Council (UN ECOSOC) (2000, 1 July–August) "Development and international cooperation in the twenty-first century: the role of information technology in the context of a knowledge-based global economy." Draft ministerial declaration of the high-level segment submitted by the President of the Economic and Social Council on the basis of informal consultations, Substantive session of 2000, New York, 5 July–1 August 2000, Agenda item 2.

United Nations Economic and Social Council (UN ECOSOC) (2000, 21 July) "United Nations contacts G-8 on information technology gap." Press release, ECOSOC/5920

PI/1263. http://www.un.org/News/Press/docs/2000/20000721.ecosoc5920.doc. html.

United Nations Educational, Scientific and Cultural Organization (1999) *Statistical Yearbook*, Paris: UNESCO. Online. Available: http://unescostat.unesco.org/en/stats/ stats0.htm (accessed 10 July 2001).

United States Congress (1996) Telecommunications Act of 1996, Public Law 104–104, 104th Congress, February 8.

United States Department of Commerce (1998, January 30) "A proposal to improve technical management of Internet names and addresses: proposed rulemaking discussion draft." Online. Available http://www.ntia.doc.gov/ntiahome/domainname/ dnsdrft.htm (accessed 9 April 2003).

United States House of Representatives, Committee on Science, Subcommittee on Basic Research and Subcommittee on Technology (1998) *The Domain Name System, Parts I-II*, 105th Congress, Serial no. 78, Washington, DC: GPO.

United States House of Representatives, Subcommittee on Courts and Intellectual Property (1999a) *Collections of Information Antipiracy Act; Vessel Hull Design Protection Act; and Internet Domain Name Trademark Protection*, 105th Congress, Serial no. 115, Washington, DC: GPO.

United States House of Representatives, Subcommittee on Oversight and Investigations, (1999b) *Domain Name System Privatization: Is ICANN Out of Control?* 106th Congress, Serial no. 106–47, Washington, DC: GPO.

Van Dijk, J. (1999) *The Network Society*, London: Sage.

Vasak, K. (1990) "Les différentes categories des droits de l'homme," in A. Lapeyre, F. de Tinguy, and K. Vasak (eds.) *Les Dimensions Universelles des Droits de l'Homme*, Bruxelles: Bruylant.

Vincenti, W. G. (1995) "The technical shaping of technology: real-world constraints and technical logic in Edison's electrical lighting system," *Social Studies of Science*, 25: 553–574.

Voth, D. E. (1989) "Evaluation for community development," in J. A. Christenson and J. Robinson (eds.) *Community Development in Perspective*, Iowa: Iowa State University Press.

Wakefield, M. *et al.* (1993) "Characteristics associated with smoking cessation during pregnancy," *Addiction*, 88, 10: 1423–1430.

Walker, J. (1983) *Free Frank: A Black Pioneer on the Antebellum Frontier*, Lexington, KY: University Press of Kentucky.

Walker, J. (2002) *Links and Power: The Political Economy of Linking on the Web*, Baltimore, MD: Hypertext 2002.

Warburton, D. (1998) "A passionate dialogue: community and sustainable development," in D. Warburton (ed.) *Community and Sustainable Development: Participation in the Future*, London: Earthscan, pp.1–39.

Warren, R. L. (1978) *The Community in America*, Boston, MA: Houghton Mifflin.

Webster, F. (1995) *Theories of The InformAtion Society*, London: Routledge.

Wellman, B. (1997) "Structural analysis: from method and metaphor to theory and substance," in B. Wellman and S. D. Berkowitz (eds.) *Social Structures: A Network Approach*, Greenwich, CT: JAI Press.

Wellman, B. (2002) "Little boxes, glocalization, and networked individualism," in M. Tanabe *et al.* (eds.) *Digital Cities II: Computational and Sociological Approaches*, [Lecture Notes in Computer Science Series 2362], Berlin: Springer-Verlag, pp.10–25.

Werry, C. (1999) "Imagined electronic community: representations of virtual community in contemporary business discourse," *First Monday*, 4, 9 (Sept.). Online. Available http://firstmonday.org/issues/issue4_9/werry/index.html (accessed 4 April 2003).

White, D. (1950) "The 'gate keeper': a case study in the selection of news," *Journalism Quarterly*, 27: 383–90.

White, S. (1999) *The Art of Facilitating Participation*, London: Sage.

Wilkinson, R. G. (1996) *Unhealthy Societies: The Afflictions of Inequality*, London: Routledge.

Williams, K. and Alkalimat, A. (2004) "A census of public computing in Toledo, Ohio," in D. Schuler and P. Day (eds.) *Shaping the Networked Society: The New Role of Civic Society in Cyberspace*, Cambridge, MA: MIT Press. Online. Available http://www.communitytechnology.org/toledo/ (accessed 17 Mar 2003).

Wingfield, N. (1996) "What's in a name? bigmoney.com." C | Net NEWS.COM, The Net. May 4. Online. Available http://news.com.com/2100–1023–211292.html (accessed 9 April 2003).

Winner, L. (1980) "Do artifacts have politics?' *Daedalus*, 109, 1: 121–135.

Wolfe, A. (1989) *Whose Keeper?: Social Science and Moral Obligation*, Berkeley: University of California Press.

World Bank (1998) *World Development Report 1998/99: Knowledge for Development*, Washington, DC: World Bank. Online. Available: http://www.worldbank.org/wdr/wdr98/index.htm (accessed 20 October 2002).

World Bank (2000) *El Salvador Data Profile*, Washington, DC: World Bank. Online. Available: http://devdata.worldbank.org/external/dgprofile.asp?rmdk=82690&w=0&L=E (accessed 20 October 2002).

World Bank and International Monetary Fund (2001) *Staff Assessment of the Macroeconomic Effects of the Earthquakes in El Salvador*, Washington, DC: World Bank, IMF. Online. Available: http://www.terremotoelsalvador.org.sv/smicentral2/www2/cepal/madrid/elsalvador.pdf (accessed 20 October 2002).

World Health Organization (1986) *The Ottawa Charter for Health Promotion,* Geneva: World Health Organization.

World Press Freedom Committee (March 6, 1997) "NWICO: an old threat returns," Newsletter of the World Press Freedom Committee for its Affiliates and Contributors and Other Media Leaders, retrieved from the World Wide Web on March 22, 2003: http://www.wpfc.org/March%252097.html (accessed 9 April 2003).

Zelip, B. (2002) "Black people's hair: the digitization of popular culture," unpublished MA thesis, University of Toledo.

Zittrain, J. and Edelman, B. (2002) "Localized Google search result exclusions," Cambridge, MA: Harvard Law School. Online. Available: http://cyber.law.harvard.edu/filtering/google/ (accessed 9 April 2003).

Index